Gender and the Boundaries of Dress in Contemporary Peru

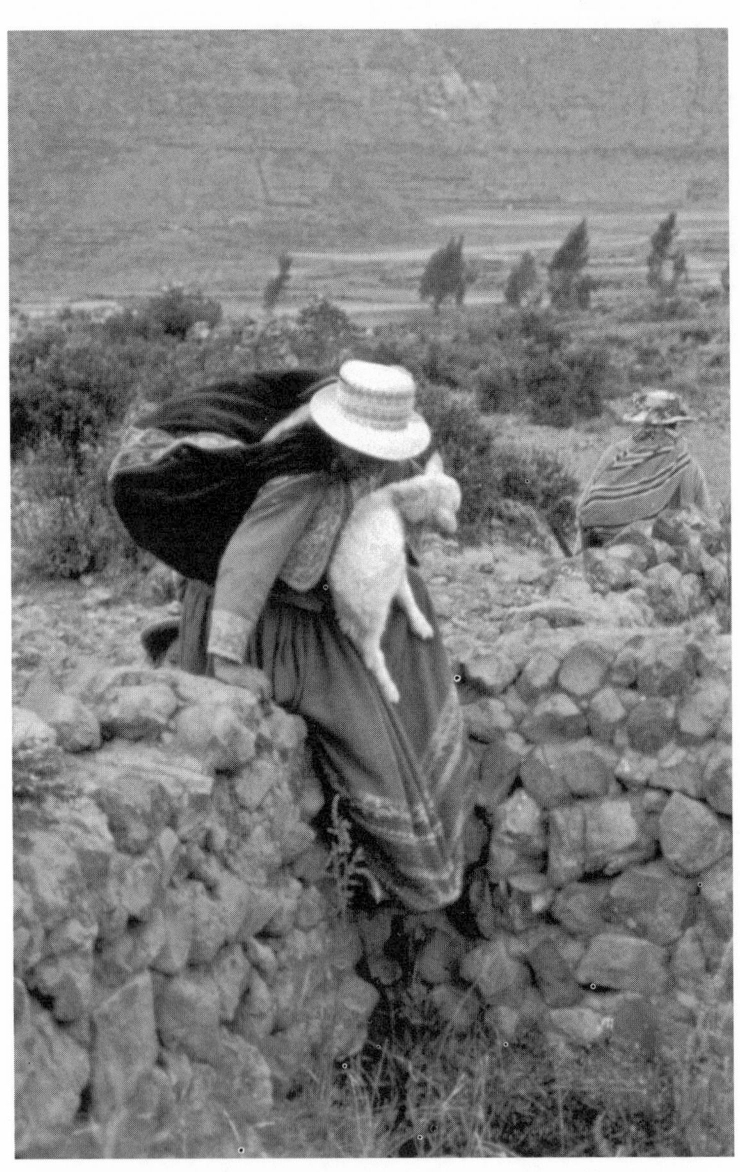

Gender and the Boundaries of Dress in Contemporary Peru

Blenda Femenías

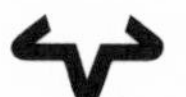 University of Texas Press, Austin

Book 6
Louann Atkins Temple Women & Culture Series
Books about women and families, and their changing role in society

The Louann Atkins Temple Women & Culture Series is supported by Allison, Doug, Taylor, and Andy Bacon; Margaret, Lawrence, Will, John, and Annie Temple; Larry Temple; the Temple-Inland Foundation; and the National Endowment for the Humanities.

Printed in the United States of America
First edition, 2005

♾ The paper used in this book meets the minimum requirements of ANSI/NISO Z39.48-1992 (R1997) (Permanence of Paper).

Library of Congress
Cataloging-in-Publication Data

Femenías, Blenda.
Gender and the boundaries of dress in contemporary Peru / Blenda Femenías.
p. cm. — (Louann Atkins Temple women & culture series ; bk. 6)
Includes bibliographical references and index.
ISBN 0-292-70543-3 (cloth : alk. paper)—
ISBN 0-292-70263-9 (pbk. : alk. paper)
1. Indian women—Clothing—Peru—Colca River Valley (Arequipa) 2. Indian textile fabrics—Peru—Colca River Valley (Arequipa) 3. Indian embroidery—Peru—Colca River Valley (Arequipa) 4. Costume—Symbolic aspects—Peru—Colca River Valley (Arequipa) 5. Costume—Psychological aspects—Peru—Colca River Valley (Arequipa) 6. Body, Human—Symbolic aspects—Peru—Colca River Valley (Arequipa) 7. Colca River Valley (Arequipa, Peru)—Social life and customs. I. Title. II. Series.
F3429.3.W7F46 2004
391′.0098532—dc22
2003026026

For my mother, Felicia Blenda Wistrom Femenias (1913–1999)

Contents

xi Acknowledgments

1 Introduction. False Borders, Embroidered Lives

35 1 Traveling

78 2 Fabricating Ethnic Frontiers: Identity in a Region at the Crossroads

103 3 Clothing the Body: Visual Domain and Cultural Process

147 4 Addressing History: Representation and the Embodiment of Memory

185 5 Dancing in Disguise: Transvestism and Festivals as Performance

215 6 Marching and Meaning: Ethnic Symbols and Gendered Demonstrations

241 7 Making Difference: Gender and Production in a Workshop System

267 8 Trading Places: Exchange, Identity, and the Commoditization of Cloth

298 Conclusion. Why Women Wear *Polleras*

305 Notes

323 Bibliography

355 Index

Maps and Figures

Maps

1. Southern Peru 4

2. The Colca Valley and surrounding areas 6

Figures

1. A woman from Maca sells *tunas* outside Chivay market. 3

2. Women and soldiers attend flag raising in Chivay. 9

3. Street market, Arequipa 11

4. The village of Coporaque 37

5. Sabancaya Volcano emits ash and vapor. 41

6. Maximiliana Terán picks dry beans. 42

7. Candelaria Bernal vaults over a wall carrying an orphaned lamb. 53

8. Layout of house compound, Colca Valley 56

9. Margarita Sullca at her stand in Chivay market 96

10. Leonardo Mejía shakes out a poncho. 99

11. Susana Bernal and Leonardo Mejía in their workshop 104

12. Woman's embroidered jacket by Tiburcio Ocsa and Vilma Mejía 111

13. Woman's embroidered vest by Susana Bernal 111

14. Chivay-style embroidered *pollera* by Susana Bernal, detail 113

15. Cabanaconde-style embroidered *pollera* by Hugo Vilcape, detail 113

16. Cabanaconde-style embroidered hat by Leonardo Mejía 114

17. Cabanaconde-style embroidered hat by Hugo Vilcape 114

18. Enadi Condori Bernal in *polleras* after her baptism, with her sister Lorena and their father, Juan Condori 120

19. Hummingbirds and flower; detail of an embroidered vest by Susana Bernal 133
20. Rows of figures, including hummingbirds and flowers, on a woven shawl by Grimalda Vega 133
21. Nilda and Candelaria Bernal's children, Marisol, Dante, and Ana Condorhuilca and Enadi Condori, with Blenda Femenías 142
22. Vendors selling around fountain, Chivay 149
23. Llama train leaving Salinas emporium, Chivay 149
24. Men of Lari 159
25. Women seated around airplane, Lari 160
26. Witite dancer 186
27. Dancers whirl about. 197
28. The Wife in *polleras* addresses the Judge. 216
29. Zenobia Taco is sworn in as president of the Women's Federation. 225
30. A march against violence 231
31. Women in *polleras* participate in a political demonstration. 234
32. Men and women voters; a woman mayor 234
33. Gerardo Vilcasán at work in his Chivay market kiosk 242
34. Chivay market and church 251
35. Juan de Dios Choquehuanca applies yarn to a *pollera*. 257
36. Vest embroidered by Juan Condori and Nilda Bernal 269
37. Nilda Bernal holds a black shawl embroidered by her and Juan Condori. 273
38. In the Coporaque cemetery, women wear black shawls and *polleras*. 276
39. Livia Sullca's store, Chivay; her daughter Jenny models *polleras*. 293

Acknowledgments

Every large project generates many debts. I begin with my family. My mother, Felicia Femenias, was the woman whose stories of living and traveling in Latin America made me aware of possibilities. My sister, Ramona Femenias, has done it all, from visiting me in Peru to planting tulips to balancing checkbooks.

My Ph.D. committee at the University of Wisconsin-Madison shaped the book's first incarnation, then prompted me to keep thinking about issues raised in graduate work. Thanks go first to advisor Frank Salomon, Andeanist extraordinaire, who guided the dissertation. Jane Collins always understands why we struggle and how to untangle complex problems. Maria Lepowsky's knowledge of gender studies is unsurpassed, Richard Flores provides insights into culture as performance, and Virginia Boyd reveals that ethnography reaches across genres.

The dissertation research phase in Peru was supported by grants from the Fulbright Commission-Institute for International Education and the Wenner-Gren Foundation for Anthropological Research. For research in the United States, the American Museum of Natural History awarded me a Collections Study Grant. Craig Morris, Senior Vice President and Dean of Science; Barbara Conklin (now retired); and Sumru Aricanli in the museum's Division of Anthropology, and Barbara Mathé, Museum Archivist and Head, Library-Special Collections; and Joel Sweimler have guided my use of photographs from the Shippee-Johnson Peruvian Expedition. I am grateful to the museum for permission to reproduce four photographs. A Research Fellowship from the National Endowment for the Humanities, a Fellowship in International Studies at the Library of Congress, and a Fulbright Research and Teaching Scholarship, which were awarded for a new project, enabled me to travel to Peru and to live in Washington, D.C., and so helped me remain involved with Andean issues. I thank the staff of the Museo Nacional de la Cultura Peruana and the Museo Nacional de Antropología, Arqueología e Historia in Lima, and the Hispanic Division at the incomparable Library of Congress.

While we were all graduate students at the UW-Madison and wrestling with dissertations, Karin Alejandra Rosemblatt and Sinclair Thomson provided stimulation, steadfast friendship, and large doses of comfort and common sense. Earlier phases were animated by the loudest women I know: Karin, Eileen Findlay, and Marisol de la Cadena. Marisol never let me forget that my thesis was about gender and power, including the power we have in ourselves. Nancy Appelbaum, Anne MacPherson, and Patrick McNamara energetically grappled with my roughest draft. In finalizing the thesis, Kay Candler's contributions stand out, Daniel Slive and María Elena García pitched in with proofreading, and Margaret Brandenburg vouchsafed its passage into the library. Other supportive friends in Madison, some of whom have since moved away, helped in many ways. Laurel Mark, I am lucky for your friendship. Thanks to Laurie Greenberg, Alberto Vargas, Mary Clark, Mark Gasiorowski, Cynthia Ofstead, Taylor Elkins, Mark Rogers, Elizabeth Marberry, Kent Mathewson, Kathleen Kennedy, Seemin Qayum, Joanne Rappaport, David Gow, Hector Parada, Deb Coltey, and René Reeves.

Many friends and colleagues read chapters and conference papers, sat on panels, and thrashed out problems. Elayne Zorn teaches me that cooperation among colleagues is not only possible but imperative; for a friendship borne of mutual love for cloth, Andean culture, and countless late-night chats, thanks always. Among my steadfast supporters, William M. Denevan and Sue Denevan occupy a special place—and where would I be without Enrique Mayer and Deborah Poole? I constantly count on Kay Candler, Clark Erickson, David Stemper, and Gloria Almeyda, and, re all things pre-Columbian, Elizabeth Benson, Susan Niles, and Ann P. Rowe. Lisa Markowitz, with her camelid concerns, surpasses even my obsession with highland matters, and David Ruccio casts an economist's eye on goods. Paul Gelles, Karsten Paerregaard, and Robbie Webber are generous with their deep knowledge of the Colca Valley. Maria Benavides shows how intellectual engagement keeps us young. In Washington, thanks to Catherine Allen, Barbara Conklin, William Conklin, and all Huaca Club members. In 2003, the Andeanist community was greatly diminished when the brilliant scholar Anne Paul died. To Anne, whose insights and generosity were unsurpassed, I owe thanks for decades of emotional and intellectual support.

Many fellow textile fanatics have converged in the Textile Society of America. To Mattiebelle Gittinger, a special debt of gratitude for years (admit it, decades) of support and unflagging confidence: you're the person who told me in the T.M. library, when you're ready to get a Ph.D., you'll know it. To Louise Mackie, former TSA President, thanks for leadership, and to Mary Dusenbury, current President, thanks for good counsel, visits, and reading and listening. Julia Burke unfailingly offers her comprehensive understanding of objects and exhibitions as well as cherished friendship. Lynne Milgram's hospitality and conference lunches keep me going too.

In Lima, the Instituto de Estudios Peruanos provided an affiliation. Special thanks to Carlos Iván Degregori, then Director. At the Lima Fulbright Commission, Henry Harman Guerra, current Director, and Marcia Koth de Paredes and Cecilia Esparza, past Directors, have supported various phases of research, which I could not have accomplished without Marcela de Harth and Ada Visag. Aroma de la Cadena provided hospitality and exquisite translations. Lissie Wahl opened her home to me, as did Adriana Soldi and Jorge Recharte. At Kuntur Huasi, Alix Bayly, John Alfredo Davis, Eleonore Davis, and Manuel del Solar share master knowledge of Andean arts. My list of people in Arequipa and the Colca Valley could fill a separate volume; the names of many *compadres, ahijados,* friends, and neighbors appear in this book. Hundreds of artisans who make *bordados* made my work possible. Antonia Kayser and Joan Toohig have the world's definitive kitchen, and the best table for writing fieldnotes; the presence of the late Sara Kaithathera remains strong, and the rest goes without saying. Valuable research assistance was provided by the very talented Flora Cutipa, Margarita Larico, and Oscar Valdivia. Pablo de la Vera Cruz, an archaeologist of the Instituto Nacional de Cultura, shared knowledge of the Colca and *chupe de camarones.* Thanks to Felix Palacios, Miguel Monroy, Lolo Mamani, and other faculty at the Universidad Nacional de San Agustín. At DESCO-Arequipa, Oscar Toro, Director, and the Chivay project staff provided many pointers and lots of rides. At CAPRODA, René Apaza, Director of the Arequipa office; advisors Herman and Frieda Swen; and Caylloma office staff facilitated my engagement in Women's Federation activities. Mauricio de Romaña and Patricia Gibson offered the comforts of Qoriña. Patricia Jurewicz shared expertise in design. Catherine Sahley, *compañera* and ecologist, helped me see the beauty in the desert and, with Jorge Torres, shared her home and the joy of the lovely Isabella. Thanks also to Lisa Paz-Murray, Miguel Paz, Sarah Chambers, and Gene

Ozansky. José Borja and his Paco Yunque puppet theater pulled me back into performing, reminding me that life is shaped by the sound of children's laughter. To Edith Cortés, thanks for talks about art and life and for luminous watercolors, and to Juan Ciro Goyzueta and other members of the Asociación Nacional de Escritores y Artistas (ANEA) for stimulating, boisterous friendship.

In 1987, at the Haffenreffer Museum of Anthropology at Brown University, I presented my first conference paper on the Colca Valley (later published in *Textile Traditions of Mesoamerica and the Andes: An Anthology*, ed. Margot B. Schevill, Janet C. Berlo, and Edward Dwyer [1996]). Little did I suspect that nine years later I would join the Brown faculty. For seven years as a visiting faculty member, fellow, and scholar, I thank the Department of Anthropology: David Kertzer, Chair; Katherine Grimaldi, Administrator; and all the faculty and staff; the Center for the Study of Race and Ethnicity; and, of course, my students. With inimitable flair, Shepard Krech III demonstrates how one combines the roles of exemplary scholar, museum director, and mentor. Nicholas Townsend cheerfully shared the junior faculty experience. Marida Hollos found me a home, where Lucie Searle's garden nourished me. At the Haffenreffer Museum, I thank Barbara Hail, now Curator Emerita; Thierry Gentis, Associate Curator; Kathleen Luke, Office Manager; and all the staff. Among many others at Brown or connected with Brown, Nancy Jacobs offers unfailing friendship and collegiality. In Latin American Studies, I owe much to Thomas Skidmore, former Director, and R. Douglas Cope. Provocative conversations with Sheila ffolliott energize my thinking about gender, history, and the arts. Anita Garey provides a peerless role model with enviable grace.

Preliminary studies and different versions of parts of this book have been published previously. The lime green part of Chapter 3 (included in the 1995 Textile Society of America Symposium Proceedings) was adapted for *Chungara,* a Chilean journal, in 1998, for which I thank Amy Oakland and Calogero Santoro, and *Contemporary Cultures and Societies of Latin America,* ed. Dwight Heath (2002). "'Why Do Gringos Like Black?'" based on Chapter 8, will appear in *The Latin American Fashion Reader,* ed. Regina Root (2004). The book's themes developed through numerous presentations. I am especially grateful to the Embassy of Peru in Washington, D.C., and to Allan Wagner, then Ambassador of Peru to the United States, for inviting me to speak in 2002. Stimulating discussion with faculty and students resulted from invited lectures, seminar presentations, and colloquia in Peru at the Museo Nacional de la Cultura Peruana (Lima) and the Universidad Nacional San Agustín (Arequipa), and in the United States at the Natural History Museum of Los Angeles County, Syracuse University, Tufts University, the University of Arizona, the University of Central Florida, and Wesleyan University. At the following conferences and annual meetings I have presented related papers: American Anthropological Association (1994, 1995, 1997, 1999, 2000), American Ethnological Society and Council for Museum Anthropology (1993 combined annual meetings), Congress of Latin Americanist Geographers (1997), and International Congress of Americanists (1991, 1997).

For tireless efforts to turn an unruly manuscript into a book, I owe much to the University of Texas Press. First and foremost, I thank Theresa May, Assistant Director and Editor-in-Chief, for seeing the spark in this project and gracefully fanning the blaze. Comments from Carol Hendrickson, Anne Paul, and an anonymous reader helped improve the manuscript. Heartfelt thanks as well to Allison Faust, Associate Editor, and Nancy Bryan, Catalog and Advertising Manager. Complementing the press, Kay Candler provided priceless help in shaping the manuscript. Catherine Allen, R. Douglas Cope, William Denevan, Mary Dusenbury, Lindsay French, María Elena García, Mattiebelle Gittinger, Shepard Krech III, Lisa Markowitz, Susan Niles, Karin Rosemblatt, and Ann P. Rowe commented on individual chapters, and María Eugenia Ulfe contributed editorial assistance. Steven Wernke created the maps, and Mattiebelle Gittinger ably consulted on all matters visual. Very special thanks are owed to Peter Heywood, and we are grateful for Wesley's smiles.

In the United States, those who are interested may find Colca Valley textiles in two collections. The Helen L. Allen Textile Collection, University of Wisconsin-Madison, contains numerous embroideries that I collected in the 1980s. At The Textile Museum, Washington, D.C., I am grateful to Ann Pollard Rowe, Curator of Western Hemisphere Textiles, and Ursula McCracken, Director, who were instrumental in encouraging me to collect woven and embroidered textiles and costumes in 2002, and for the support of the Latin American Research Fund.

To any supporters I have inadvertently omitted, thank you, too.

John Treacy first took me to Coporaque, and parts of both of us are still there.

Introduction

False Borders, Embroidered Lives

Ambulantes flood the streets of downtown Arequipa. Fanning out from the commercial hub of San Camilo market, these independent vendors stake out tiny patches of pavement. Throughout the center of this city of one million, near plaza and bus stop and railroad station, no matter which way you turn, their boxes, bags, stands, carts, cloths, and baskets jumble together in a frenzied kaleidoscope of things. Here shoppers can find anything; here thieves prey on the careless. From basic foodstuffs to imported commodities, commerce is largely informal, an affair of the streets or bazaars tucked into rickety buildings. On sites where centuries-old stone structures have been demolished in the name of progress, optimistic developers erect elegant new shopping centers. Few retailers can afford the high rents, so the centers resemble ghost towns. Few consumers can afford the imported luxury goods, saddled with 30 percent duties, sold there. The *ambulantes* are the ones who provide the desired goods at affordable prices. Most vendors are recent migrants from rural communities throughout southern Peru; long-term residents of Arequipa lump them together as "Indians" and denounce them as unwelcome invaders.[1]

In Maca, a village of 1,500 one hundred miles away, women load baskets of fruit onto overcrowded buses. A thirst-quenching snack, the fruit of the prickly pear cactus (*tuna*) tastes like kiwi crossed with honeydew. When the *tuna* fruit is fully ripe in February (midsummer in Peru), dozens of women leave their villages to sell it in Arequipa. Arriving in the metropolis, they claim places amidst the other sidewalk vendors. Prickly pears grow in Arequipa as well, but Maca is known for its delicious *tuna*. Maca and other villages in Caylloma Province are also known for their women's stylish clothes, called *bordados* (embroideries) or *polleras* (skirts), adorned with intricate multicolored motifs embroidered on sewing machines (Figure 1). Attracted by these markers of Caylloma, buyers stop to buy the fruit.

Today I pick a careful path through the melee that is downtown Arequipa. The city is highly centralized, so most errands must be done downtown. For the last few months, since I was almost robbed when a team of four thieves surrounded me, I have avoided this district. But I must travel to Chivay, the capital of Caylloma, and I can buy the ticket only at the bus company office.

I will visit Caylloma to continue fieldwork on a project addressing identity formation through daily life experience in several villages near Maca. Caylloma's 39,000 residents, mostly farmers and herders, are clustered in fifteen villages in the Colca River Valley.[2] My investigation concerns the ways they use objects to represent and construct their identities as women, men, and Cayllominos (people from Caylloma). Gender and ethnicity, I believe, are the most powerful forces shaping identity as more people migrate to Arequipa and as Caylloma's regional and national importance fluctuates. *Bordados* provide an ideal focal point because women wear them, but both men and women make and sell these distinctive emblems. *Bordados* literally means "embroideries" in Spanish, and *polleras* means "skirts," but the entire ensemble of blouse, vest, jacket, skirts, and hat is usually referred to by either term interchangeably.[3]

On my way to the bus company, I see a woman selling *tuna* fruits on a crowded corner. The colors and forms of her *bordados* indicate that she hails from a rural Caylloma village. On a hot February afternoon, almost 80°F, she wears a blouse and a jacket, both long-sleeved, with several ankle-length skirts that flow around her onto the sidewalk as she sits on a tiny stool. Another marker is her hat, made of tan felt with a wide embroidered brim and plain crown. It narrows the range of her origin to two or three communities. The basket of *tuna* beside her provides another clue that she is a Maqueña (woman from Maca). Stopping to chat, I buy a few fruits, three for the equivalent of about ten cents U.S. As she peels and passes them to me, we discuss the current state of affairs.

She confirms that she is from Maca. Things are very hard back home in this second year of drought. Corn and barley—the standard subsistence crops—are failing; in fact, only *tuna* is doing well, as cactus requires no watering. Thousands of llamas and alpacas are dying for lack of pasture. I decide to stay and converse longer, postponing my errand for a while. Fieldwork is where you find it. Also, Maca is a special case; it suffered a serious earthquake the previous year, so I usually ask Maqueños about the

1 A WOMAN FROM MACA SELLS *TUNAS* OUTSIDE CHIVAY MARKET.

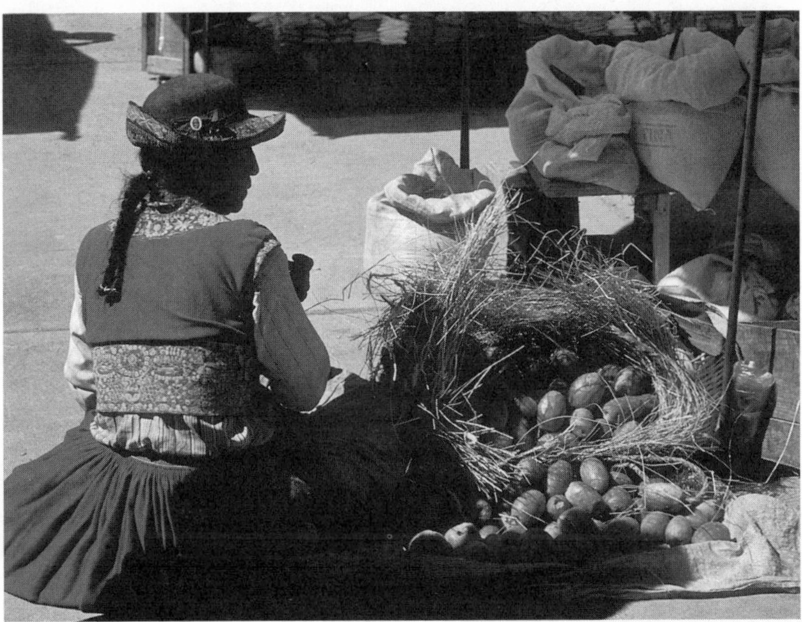

Map 1. Southern Peru

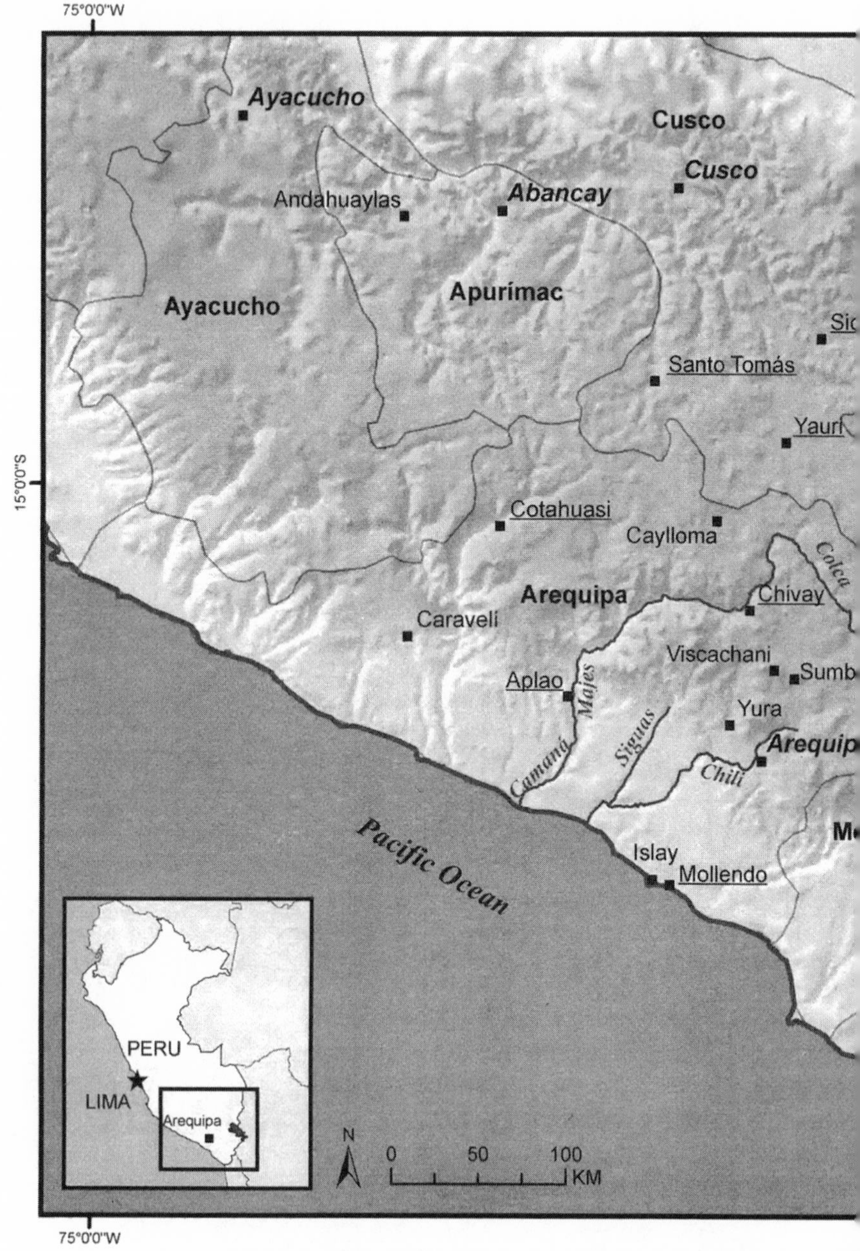

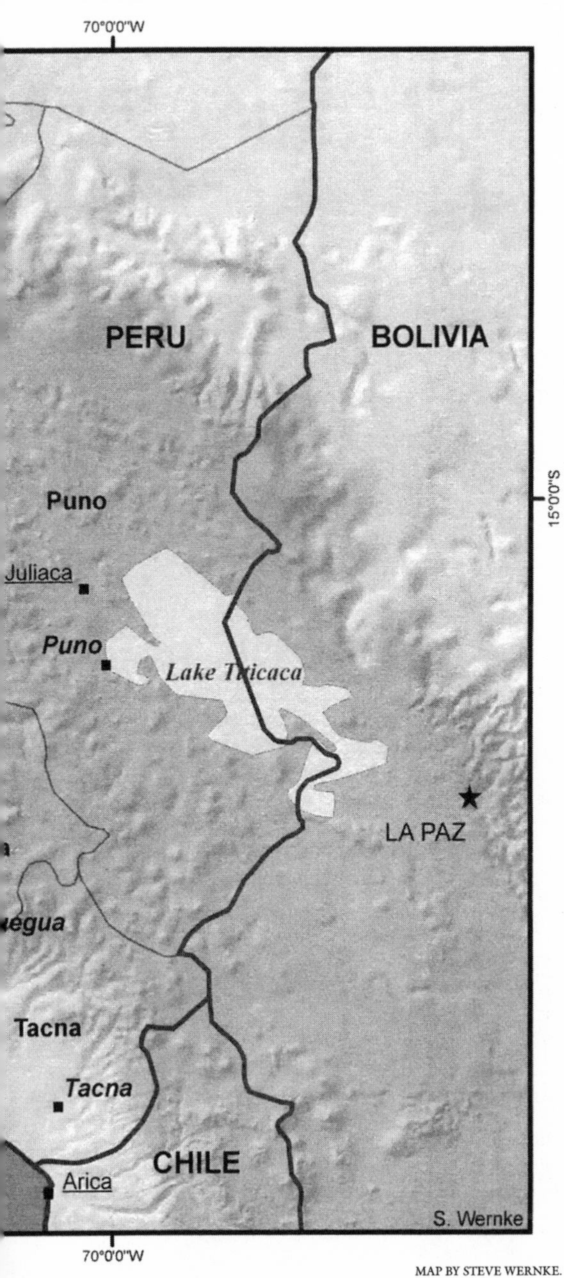

MAP BY STEVE WERNKE.

MAP 2. THE COLCA VALLEY AND SURROUNDING AREAS

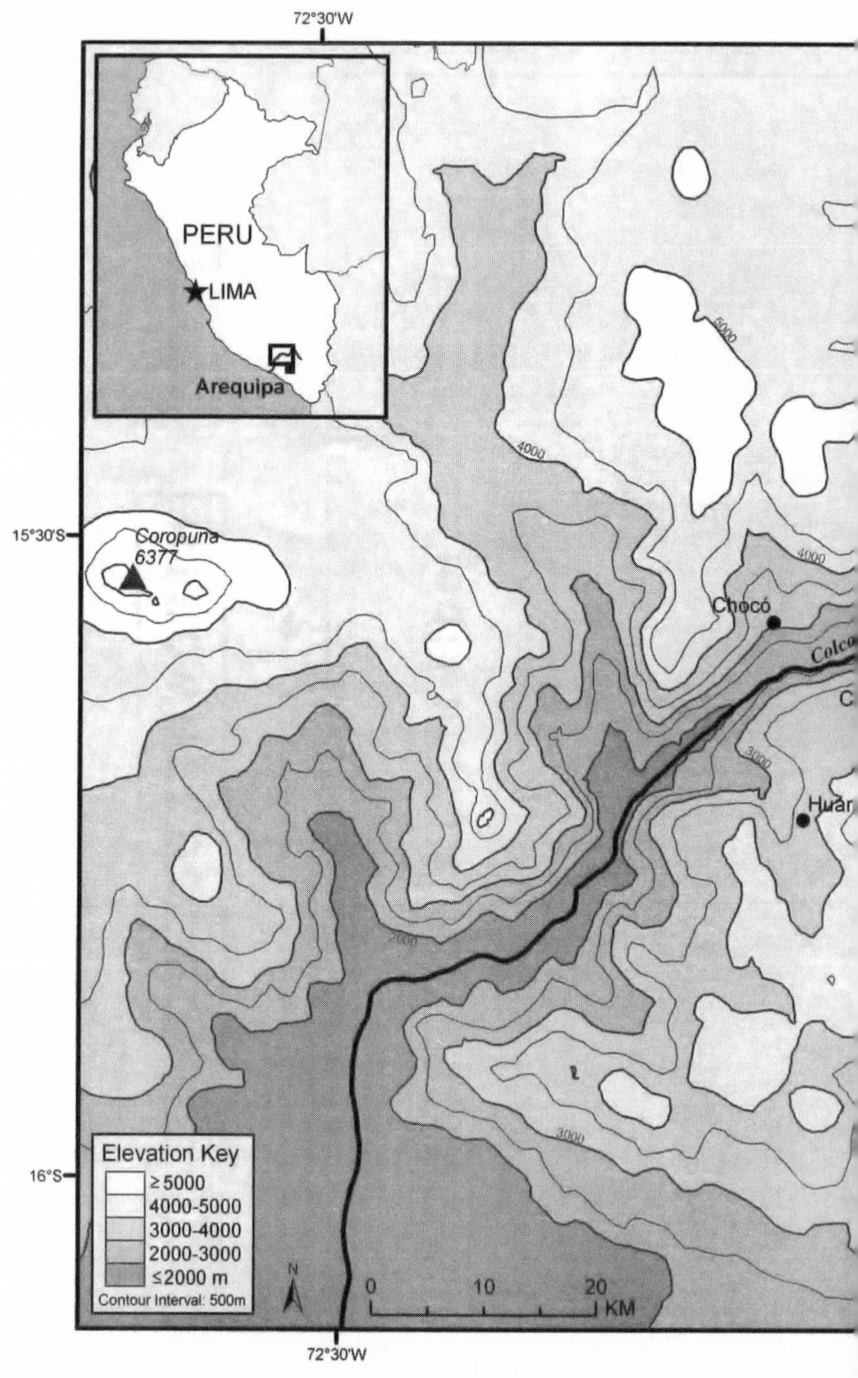

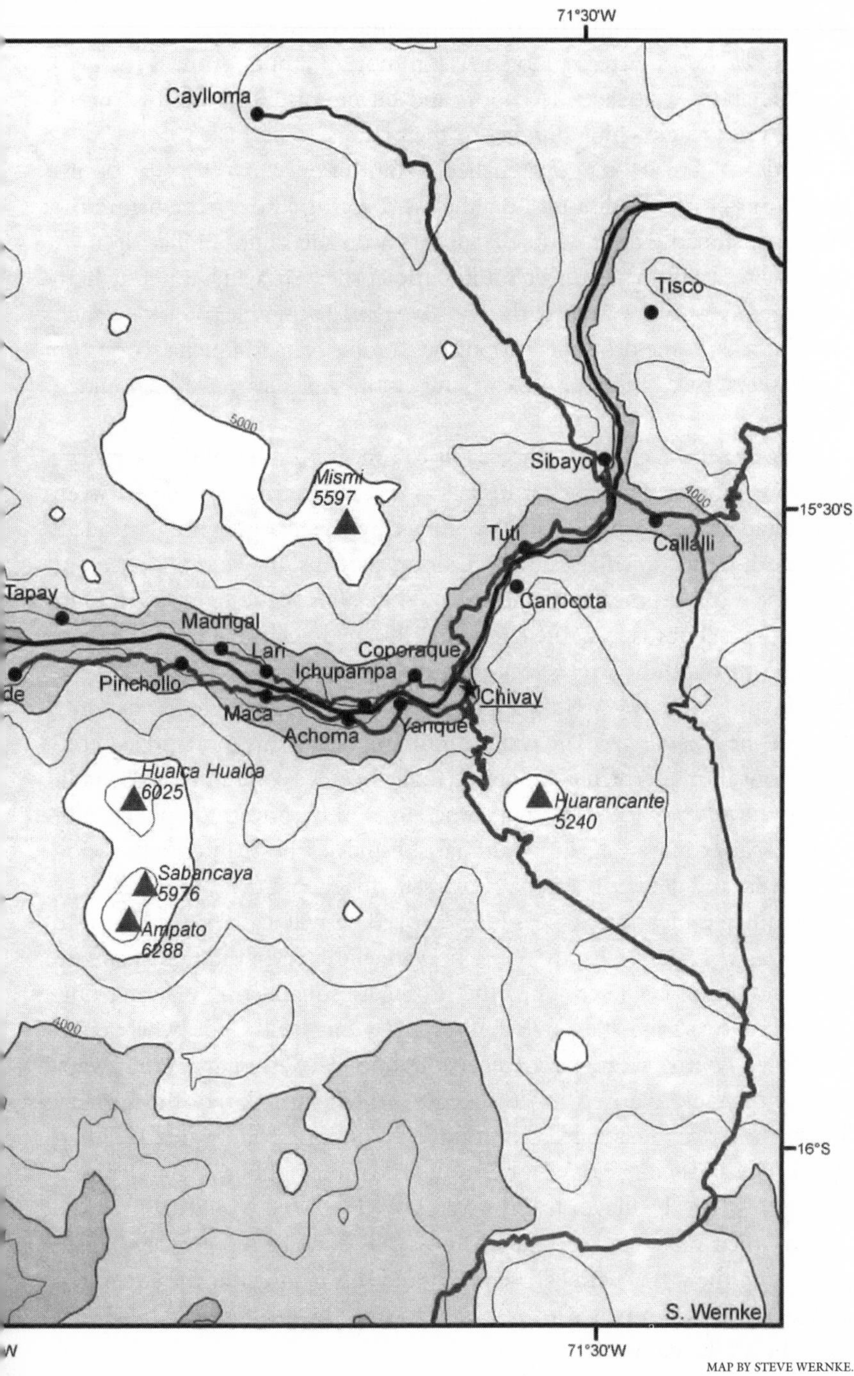

MAP BY STEVE WERNKE.

village's recovery. And perhaps this vendor will want to talk about her *bordados.* I tell her my name, but she has no time to tell me hers.

"*¡Rochabús!*" (Water cannon!) A commotion erupts. Amidst the general hue and cry, a wave of vendors and buyers rushes frantically toward us, the vendors clutching bundles to their chests.

Hide! Where? Don't get drenched, I think at once. An everyday occurrence, this cry spells disaster nonetheless. I spring into a store before the clerk can shut the door. Outside appears a dreaded but familiar sight. A truck with a tall metal turret rounds the corner, spraying water at high pressure on everyone in its path. The *ambulantes* scramble to pick up their small stocks; some drop their goods or stumble. The Maqueña scoops up her baskets, tucks them into a carrying cloth, slings it over one shoulder, and flees.

The *ambulantes* have no choice but to run. It is doubtful that any store owner would let them shelter inside, as the competitive enmity between stores and hawkers runs deep. My presence in the store goes unquestioned. The clerk slams down a solid metal door. Safe inside, we cannot see out but hear water drum against the door. When all is silent, he raises it. Outside, not a vendor is in sight. The sidewalks are drenched, and the torrents gushing through the streets reek of kerosene.

Mayor Cáceres of Arequipa has made good his word. He has declared war on the *ambulantes.* The water cannon is one of his most prized contributions to modernizing Arequipa. Luis Cáceres's commitment to eradicating the *ambulantes* has been a cornerstone of his governing policy. Not only do they compete against legitimate businesses, he maintains, they clog the streets and detract from the clean, safe image that the "White City"—as Arequipa is nicknamed—has long enjoyed. "I will wash the streets clean of *ambulantes*!" he declared. Cáceres's evangelical fervor did not square up with the questionable ethics of the profligate squandering of water during the century's worst drought.[4] Inspired by Lima and Chile, where tanks are crowd-control weapons, Cáceres bought one for Arequipa. While waiting for the tank to arrive, he deployed a makeshift truck. For the first few weeks the *rochabús* patrolled the city streets shooting plain water. It did no good. The *ambulantes* got wet, ran away, and came right back. Accelerating the aggression, the mayor had the water dyed red so it would stain as well as soak their merchandise, again to no avail. Now he has escalated again by mixing the water with kerosene. Should this fail to clear the streets, he threatens, he will mix it with pesticide to ruin the merchandise—the vendors' health be damned.

All this the woman from Maca risks to sell cactus fruits three for a dime. To do so she wears an outfit that cost more than a hundred dollars.

Real life in Peru was hard and scary. When I began fieldwork, political and economic tensions had strained the nation for more than a decade. These were years of civil war. Power struggles between the state and insurgent groups, including the Shining Path (Sendero Luminoso, SL), were enacted daily on the bodies of the powerless.[5] Combining military force and neoliberal reform, President Alberto Fujimori's government struggled to retain control. From 1991 to 1993, I lived in urban Arequipa and rural Caylloma Province, constantly traveling those hundred miles between city and country. Danger was on everyone's mind. Remarkably, Arequipa was spared the major war activities that decimated Ayacucho and central Peru, ravaged the eastern jungle, and severely depopulated the Puno countryside. Because Arequipa is Peru's second largest city—after Lima, the capital—its continued security became a national priority. Beginning in 1990, army troops were stationed in Arequipa's highlands; soldiers patrolled the villages and surrounding mountains. The national government declared a "state of emergency," placing Caylloma and several neighboring provinces under military occupation (Figure 2). Because Arequipa seemed safe, it

2 Women and soldiers attend flag raising in Chivay.

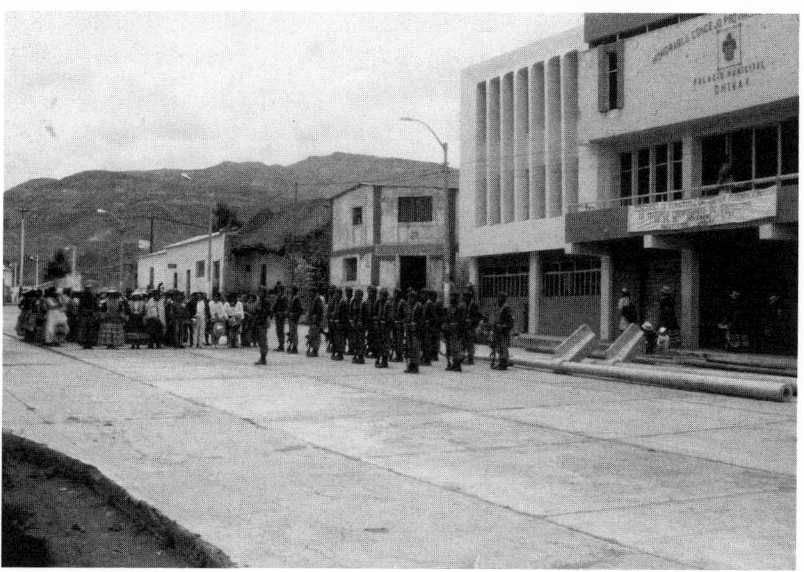

became a magnet for refugees from all over southern Peru. Nevertheless, Mayor Cáceres's little local war against the *ambulantes* echoed the larger national war. The problems the Maca vendor faced were Arequipa's daily fare: poverty, unemployment, petty crime, racism, and class struggle.

Some days the war came closer. In the Plaza de Armas, Arequipa's main square, police teargassed schoolteachers demonstrating during their union's six-month-long strike. Two national insurgent groups were operating in Arequipa: a cell of the Tupac Amaru Revolutionary Movement (Movimiento Revolucionario Túpac Amaru, MRTA) was uncovered in the university, and a local intellectual was detained by police as a suspected Sendero sympathizer.[6] Even in Arequipa, the climate of terror and the ubiquity of civil war were constant companions. Unsettling thoughts and unspoken threats were deep rivers indeed. One scarcely needed to verbalize them.

It was hard to do research in this climate. As a graduate student in the United States, I had planned to explore the "symbolic economy": examining the material dimensions of objects to discover how they communicate abstract ideas and affect cultural and economic values. Once in Peru, I found that the harsh realities of war made questions of meaning even more urgent and compelling. In particular, I became convinced that *bordados* are a uniquely powerful kind of clothes—emblems of gender and ethnicity that Cayllominos use in every phase of the life experience and have used for decades. To explore Cayllomino clothing use, production, and exchange, I needed to understand both the rural and the urban situations which they constantly negotiate. This kept me on the go.

It was hard to get to know Arequipa. Setting out every day from Umacollo, my middle-class neighborhood, following roads leading away from the central Chili River Valley, I traced the bulging contours of a city racked by growth. In 1540 Spaniards plotted a town along the Chili's fertile banks to accommodate a few hundred colonists and pull together the dispersed indigenous settlements. Now almost a million souls call the mushrooming metropolis home, testing the limits of the oasis's powers to provide. Bus service reached only so far; even in the city, I had to walk a lot. Almost daily I took half-hour bus rides to Alto Cayma and La Tomilla, established neighborhoods (*urbanizaciones*) where migrants from Caylloma cluster (Figure 3). I made periodic sojourns to new shantytowns (*pueblos jóvenes*) in the barren foothills of Misti Volcano; there were only two buses a day, and from the last stop I walked another hour. Tromping up dusty hills and across rocky ravines; circulating among rich and poor neighborhoods, the university, the art school, markets, and meetings of the clubs; getting to know many different Arequipas, I too became a sort of *ambulante*.

It was harder for the Caylloma-based travelers and migrants to grapple with all those Arequipas. While some had moved permanently from Caylloma to new Arequipa homes, others came to the city often to do business, and still others visited only once a year. Some had lived in the city for almost their whole lives, so their natal province was a dim memory of mountains, cornfields, and alpaca herds. The newly arrived, bound and determined to make a living, hoped that one of the city's large industries—milk-canning plant, brewery, and textile factories—or the state bureaucracy would hire them. Meanwhile, they sewed blouses, sold contraband radios, raised rabbits, or brought cactus fruit or corn to sell—whatever it took to put food on the table as prices skyrocketed through structural adjustment programs. Their Caylloma identity, which helped them parlay connections with other migrants into multiple social networks, was crucial to their survival.

3 STREET MARKET, AREQUIPA

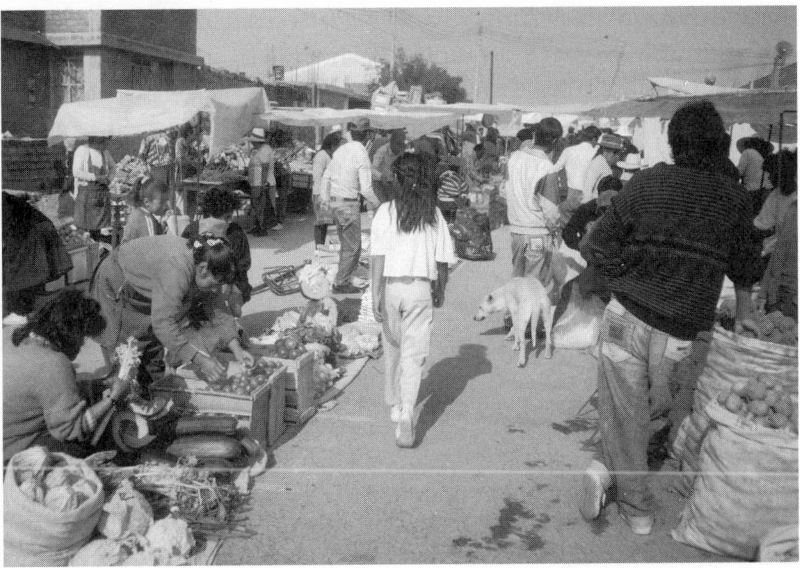

It was hard to do my project. Sometimes it seemed hard just to explain it. What is your research about? "*La mujer*" (women), "*la artesanía*" (crafts), or, if I knew a person better, "*el poder*" (power), I would reply. Launching into my well-rehearsed rap, I seldom got far, for people interrupted with their opinions. It proved more interesting to hear their interpretations than to explain my project. Many people encouraged me to learn about Caylloma lifeways or offered sympathetic anecdotes about their own rural living experiences. Others, despite good intentions, provided erroneous "facts" about *bordados* and the people who wore them. All and sundry freely advised me on my proper role. Some urban elites suggested that I develop and market crafts for the improvement of the poor. Others, assuming I was with a development agency, told me not to waste my time trying to help "those Indians," because they were too lazy to work. At first, my reactions to similar comments—usually paternalistic but sometimes blatantly racist, even genocidal—embroiled me in many arguments. Eventually, I got better at biting my tongue, but it always took effort not to get riled. I had to remind myself constantly that discussion would be futile and that I was a foreigner and a guest, in potential danger.

In April 1992 we had a coup. President Alberto Fujimori staged an *autogolpe* (self-inflicted coup): he suspended civil liberties, dissolved the national Congress and Supreme Court, and declared the Constitution null and void. In imposing autocratic rule, he disrupted the fragile democratic process through which Alan García Pérez had passed him the reins of government not even two years earlier. Fujimori's election had confounded the pundits, who failed to anticipate that this Japanese-Peruvian upstart would steal the thunder of the white elite favorite, Mario Vargas Llosa, originally from Arequipa, as well as end the domination of García's party, APRA (Alianza Popular Revolucionario Americano). The *autogolpe* seemed but one more phase in learning to expect the unexpected.

The coup shook me up. I had no idea what would happen. I kept working in Arequipa rather than travel to Chivay. In the evenings, I, like the rest of the country, was glued to the television news. I read all the newspapers and magazines; I listened to endless rumors and gossip. What next? Would the country be rocked by waves of increasing violence? Would Peru become the next Cambodia? In fact, the scope of the war did not escalate, but the violence, although less visible, became more insidious and deeply ingrained. Fed up with war and corruption, many Peruvians demanded harsh solutions to complex problems. Fujimori's strong hand was approved in many sectors, but his blatant violations of civil rights and due process were vigorously protested in others. Demonstrations of popular support alternated with widespread debate about the military's role in the coup. Was Fujimori a dictator or a puppet?[7]

My own daily routine was remarkably uneventful. I kept right on doing fieldwork. With only four months remaining of my eighteen-month research period, I needed to accelerate in the homestretch. My colleague, Flora Cutipa, and I met hundreds of Cayllomino migrants, primarily in markets, Mothers' Clubs, and the Caylloma Provincial Association. Many of these migrants were women, and almost all of them were poor. More often than I would have predicted, they told me of their hardships. Women recounted the complicated juggling acts of their lives: holding down two jobs, staffing the soup kitchens of a women's group, organizing locally to get electricity in their *urbanización,* coordinating schedules with their husbands, and, all too often, enduring domestic abuse in order to protect their children and keep the family together.

In Cayllominos' lives, even in the city, artistic production and handwork were conspicuously central. When I talked about "crafts" or knitted, people showed me textiles old and new. Cherished, woven heirlooms from Caylloma helped them feel at home in the city. *Bordados* had particular currency in contemporary urban life. Women donned those clothes to sell produce like *tuna* fruit, to join with other migrants in social clubs and festivals, and to engage in political activism on behalf of Cayllominos. In makeshift shops set up in houses that were no more than stacks of rough volcanic blocks, embroidery artisans made beautiful things and patiently explained their work to me. City workshops were few, however, compared to the number in Caylloma. My investigation of production and exchange was centered in Chivay, a market town of five thousand people. I spent considerable time there, interacting with more than one hundred artisans who labored in about fifty embroidery workshops.

About a month after the *autogolpe,* a violent incident occurred in Caylloma. Late one night, a bomb ripped open the Armed Forces Recruiting Office in downtown Chivay. No one was injured or killed; two buildings were damaged. The incident proved isolated. The bombing was neither claimed by Sendero nor accompanied by pro-Sendero graffiti. I was in Arequipa and, after I heard, postponed a scheduled trip to Chivay. Two weeks later I went. A few people willingly discussed the bombing, but I learned little beyond the fact that no one was ever arrested.

During that week I walked around Chivay as usual, focusing on a particular research task or just going to grab lunch in a restaurant. Typically, I spent several hours each day with artisans in a workshop, where they assembled the multicolored garments and embroidered birds and flowers on them. About forty workshops are clustered in the market, and several others are scattered around the side streets. Going anywhere in town, I would invariably pass at least one. As I walked by, the whir and clunk of treadle sewing machines poured out of open doors. Often I poked my head inside to greet a friend. Such was the rhythm of daily life, the well-worn path of fieldwork.

Every day I had to pass the bombed-out recruiting office, just two blocks from my house. The door blown off its hinges had been replaced by the time I reached Chivay. The damaged roof of the jail behind it had not. Twisted edges of corrugated metal spiraled skyward and trailed off like thin tongues of flame. The first time I walked past, I gawked at the grotesque sight. No one else even glanced that way.

Someone was out of touch with reality. But who? Was it me, intently tracing every step it took to make and sell *bordados*? Was it the Caylloминos, dedicating dozens of hours a week to embroidering beautiful clothes? After a bomb went off one night, how could people sew hummingbirds the next day? To what lengths would they go to put the war out of their minds? How could the creative process matter amidst violent conflicts? In the quagmire of a civil war, what did a "symbolic economy" mean?

Beyond the doubts that bedevil every large project, my doubts were honed by the war that surrounded me and affected the lives of people with whom I worked and lived. Sally Ness, an anthropologist studying a popular dance-drama in the Philippines during troubled times, wondered about the value of analyzing what people constantly told her was a "meaningless event" (Ness 1992:24–25). And embroidery? Likewise, I wondered about the value of something so decorative, so superficial, and perhaps so frivolous. Resisting the temptation to dismiss embroidery as an excessively trivial occupation, I found the serious questions buried deep within my doubts. Who was trivializing this activity? And why?

Trying to reconcile bombing with embroidering made me stop, step back from the details, and reconsider what I knew about *bordados* and their roles in Cayllominos' lives. That is how I came to view them as a genre, a unified form of cultural expression. Now I could understand how artisans were encoding important messages. Their work has been trivialized because they employ "a form, mode, or genre that the dominant culture considers unimportant, innocuous, or irrelevant" (Radner and Lanser 1993: 19), and thus apparently weaken the importance of the message that form carries. Yet when a nonthreatening form is used, its message or transcript can be more meaningful to its creators and users, precisely because it is discounted by, or hidden from, the dominant culture (Scott 1990). *Bordados* are this kind of creative work. The gendered and ethnic messages they encode, while threatening in other contexts, may seem trivial because of the medium. Historically, embroidery has frequently been "characterized as mindless, decorative and delicate; like the icing on the cake, good to look at, adding taste and status, but devoid of significant content" (Parker 1986:6). In this medium in particular, meaning is all too often disguised or obscured (ibid.:13).

"Symbolic economy," far from being trivial, proved to be a more useful concept than I anticipated. It acquired new resonance and depth in Peru at war. My analysis of "symbolism" came to center on one symbolic domain, *bordados,* in its political and economic contexts, both contemporary and historical. *Bordados* were an important subject because gendered ideologies dominated their symbolism. This is the case not only because women wear them, but because all clothes are often glossed as female. At least in western society, fashion and dress form a category so closely associated with the feminine that "male fashion" seems an oxymoron (Hollander 1994:10–11). *Bordados*' decorative surface apparently intensifies their female associations because embroidery is a feminine category (Parker 1986). But would these gendered associations hold in Caylloma, where men as well as women make, and even sometimes wear, *bordados*?

The "economy" side of the symbolic economy concept had also troubled me; it seemed too grand a term to describe the hardscrabble existence of twenty-two million struggling souls. Although subsistence agriculture plays a crucial role for rural Peruvians, it coexists with capitalist extraction, multinational development, and a vast informal sector. But "subsistence" and every other label I applied to economic activity called into question the symbolic dimensions of economy. Rethinking "economy" preceded understanding the workshop organization of *bordado* production, which does not set neatly within any single economic system. While the men, women, and sometimes children who make embroidered clothes are workers, with a stake in the financial outcome of their labors, they are often kin who give as well as sell their products.

Contradictory values and categorizations, I came to see, were not extraneous appendages to cut off the body of the project nor were they distractions to ignore. These political issues were precisely the substance of the problem. The symbolic and the economic, the art and the work, the urban and the rural—these divisions were false borders that did not represent the world I saw around me. The ambiguity of these emblems, especially the gendered and ethnic concepts they embody, contains the irreducible tensions in which their value lies. Questions of meaning are questions of power. Objects do not float detached from cultural values, but acquire their meanings as the products of human creativity and labor. The *bordados* themselves contain the stories of the people who wear them and the artists who create them. They hold embroidered lives.[8]

By 1991, when I went to live in Peru, I had already visited several times. Although life during wartime would be hard, the everyday dangers of urban life should come as no surprise. For many years I lived in Washington, D.C., where urban street crime was familiar fare. Military occupation, with U.S. army tanks patrolling the streets, figured in my adolescent rites of passage during the Vietnam War. Years in safe, sane Wisconsin had dulled my instincts, but when I moved to Peru, my street smarts snapped back sharper than ever. It was only prudent to stay alert on the street, where water cannons rumbled along, thieves flashed razors, and police lobbed tear gas.

What threw me was different: Terror, not terrorism per se. Violence, not the violent acts themselves. The expectation, normalizing, and routinizing of violence—that was terror. Failure to anticipate a violent event could lead to inconvenience, such as drenching by the water cannon, or to catastrophe. In fleeing the *rochabús,* the *ambulantes* and I momentarily shared a problem. That day, I found safety. None of us was immune, however, to random, capricious chance. Anticipating violence could not prevent it. Victims of the war were in the wrong place, trapped inside a building that was bombed or caught in the crossfire of a police sweep. Assassinations, massacres, and disappearances claimed the lion's share of media attention and international human rights outrage.[9] But the climate of terror was worse. Fostered by the small daily violence of routine hostile encounters such as the water cannon's sorties, this climate inured the soul to acts of violence and enabled the acts to multiply.[10]

War is not what you think it is unless you have lived in it. Daily life goes on, but it takes unexpected turns. Terror feeds into an escalating spiral of violence, but it also brings alienation, the breakdown of civil society, and the paralysis of anomie. Even so, the climate of violence sparks people to create as well as to destroy. What does it take to galvanize people into action? What kinds of acts are sane in an atmosphere of lunacy? Whence springs the energy to create and stave off the destruction?

In Peru during the years of crisis, loss of faith in action and hopeless despair were the silent accomplices to the fiery rage of war. All around me, however, people interrogated both violence and passivity. Gender identity was a vital factor shaping how women and men deployed cultural forms to navigate the suspect terrain their daily lives occupied. And racial heritage and ethnic pride played crucial roles in helping migrants from rural communities search for a modicum of security and some kind of livable space (Turino 1993:3). With the bombs' destruction, explosions of another kind surged forth. Art, craft, literature, theater, music, festivals—all kinds of popular cultural expressions multiplied and regenerated.[11] More than a painting, in the way of a song, Caylloma *bordados* are such an expression. "Eruptions of creativity within cultural performances comment upon, just as they often reformulate, the dilemmas a society faces at a particular historical moment," observed Rosaldo, Lavie, and Narayan (1993:6). Against the normalization of violence, continuing daily life was the quintessence of creativity in action. That is how Peruvians struggled with those dilemmas. Creativity during crisis, the fraying and mending of the fabric of culture, and the embodied power of gender and ethnicity in such troubled times are issues with which I grapple in this book.

Ambiguous Emblems

> *When I'm in Arequipa and I see a lady in embroidered clothes, I always greet her. She's from my land, she's my compatriot. . . .* — LEONARDO MEJÍA
> (Interview, Chivay, February 1992)

When the Maca fruit vendor set out for Arequipa, she could assume that Arequipeños would identify her with Caylloma, and that dressing in *polleras* would boost sales. When Leonardo Mejía walked through the streets of Arequipa, he could be sure that a woman in *bordados* was his *paisana* (compatriot). For Mejía as a Cayllomino, even far from his hometown of Coporaque, embroidered garments would signal that the woman wearing them was from the same land (*tierra*), prompting him to greet her. For him as an experienced embroidery artisan, the *bordados* would have personal and professional meaning. A closer look would determine if he himself had made them. *Bordados* inspire recognition, but they also circulate in other spheres of meaning.

On the streets of Arequipa, I sometimes met and greeted women in beautiful, luxurious *bordados*. In Caylloma I was surrounded by them. But there were no published studies that explained why this was so: no studies centering on *bordados*, any type of Cayllomino textiles, or gender in Caylloma. In the sizeable literature on Caylloma, scholars made only a cursory mention of women's dress, and no one addressed the economic importance of the workshops. Convinced that *bordados* constituted a genre, I soon realized that they should occupy the center of my study of gender.

This ethnography of the clothed body is the first book to analyze a Peruvian creative domain primarily through the lens of gender. One central theme is that unequal power relations make, rather than reflect, gendered and ethnic difference. Caylloma *bordados* are the primary domain of representation through which I explore that theme. These ambiguous emblems are simultaneously gendered symbols, ethnic markers, class statements, emblems of resistance to racism, works of art, and elements in production and exchange practices. *Bordados* mark place: they are the exclusive products of the Peruvian nation, the Arequipa region, the province of Caylloma, the valley of the Colca River, and a few villages. *Bordados* mark time: points in personal life courses, annual calendars, and historical epochs. They are contemporary allegories of vibrant traditions based in the past, but their characteristic embroidery originated no earlier than the 1930s. Their power as key symbols inheres not only in their precision as markers but in their very ambiguity.

Every day several thousand Cayllominas wear *bordados*, and during her lifetime, each woman will spend several thousand dollars on elaborate outfits. Though a modestly priced complete ensemble may cost less than $100, one spectacular skirt may cost three times that amount. Women take pride in dressing well, and men and women artisans take pride in making the intricate work skillfully. But the burden of representation is unevenly gendered, as different values, tasks, and images are assigned to female and male —both actual persons and conceptual categories. Although in daily life only Caylloma women wear *bordados*, on numerous ritual occasions men wear them. In these contradictions lies the ambiguity of *bordados* as gendered emblems. In contrast to Cayllominos' pride, national society marginalizes people who dress in *bordados*, and elites denigrate these symbols of the "Indian." In this lies their ambiguity as ethnic emblems. Women in *polleras* are seldom well-to-do, yet they spend considerable sums to purchase the locally made garments. In this lies their ambiguity as class emblems.

In the hierarchical, patriarchal society of contemporary Peru, indigenous women are often painted as powerless and invisible. At the same time, they are exalted as emblems of ethnicity, motherhood, and beauty. Forced to absorb the burden of racist and domestic violence, they are also charged with the embodiment of moral and aesthetic values. Why do women's bodies carry such a heavy physical and symbolic weight? Why do women embellish their appearance, attracting the eyes of others to their bodies? In a modern nation that censures "Indian" appearance, why do ethnic traditions remain vital? Embroidery production flourishes in family workshops throughout Caylloma. In economically depressed times, why do artisans make *bordados*? If the people are so poor, why do they dress so fancy? Why do women wear *polleras*?

These questions stare ambiguity in the face rather than shy away from it. To answer them, I analyze representation primarily as a productive practice. Employing a practice-centered approach (Bourdieu 1977), I privilege the process of clothing the body as a performative realm in which people represent their identities.[12] "Clothing" is an active verb, a process. Because human actions simultaneously construct and express identity, clothes do not merely display or reflect an identity formed through other processes. Rather, *wearing* garments produces persons. In Caylloma, this identity-formation process is linked in myriad ways to the garment-production process. *Making* clothes also produces persons.[13]

Dancing with Cayllominos in festivals, harvesting in the fields, putting on my own *polleras*—all these practices led me to understand that symbolism is more material than abstract. Identity is embodied, and *bordados* incorporate meanings into gendered bodies. People dress together as they act together in communities of practice. Wearing *bordados* transforms exterior pressures, yielding an internalized, cultural sense of the person. While centered in the individual, this sense derives meaning, and ultimately power, from the person's connections to larger groups. Clothes are a primary means of making these connections.

Sewing with Cayllominos in workshops, buying fabric in Chivay market, negotiating the price of a hat—other practices attested that the producing and marketing of clothes are also important representational practices. *Bordados* are commodities. About 150 specialists in eighty workshops make embroidered clothes. On an average day, ten thousand women may wear them and hundreds of people may buy them from the artisans or merchants. *Bordados* are expensive. A luxurious set can cost $500, whereas a set of industrially manufactured "Western" clothes can be had for $20. *Bordados* are investments. As symbolic and economic capital (see Bourdieu 1977:179–180), they bring prestige and renown. The makers strive to market expensive goods and to increase the value of their work; the wearers don, display, and treasure their finest *polleras* for years.

Even casual observers are fascinated by the beauty and technical complexity of Andean textiles. Yet two stereotypes thoroughly dominate popular thought and influence scholarship (Femenías 1987). The first is that women make them at home for their families; the second, that women weave them by hand on "frame" or "backstrap" looms. Neither is true of *bordados.* They are made in workshops, sewn and embroidered on treadle machines. My focus on *bordados* pushes us out of the stereotypes to encompass workshop-produced, machine embroidery. The importance of the workshop system centered in Chivay extends beyond Caylloma, as it echoes the petty commodity system in medium-size towns throughout Peru, a vital part of the national economy. This local phenomenon, then, also compels us to confront the magnitude and variety of production and exchange systems, previously under-represented, that yield Andean textiles and occupy Andean people.[14]

Cayllominos, especially women, do weave fine textiles, which they use and sell.[15] Caylloma's documented, five-century association with cloth was one reason I chose to do research there. Alpacas abound in Caylloma; their fiber is highly prized. During the "wool boom" of the late nineteenth through early twentieth century, power struggles pivoting on cloth and fiber linked southern Peru to global markets. National and foreign schemes to extract resources and introduce commodities expanded exponentially. As alpaca went out, foreign materials came in. Even as Cayllominos resisted outside authority and racial domination, they appropriated new materials, technologies, ideologies, and productive strategies—and turned them into *bordados.*

Delving into the genesis of *bordados* offers many insights into Caylloma's fluctuating importance in Peruvian ideology and political economy. These oscillations, in turn, prove significant in understanding how and why *bordados* came to be so misunderstood. Confronting the inaccuracy of the prevailing assumptions raises serious questions about value as a political system. To understand the power embodied in *polleras,* we must address how people produce and use objects of economic and cultural value (Appadurai 1986; Myers, ed. 2001; Phillips and Steiner, eds. 1999). Throughout this book, I analyze the politics of value primarily through the close association between gender and cloth/clothes, and secondarily, between ethnicity and cloth/clothes. I also analyze gender and ethnicity separately and uncover how they are mutually dependent.

I maintain that to ascertain norms of representation through dress, whether gendered or ethnic, we need to identify what people wear on a daily basis and how that fits with other quotidian aspects of identity formation. We also need to examine how dress for special occasions and rituals differs from that for quotidian ones, how these occasions correspond to points in the life course, and how Cayllominos use such events instrumentally. This attention to practice enables us to understand how ideologies that characterize particular activities as male or female are embodied, reproduced, and changed.

My first argument regarding gender is that *bordados* mark gender identity because they are worn almost exclusively by women. Within all Cayllomino ethnic groups and classes, the clear gendered marking in dress generally means that women wear skirts and men wear pants; unisex and unmarked clothes are uncommon. The gendered marking in *bordados* specifically also means that women's bodies are the focus of ethnic differentiation through dress, while men's bodies rarely are. In concrete terms, most Cayllominas who wear *polleras* are farmers and herders. As they work in the fields, layers of clothes envelop them from neck to ankle. Their long full skirts blaze with hummingbirds and fuchsia blossoms. But the men working alongside them look drab in monochrome jeans and shirts. Because men have no daily dress that comparably expresses ethnic difference, their quotidian self-representation is qualitatively different. There are, significantly, several exceptions to the decorated, skirt/female: unadorned, pants/male norm. In particular, men wear women's skirts in rituals. I attend closely to the effects and meanings of such apparent subversions of conventional gender norms.

A second premise undergirds my analysis of the gender-cloth/clothes association: *bordados* are gendered work. A strong gendered division of labor structures the *bordado* system, although almost equal numbers of women and men participate, often side by side, in embroidery production and exchange. Even as I contend that ideologies of female domesticity significantly constrain women, I also insist that such assumptions facilitate empowerment. Understanding gendered work requires attention to creativity, ownership, control over resources, control over labor, and kinship. Men frequently privilege their roles as artists, workshop heads, and workers. Women tend to underplay or deny these roles, sometimes saying they do not work but just help their families. Profiles of individual embroiderers, mostly men, whose work is highly esteemed for aesthetics persuaded me that gender strongly affects artistic aspiration and achievement. Here, too, exceptions to gendered norms matter. Female leaders in the *bordados* business, for example, merit scrutiny for the ways they parlay home-based activities into outside income-generating opportunities.

To explore the ethnicity-cloth/clothes association, I work from the premise that ethnicity is primarily a problem of relational identities. Again emphasizing the performative dimensions of everyday life, I contend that ethnic groups are basically communities constituted through "ethnic practices" (Bentley 1987). Analyzing how similar actions draw differently positioned subjects together also requires analyzing how those actions influence ideologies; they do both as they establish, confirm, and test boundaries between groups. This approach rejects the idea that ethnic groups are primarily sets of people with common interests indicated by common markers, because treating those attributes as fixed implies that culture is static. Instead, I examine why and how particular markers become associated with ethnicity as well as the consequences of creating and reinforcing those associations.

Among the ways that Peruvians form and characterize identity, I focus on matters of Indian identity. I question why others identify Indians through association with "handmade" crafts, especially cloth, and with "costume." More broadly, I inquire why nonindustrial, premodern lifeways and technologies are such common markers of ethnic and racial difference. The categories of "Indian" (*indio, indígena*), "white" (*blanco*), and "mixed" (*mestizo*) still dominate the complex system of race, ethnicity, and class that operates in today's Peru. Many Peruvians trace their heritage to ancestors who inhabited the land before Spaniards arrived. Their names for themselves include references to their contemporary community of origin and pre-Columbian polities. They rarely claim to be Indians. In Peru, it is always the Other who is native.[16]

My analysis further depends on disentangling race and locality as integral, but incompatible, components of ethnicity. Because people who do not wear "handmade" clothes widely believe that those who do are Indians and live in rural areas, especially the mountains, they characterize all *polleras* as fundamentally the same. Yet Cayllominos distinguish sharply between styles made in different parts of the province, using precise markers to identify locations only a few miles apart. Examining the relationship between use of generalized, "ethnic" dress and the variant characterizing a specific location is key to understanding how dress is maneuvered for political unity and division. Primary among *polleras'* explicitly political arenas are women's organizations, in which female political leaders appear in *bordados.* By focusing on such public expressions, we see how ethnic identification can help women gain power, so elusive in a country where official channels of power, especially public office, are rarely open to women.[17]

Furthermore, I consider craft production as a vehicle for both genders, but especially men, to gain prestige and even fame, and I inquire how this mobility may translate into broader advantage and power. Artisans play important roles beyond Caylloma in promoting a positive image of their community, but they are rewarded with success only within the narrowly demarcated realm of folklore—a category that gained currency along with the rise of the modern nation.

Unraveling *bordados'* multiple meanings makes clear how markers of Indian identity, no matter how beautiful and exalted, are circumscribed by the racism in everyday life, which subordinates people identified as indigenous by linking them to nature, tradition, and the past. When not outright ignored, *bordados* have been dismissed as domestic crafts and maligned or romanticized as archaic holdouts against the onslaught of modern capitalism. My research strongly suggests otherwise. Neither anachronistic nor unthinkingly "handed down," Caylloma traditional dress stands firm as the paradigm of all traditions: profoundly contemporary and re-invented in each new generation.[18] As garments that are simultaneously modern and traditional, *bordados* exemplify the contradictory effects and desires of Peruvian society. Confronting the connections between creativity and ethnicity played out in this commonly trivialized domain compounded my awareness of the ambiguities surrounding gender, ethnicity, cloth, and embroidery.

After two years of intensive research on Caylloma and its *bordados,* I began to write this book. As I wrote, repeating the word "embroidery" so frequently became tiresome. The thesaurus yielded only one literal synonym: "needlework." But M. Roget obliged with other synonyms for "embroider": "ornament," "embellish," "disguise," "pervert," "distort," "misrepresent," and "falsify." This was hardly reassuring. Here embroidery was labeled not merely superficial, but actually untrue. One embroiders on the truth. Over the course of my research, as I learned how much *bordados* meant, my concerns about triviality had diminished. Now a new worry surfaced. Even if my study of embroidered clothes proved substantial, would it, like embroidery itself, distort the substance it embellished? No. It could not be. For people who make and use the clothes, embroidery is not superficial. But because it is creative, it is embellishment, and because it expresses ideas and interpretations, it is a kind of representation. Thus, embroidery has the capacity to misrepresent and to falsify but also to provide a model for the broader creative processes of everyday life and a metaphor for creativity. And this book about embroidery is an ethnography—the product of one person's research in one time and place—so it can do those things as well.

The *bordados* of Caylloma, the primary subject of this study, are a kind of cultural production that often has been observed, collected, gazed at, and recorded, but seldom analyzed. The subject of this study is, however, also an object. As a thing charged with meaning, the garment condenses signification; it illuminates rather than obscures the milieu in which it is inserted and from which it derives and departs. In one sense, I retain an old-fashioned focus on the object, considering its concrete physical properties to be meaningful and not arbitrary. But in another sense, that focus dissolves as I analyze the object as simultaneous latency and actualization. The object is the thing in the process of becoming as well as the thing that is. We must consider both product and process if we are to understand the ambiguities of gender and representation in Caylloma, and why Caylloma matters in the broader scheme of things.

The Garment of Culture: Theoretical Considerations of Gender, Practice, and Performance

> *But it was fitting me like a tight chemise. I couldn't see it for wearing it. It was only when I was off in college, away from my native surroundings, that I could see myself like somebody else and stand off and look at my garment. Then I had to have the spy-glass of Anthropology to look through at that.*
> — ZORA NEALE HURSTON (1990 [1935]:1)

The gendered and ethnic ambiguities of one kind of dress matter, in part, because of what they tell us about dress more generally. I argue that clothes are the whole: the emblem of culture itself. Clothes are powerful symbols of culture because they work both as metaphor and as synecdoche. As metaphor, clothes equal culture in a relationship of whole to whole: the process of clothing one's body equals that of learning one's culture. As synecdoche, clothes are part of culture in a metonymic relationship of condensed signification in which the part stands for the whole.[19]

Zora Neale Hurston compared dress to culture long ago. In *Mules and Men,* she portrayed culture as a garment that fit "like a tight chemise." Worn habitually, the garment of culture became invisible: "I couldn't see it for wearing it." Yet habituation was not total. She was aware that the garment was different from herself: "it was fitting . . . tight. . . ." The passage, as it engages the clothes:culture metaphor, offers a felicitous entry into theoretical and epistemological issues. Hurston's examination of her culture emphasized its visuality: "I could see myself . . . and look at my garment." Invoking the "spy-glass of Anthropology," she added a narrow, voyeuristic aura to this examination; she made of it a gaze. And while it was her gaze, it was not primarily reflexive, because "I could see myself like somebody else. . . ." The invisible, internalized garment of culture required a move "away from my native surroundings" to become visible. Hurston must "stand off and look at my garment."

When anthropologists turn a spy-glass on the metaphorical garment of culture, what do we see? When we look at ourselves within culture and at the same time from outside it, how does the garment fit? When we take the metaphor literally and examine actual garments, what do we learn about culture?

In "Clothes Make the Man," Marjorie Garber (1992) explores transvestism as a primary means of producing culture in both literal and metaphorical ways. "Do Clothes Make the Woman?" counters Kath Weston (1993) in regard to dress and eroticism. Both authors address the constitutive aspects of dress, but Weston's analysis of gender identity through lesbian fashion statements also confronts some tenets of performance theory. These works, among other recent studies of dress and gender, center on cultural constructions of persons.[20] In analyzing the constitutive and performative aspects of clothes, many such works focus on cross-dressing. But what borders are crossed in dressing? How can performance theory help us understand how—or even if—clothes make the man a man and the woman a woman? My approach, likening clothes to culture as metaphor and as synecdoche, provides several paths to learning how clothes make gendered persons. Juxtaposing the literal and figurative qualities of dress reminds us that questions of practice are always questions of power. Emphasizing the materiality of the clothing experience and the concreteness of acted-out events, my formulation of practice as performance stresses the embodiment of discourse in lived experience.

Marjorie Garber and Judith Butler have helped me think through troubling questions of gender, clothes, and culture. Transvestism creates culture, Garber maintains. Examining the ways that "clothing constructs (and de-constructs) gender and gender differences . . . [and] the role of cross-dressing in the construction of culture itself" (1992:3), she notes that cross-dressing challenges binarity, requiring us to critique the categories "female" and "male" (ibid.:10–11). Because transvestism directs attention to the boundaries between categories, and thus to the norms the boundaries mark, it "is a space of possibility structuring and confounding culture" (ibid.:17). In sum, you have to know where the boundaries are before you can cross them, and that knowledge is part of what makes the boundaries.

All gender is drag, Judith Butler suggests. Her approach emphasizes the fluidity of categories more than the boundaries between them. Stressing the construction of gender as discourse, Butler points out that "*woman* itself is a term in process, a becoming, a constructing that cannot rightly be said to originate or to end" (1990:33). The open resignification of discursive practice makes gender "a kind of persistent impersonation that passes as the real. . . . Is drag the imitation of gender, or does it dramatize the signifying gestures through which gender itself is established?" (ibid.:viii). Questions of cause and effect arise as gender is reified in and imposed on the body, and as it is regulated and policed.[21] The troubled significations in the terms "female" and "woman," Butler insists, encourage us to analyze how "language itself produce[s] the fictive construction of 'sex'" (ibid.:ix). In sum, only when you name the boundary do you construct it, and because the boundaries are constantly constructed and reconstructed, they are ideal and never real.

Performative approaches to gender both depart from and build on anthropological approaches to performance. Victor Turner, observing that social time has a form that is essentially dramatic, persuasively demonstrated how social dramas mutually constitute person and society (1974:32). In emphasizing rituals as the dramatic essence of social expression, however, Turner's approach tended to be functionalist and teleological. Viewing rites as always moving toward equilibrium, punctuated by breach and resolution, he treated real life as episodes in the plot of a play. The life course unfolds, however, as much through daily practices as through points of condensation and interruption. Performative approaches to anthropology (Kondo 1997; Schechner 1988) have been enriched by attention to practice, following the "logic" elaborated by Pierre Bourdieu (1977, 1984, 1990). Stressing that the constitution of habitus and identity is ongoing, rather than defined only by hypermeaningful episodes, Michel de Certeau (1984) has emphasized that practice is what happens in mundane activities. Thus we learn to walk the walk.

In recent years, performance theory has been applied in the analysis of gender (Case 1990), and performance approaches in anthropology, influenced by Bourdieu's works, pay increasing attention to habituation as it operates in processes of embodiment. Shifting from viewing cultural productions as enactments that occur in ritual breaches to understanding them as actions that are intertwined with quotidian concerns helps us avoid overprivileging the outcome of a process.

Maybe Judith Butler (1990) said it best: gender is trouble. Gender gets us into trouble, and trying to explain gender never ceases to cause trouble. Performance theory seems to offer a resolution to that trouble. Is gender "all made up"? So Rosalind Morris's (1995) title suggests. Or, as Weston (1993) alludes, is performance theory all dressed up with no place to go? Performance theory cannot resolve all gender trouble, and it causes some troubles of its own. The cultural anxiety of the postmodern condition, of which Garber writes, is revealed, but not alleviated, by unveiling the constructedness of gender identities. Gender is real. Focusing only on discourse can make us forget that fact. As I investigate expression through dress, I return always to the limits of such expression. "Gender no more resides in gesture or apparel than it lies buried in bodies and psyches" (Weston 1993:16). When we break gender loose from essential categories, Morris notes, we must take care, for such rupture may "entail the ironic effacement of gender itself, . . . [creating a] principle of 'genderal' emptiness" (1995:583–584), which could blind us to the historical and political meanings of gender. Although categories are continuously resignified and identity is fluid, those processes do not happen randomly, and they do not happen in ways that render all identities equivalent. Signification does not have free play in our material world. "[B]odies are not passively inscribed by signs, they are inscribed by people who select items of material culture from a restricted range of options and arrange them according to imaginations that are shaped by historical developments" (Weston 1993:13–14; Connerton 1989:72 also discusses inscribing practices).

Because gender is real, I insist on paying attention to the body, the object, the realities of everyday life, and the imbalances of power. Like other feminist scholars, I am concerned with contradictory effects and desires entailed by garments that are simultaneously modern and traditional, such as the Muslim women's veil (El Guindi 1999). In contemporary urban Cairo, Arlene MacLeod (1991) notes, lower-middle-class women begin to veil as they enter the waged work force, not because they are removed from it. Among Egyptian Bedouins, Lila Abu-Lughod (1986) observes, veiling provides women with self-assurance, marks their position in a cultural group, and offers personal privacy in a demandingly collective environment. When Cayllominas select *polleras* from a wide range of available clothing options, they appropriate and transform the traditional *and* the modern. Like veils, *polleras* are distinctively gendered, politically charged ethnic emblems. They have been invested with symbolic weight as they have evolved over the centuries. Their meanings have helped create and have been created by the political and ethnic troubles in which Caylloma has long been immersed, and thus are not detachable from those troubles.

The garment of gendered culture often does fit tight. Idealized norms of gender do exist, and they are policed by practices that regulate sexuality and sexual behavior. Ethnic identity and expression are also controlled through gendered discourses. Clothes make the gendered person, and the weight and force that clothes place on the body is not "merely" symbolic. *Polleras* are heavy! In Caylloma, where male and female persons use recognizably different dress, gender trouble rarely stems from confusion about appropriate male or female garb. Gender identity is constructed through clothes over the life course, but not in predetermined ways; gendering is not reducible to filling one individual's colors inside the lines of gendered structures.

Dress in Caylloma both makes and crosses borders. *Bordados* generally construct and conform to binary male and female patterns of identification: *bordados* are women's clothes, not men's. But cross-dressing abounds in ritual performances, in which men wear women's skirts: *bordados* are women's clothes, appropriated by men. Ritual transvestism in Caylloma, therefore, far from only challenging binary male-female distinctions, also serves to buttress them. Discourses about male appropriation of female dress, concerned with sexuality, potency, desire, and danger, express cultural beliefs in the need to control female power. Gender is also performed in the domains of artistic creativity and commercial production. Recall that Leonardo Mejía said, "When I see a woman in *polleras,* I always call out a greeting. She is from my place." But she is also wearing his clothes—the clothes he made. *Bordados* are men's clothes too. By watching women, by making gendered bodies their business, and by making women's bodily surface their artistic corpus, Caylloma men claim a stake in producing gendered persons. And by wearing *bordados,* women participate in the ongoing construction of their gendered identities as active subjects, despite *and* because of the ways they represent themselves as adorned objects.

As an ethnographer, I also claim a stake. My own gaze is leveled on Caylloma *bordados* as a domain of representation that depends on the intimate relationship between clothes and gendered bodies. I have tried not to substitute my analysis for the perceptions of the people with whom I have worked. In viewing *bordados* through the spy-glass of anthropology, I came to recognize that their ambiguities are primarily questions of power. Clothes have power as shield and as sign: power to represent norms of femininity and masculinity, and to dissent from them; power to express ethnic identity, and to repress it; and power to protect the fragile body beneath the dress, and to project a visual image of defiant pride.

Methods, Evidence, and Stories

Methodology depends on epistemology, as theory and method intertwine in performing ethnography. The performative aspects of gendered and personal self-construction were integral to my methods, not only a theoretical perspective that informed what I observed of others. The methodology I employed and the kinds of evidence from which I formed this book are interdependent with its goals. Visual, oral, and textual data include documents and memories, fieldnotes and "headnotes," photographs and mental images. There were garments and accessories, purchased or received as gifts; interviews with artisans and other Cayllominos; and documents from the Coporaque district council archives. A Peruvian anthropologist, Flora Cutipa, worked with me regularly for almost a year. Assisted by Cutipa, Margarita Larico, and several fieldworkers, I conducted surveys of 110 Colca Valley artisans, both male and female.[22] I almost always spoke Spanish. Cutipa and Larico interpreted Quechua when necessary. The three of us transcribed the audiotapes. I did all Spanish to English translations in the book unless otherwise indicated.

This book is about visual domains of representation, and photographs and drawings incorporated in the text are essential to my analysis, not merely illustrative of points made by the text. Visual domains are also political domains of representation. Not only the clothes themselves are such domains, but photographs of them and of people wearing them. Visual stimuli, especially images of clothed persons in other media, led viewers to reflect on the past. Dozens of photographs from the 1931 Shippee-Johnson Peruvian Expedition, archived in the American Museum of Natural History, were influential; four are reproduced in Chapter 4. All other photographs are my own unless otherwise noted.

Leonardo Mejía is only one of the many artisans from whom I learned the basics of *bordado* design, construction, and technique. During the course of fieldwork, my friendship with Leonardo and his wife, Susana Bernal Suni, deepened. Their story is one that I follow through several generations. Another story is shared among the families of Candelaria and Nilda Bernal Terán, two sisters who are my *comadres,* and their husbands, Epifanio Condorhuilca and Juan Condori, my *compadres.*

Although participant observation is the nuts and bolts of ethnographic method, no hard-and-fast line separates it from apprenticeship. In both, you learn by doing. I spent hundreds, perhaps thousands, of hours peering at objects as they emerged from hands and sewing machines. I observed embroiderers, seamstresses and "seamsters," weavers, and knitters at various stages in creative and technical processes. Observing in itself was part of my apprenticeship. Watching became an activity in its own right, a kind of performance and participation. My twenty-five years of sewing experience helped me talk about and learn design, construction, and techniques. Some tasks I took on deliberately, as an apprentice, and many others I absorbed less consciously, learning without being "taught." I stopped feeling like an intruder once I could help artisans in small ways while we talked. As long as I could contribute, I felt I had a spot in the shop.

My fieldwork depended on eliciting all kinds of discourses from friends, acquaintances, and strangers. I'm shy. I hesitated to intrude and ask bluntly about delicate topics. Even in studying gender, it was difficult to imagine directly questioning someone about sexuality. Because I was a friend and *comadre* of both men and women, I did not want to intervene in domestic disagreements. And with the Peruvian political situation so volatile, I tried my utmost not to alarm or endanger anyone by probing into political affiliations.

At first, my caution frustrated my ambitions to "collect good data," but I found it impossible to manage daily life, much less fieldwork, unless I interacted in ways that felt comfortable and natural to me. Only when I realized this was I able to hear the different ethnic and gendered discourses;

the more I relaxed into "data collection" methods that felt right to me, the clearer these discourses sounded (see also Abu-Lughod 1986). And once I learned how to avoid imposing structures of visual representation on what I saw, my view of the emblems, not only their certainties but their emphatic ambiguities as well, became clearer.

The initial borders of culture and strangeness were occasionally difficult but rarely impossible to get past. Very few people refused to talk to me at all; a handful stopped at perfunctory responses. Instead, countless people opened up and told me their stories (*cuentos,* Spanish). And how they told them! So eloquently, so forcefully, so wistfully—we might yield to tears or succumb to guffaws. In the end, jogging people's memories and getting them to talk did not prove so difficult. Sometimes the stories did not stop when I felt I had heard enough, so I listened on and on. In order to do my job as an ethnographer, I first had to learn to trust my instincts as a person.

My language use, as surely as my looks and clothes, marked me as an outsider but proved an important mediator as well. Not only is English my first language, but even when speaking Spanish, I do not sound like a Peruvian of any identifiable class or place. People in Caylloma seemed reassured by assigning me to one of their identity categories. It confused them that I was bilingual, so I tried to explain my heritage: my mother is from the United States, my father from Chile; I learned Spanish in school, not at home; and so forth. When this discourse proved too long, I abbreviated it: I speak Spanish because my father is Chilean. "Aaaaah, you're a *chilena*! That's why then." This coincidence of identity proved fortuitous. The "*chilena*" category had little to do with my father's origin but applied because I am a "*gringa,*" a white foreigner, and I speak Spanish; in southern Peru this combination defines the category of "*chileno/a*." More than once, a Cayllomina with black hair, coppery skin, and elegantly sculpted cheekbones—the phenotypical "Indian" stereotype—seized upon this evidence of our similarity. "My uncle was a '*chileno*' too," she might reflect. My *comadre* Nilda told me her grandfather was "Spanish" and from Chile: an "*español chileno*"—doubly foreign, doubly white.

Eventually it became clear that to learn how the garment of another culture fit, I needed to put on *polleras.* When I told Leonardo and Susana that I planned to obtain a full set, he commented that dressed that way I would look like a *chivayeña,* woman of Chivay. However, one thing would remain: I would have to learn Quechua.[23] My language use allowed participation, but not full membership, in Caylloma's bilingual Quechua-Spanish speech community. I communicated with the few elderly monolingual Quechua speakers through third-person mediation (and often fourth- and fifth-person assistance, with raucous results). Because our medium of communication was Spanish, a second language for most of us, Cayllominos and I created a new type of speech community, one of intersecting bilingualism.

A "Chilena" in Peru, a "Latina" in the United States, I still walk the walk and talk the talk of my American upbringing. As my ear improved, I came to recognize the contours of several story styles, but never will I learn to *contar cuentos* as Cayllominas do. In long, lively conversations with friends and *comadres,* I came close. Being another storyteller among storytellers was a way to create community, but my membership in that speech community was as partial as my membership in the larger community of practice. Secrecy was also there, our silent companion in a land at war. There were questions that could not be answered, stories that could not be told.

"Every passion borders on the chaotic, but the collector's passion borders on the chaos of memories" (Benjamin 1968:60). Walter Benjamin's observation about book collectors applies as well to the collectors called ethnographers. I acquired documents and objects in the field; some things I took back to the States, others I could not. I also acquired memories and ideas, some of which I did not know were with me until later. The data we collect borders on, as well as contains, the chaos of memories.

As Rosalind Morris (1995:574) notes, "ethnographies are as much about performing gender as are the cultures about which they speak." For me, performing gender in ethnography meant learning by doing things that women do and by sharing with Caylloma people: sharing their clothes, work, food, language, and stories. Performing gender in ethnography also meant learning by writing those stories in other forms. Always a *gringa,* I still tell my *gringa* tales, perhaps in more exaggeratedly *gringa* fashion than ever. Who can say, though, whether my style now bears the marks of Caylloma people's storytelling? Who can say how tight the garment of Caylloma culture fits? And who can say how the contours of those clothes have shaped the borders of our embroidered lives?

Organization of the Book

Chapter 1, "Traveling," situates the actors: families, friends, *comadres,* and *compadres,* among them several embroiderers, with whom I worked closely.

Emphasizing the dynamics of coming and going, and contrasting them with the emotional bonds of community and home, I show how these individuals negotiate within and among multiple places: Coporaque, a village; Chivay, a market town; and Arequipa, a metropolis. In locating myself theoretically and ethnographically, I pay special attention to explorations in feminist ethnography that have informed my approach to gender and representation.

Chapter 2, "Fabricating Ethnic Frontiers," discusses how racial and ethnic identity is constructed through dress. In particular, I show how textile production and exchange, especially involving alpaca fiber, create a unique regional configuration. Analyzing concrete forms of unequal ethnic relations, I explore the construction of Indian identity through its association with rural highland environments. Moreover, I situate this region within the larger Peruvian context and the global economy.

The next two chapters place *bordados* in the present and the past. Chapter 3, "Clothing the Body," stresses contemporary visual representations of Caylloma people. Examining fashion and style, I relate the visual and formal qualities of clothes to their configuration as art works and means of communication, and analyze changing power relations between wearer and viewer. Focusing on clothing the body over the life course, I document the steps in acquiring clothes and trace the meanings of this process for artisans, consumers, and anthropologists.

Chapter 4, "Addressing History," relates *bordados* to discourses and images of the past. I link visual representations of Cayllominos in photographs to oral history and documentary evidence. Through analysis of several embroidery artisans' biographies and of stories about the origin of embroidery, I demonstrate that these competing discourses are closely associated with gender and ethnic conflicts in Caylloma's historical process of racial mixing (*mestizaje*). The chapter shows how attitudes about the past, encompassed in the terms "tradition" and "custom," connect emotional attachments to family, mother, and home to broader Peruvian political and economic trends.

Public contexts are stressed in Chapters 5 and 6. Chapter 5, "Dancing in Disguise," explores festivals as public performance. By focusing on the Witite, a male character who dances cross-dressed in a woman's *polleras,* I connect the performance of gender to the multiple ways that Carnival and other festivals form identity. By situating the Witite within his contemporary context and tracing the history of the dancer and the dance, I unmask transvestism as an emblem of cultural pride that derives from ethnic conflict. Although the public displays in fiestas ostensibly celebrate male political authority, they also represent women's work as the social and economic resource base of fiestas.

Chapter 6, "Marching and Meaning," charts politics and gender through dress. Focusing on women's participation in explicitly political public displays, I examine the relationship between new political organizations and traditional power structures. Of particular interest are nonviolent events held in Chivay which encourage women to appropriate public space, protest gender inequality, and promote female solidarity. I explore how women use *bordados* as ceremonial regalia which signifies community membership, indigenous authenticity, and maternal authority.

Chapters 7 and 8 consider issues of production and exchange. Chapter 7, "Making Difference," analyzes the embroidered clothing production system and its role in creating gendered persons. Presenting the artisans as workers within petty commodity production, I question how the local production system articulates family concerns with larger capitalist structures. Concentrating on the dynamics of gender, age, kinship, and paid and unpaid labor within workshops, I address gendered patterns of designing and tailoring, and analyze how gender relates to skill, economic well-being, and attitudes toward family and work.

Chapter 8, "Trading Places," probes identity and the marketing of ethnicity through clothes. Detailing artisans' economic roles as they buy, sell, barter, and trade in regional circuits, I examine the experiences of traveling vendors in various market contexts, especially their use of *bordados* to leverage commercial transactions. Zeroing in on black clothes, as transformed from sacred symbols of mourning to commodities for sale, I show how tourism affects the marketing not only of ethnic clothes but of ethnicity as it intensifies the commoditization of Indianness.

In the Conclusion, "Why Women Wear *Polleras,*" I return to that central question, rephrasing it in specific gendered and racial terms. Why do men as well as women sometimes wear *polleras*? Why are *bordados* widely considered to be Indian dress rather than white or *mestizo*? Reflecting on the role of truth and subjectivity in anthropology, I address connections between the practices of embroidery and those of ethnography, and show how Caylloma *bordados* reconfigure our understanding of gender, race, and culture because they embody creativity in action.

1

Traveling

The Day I Left Town

This morning I am packing up my stuff. Moving means packing, and it seems like lately that is all I do. As I prepare to leave the thatch-roofed room that has been my home, I evaluate each object in it. For the trip to Arequipa tomorrow, my denim skirt will have to serve. The rest of my field clothes, old beat-up jeans and stretched-out turtlenecks, go into a suitcase to store here in Coporaque. On top of them I place my embroidered, Caylloma-style garments, handmade and tailored for me; when I come back I will need them. My friend Susana Bernal sewed the two long skirts, and my *comadre* Nilda Bernal taught me how to finish every detail. Each stitch embeds a memory of long hours learning how to make my skirts as accurate and true as my foreign fingers could approximate. Vilma Mejía and Tiburcio Ocsa fashioned the thick wool jacket. Each garment brings to my mind's eye the face and hands of the artisan who created it. Rolling up the last belt and squeezing it into the bulging suitcase settles the clothes issue. My written data is already packed away. Notebooks and photographs will travel with me in the backpack. So much else remains to sort. Ideas and memories do not fit into the mind as easily as books into a box.

On and on it goes all morning. I maneuver around the cluttered room. Take a break, step outside, check the weather. Squint at the sun—now at midmorning, high in the sky. *Quema pero no calienta,* "it burns but does not warm you," people say. Back inside, more tasks, eat lunch. If the winter afternoon turns out bright but temperate, then I will head out for one last foray on this, my last day of fieldwork in Coporaque.

The walks I took around town sometimes led me through the plaza and down the narrow lanes. Four streets flank each side of the plaza; sixteen square blocks form the village. On some days the rectilinear grid comforted me, and I was content to stray no farther than my *comadre*'s kitchen. On other days the form was too confining, and the streets and plaza only mocked urbanity. If friends were not home when I went visiting, surely they were out working in the *chacra* (field). A palpable emptiness emanated from the buildings, and I would flee the stillness in the air. I needed to be with people, joining in what they were doing, planting or harvesting as the season required. Then other walks would take me away from town, into the fields, hills, and ravines that comprise the community. Or I might choose an arbitrary destination, a pretext for just walking around the countryside, continuing the process of getting acquainted with all that was Coporaque.

I'm a walker. I walk whenever and wherever I can. In sneakers or hiking boots, striding, strolling, or ambling, this form of locomotion is the way to get to know your place. I did not have a vehicle for most of my fieldwork. Hardly anyone in Caylloma does. Rare is the man who owns a horse; most families have only burros.[1] Everyone walks. During the years I lived in the Colca Valley, I walked more than at any other time in my life. I soon learned Coporaque's main paths: up the hills, down toward the river, and along the road that stretches east to Chivay. One preferred jaunt was to San Antonio, a knobby hill filled with pre-Columbian ruins; but on the banks of the Colca River, reached by a short but steep descent, thermal baths beckoned on sleepy Sundays.

Coporaque is fortunate, people say, because it is "cornered" (*rinconada*) in a notch between two mountains (Figure 4). Shielded from cold nights and the winds that sweep through the valley, the village is a bit warmer than its neighbors. When I climbed into the hills, I would look back toward town and appreciate that sheltered situation. Coporaque's companions in the fifty-kilometer-long valley are fourteen other villages that dot the banks of the Colca River, which extends westward through a deep, narrow canyon. All are dwarfed by looming snow-capped mountain peaks. Again and again it astonished me that human beings make a living there in the valley and on the surrounding slopes and *puna* (high plains).

In June 1992, packing, sorting, and reflecting on that phase of my life, I prepared to leave Caylloma for six months. My fieldwork nearly complete, I was heading back to Arequipa to wrap up my activities there and return to Wisconsin, where I would teach anthropology in the fall semester. Although I would come back to Coporaque the following January to finish archival research and fieldwork, there was still a sense of closure. I had come to feel grounded in Coporaque, which I treasured as a hometown where I shared community. Leaving my adopted home for half a year

4 The village of Coporaque

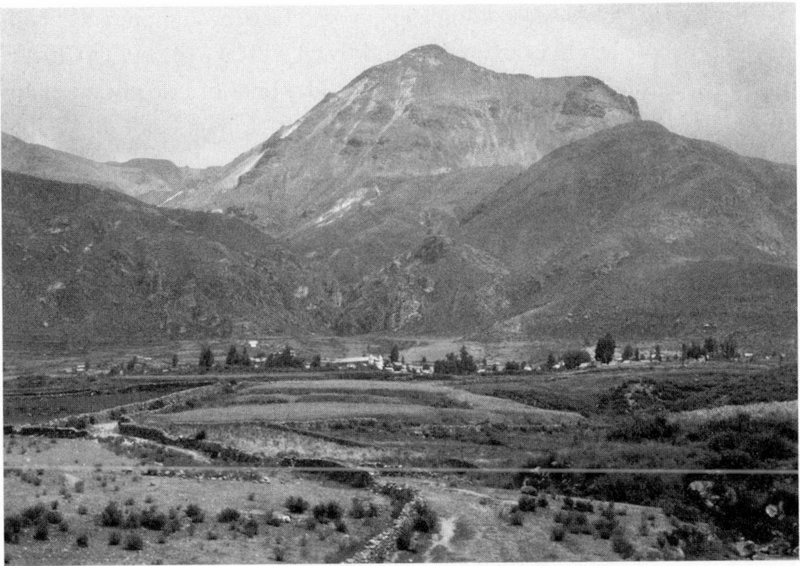

would tear those social bonds. How could they ever mend? The fact is, I am an outsider. Everyone there knew it, and none of us either denied that fact or fully overcame it. The other inescapable fact is, I was usually around. By now I knew people and places, and I had repeated mundane tasks so many times I no longer had to think about them. The first year I often sensed that I did not fit in; those feelings faded almost as fast as my clothes. Sometimes I felt like I, too, had been plunged into icy water, scrubbed raw, wrung out, and hung up to dry in the hot sun and chill wind. And so I, too, was broken in.

Comfort is a hard-won luxury that anthropologists often abjure. Is it curiosity or caprice that nudges us? Go out, investigate, do not be lured into comfort with what you already know. So on this June afternoon, the day before I leave, I set out to say goodbye to Coporaque and learn something new from it. I do not pause in town to seek a walking companion. I have already chosen a destination, a sector of *chacras* still unknown to me. In a few hours it will be dark. Now, well into winter, night will fall by six o'clock. Once the sun descends behind the mountain on the village's western flank, the sky remains light only briefly. Quirky and unpredictable, the afternoon light yields startling colors that create indelible visual memories and, with luck, almost-as-vivid photographs.

Today's trek takes me east along the only road out of town. If I kept walking down this rutted track, I would reach the next town, Chivay. That familiar journey, only seven kilometers, would take me an hour and a half, and local people less than an hour. Tomorrow I will take the bus to Chivay, stopping overnight en route to Arequipa; today on foot I do not intend to go so far. My destination is an expanse of gently sloping lands divided by stone walls into large flat fields (*pampas*). A ledge overhanging the Colca River will provide a new vantage point from which to observe and photograph the village and its surroundings.

Strolling along the road, I glance into the adjoining fields. This year the drought has taken its toll. The *chacras* after harvest have a somber, vacant tone; the pastures are baked bare ground with a few sparse tufts of grass. Here and there people are squeezing in final harvest tasks. All farmer families in Coporaque have lands in numerous, widely separated sectors, so in almost any area I encounter an acquaintance. Only ten minutes away from the plaza I am delighted to recognize my friend Maximiliana Terán and her family working in a field, and decide to pause and visit. I climb through a low break in the meter-high stone wall surrounding the field. Only minor damage results when cactus snags my skirt and I kick out some stones.

Greetings, handshakes, and pleasantries ensue. We speak in Spanish. With Maximiliana is her youngest child, Luisa, nearly two years old, who almost became my godchild. Also accompanying her are her oldest son, Carlos Malcohuaccha, and his wife, Juana, both about twenty, and their infant son. This baby makes Maxi a grandmother at age forty-eight. Maxi has five other children, three of them in high school in Arequipa. I know her family well, for her aunt Luisa Adriazola owns the house where I live in Coporaque; it was built by Luisa's husband, Edilberto Terán, now deceased. Maxi and her husband, Fernando Malcohuaccha, take care of it while the elderly aunt stays in Arequipa.[2] I am doubly pleased to meet Maxi here, as I am fond of her and had planned to visit her house later. Not only do I want to say goodbye, I need to consult her about looking after my room.

"Where are you going?" Maxi asks.

"I'm leaving," I begin. She scrutinizes me, puzzled, evaluating my ability to reach any distant destination with a small daypack holding meager provisions. And midafternoon is no time to embark on any journey, especially alone.

"Tomorrow. Remember? Tomorrow is the day I'm going to the United States for six months," I continue. "Right now I'm walking over toward . . . ," waving vaguely eastward.

"Wayna Lama," she suggests helpfully, naming the sector.

"Must be," I concur. "I've never come over here. I thought I'd take some photos of this side of town and of Yanque across the river. To remember."

We stand silently looking at each other. Thinking about my leaving. Knowing I might never return. Would six months turn into forever? Several foreigners have lived in Coporaque. Most of them never came back. My husband was one of them.

I break away from her gaze and look around the empty-looking field. Only a few clumps of dry broad-bean plants (*habas*) and wispy quinoa stalks still stand. June is late for harvesting. The family's activity is more like gleaning but will require an afternoon's work for three adults. After Maxi and Juana handpick the last bean pods, Carlitos cuts down the stalks with a sickle. Once they finish clearing, they will remove several stone walls, opening the fields for cattle to graze on stubble.

I get the urge to lend a hand, but, for the moment, observer wins out over participant. Aware that the light will soon fade, I decide to walk on, take my photographs, and pursue my private leave-taking while the mood is with me. Later, returning from Wayna Lama while there is still enough light to work by, I will rejoin Maxi's group and pitch in with the harvest.

During fieldwork I actively sought invitations to do agricultural work. Learning farming firsthand was central to understanding Caylloma culture because it is the substance of daily life, occupying the lion's share of time and effort for both men and women in central Colca Valley villages.[3] Tractors and combines do not appear in these highland fields. Almost all farming is done by hand, using a footplow (*chaquitaclla*), or with bulls and wooden plows. At best, it is time-consuming, tedious stoop labor, as a farmer works her way down row after row of beans. At worst, it is bone-achingly rigorous and dangerous, as a man guiding two young, none-too-tame bulls plows a furrow. I felt satisfied when I adequately performed any task suitable for an eight-year-old. I even perversely enjoyed the inevitable backaches and scratched hands, an exaggerated version of pains incurred in my vegetable garden in Wisconsin. Dabbling at chores, however, was a far cry from persevering in a farmer's daily life.

Working with Maxi and her family that day was a sobering experience. All year I had seen the drought's effects as farmers struggled to coax the land to produce the same glowing green crops with less than half the usual water. At the end of the growing season, the landscape always returns to grays and browns, but two years of drought had greatly accelerated this transformation. In a normal year, families sell and trade part of their harvest but aim to store much of it to consume throughout the year.[4] The first year of drought caused a substandard harvest, leaving little to store. The second year was even worse, so people intensified their usual extreme care in harvesting; not one grain could go to waste. Conscious of the scarcity and high cost of food, Maxi and her family invested the extra effort to glean the last few beans.

In addition to drought, volcanic activity damaged the crops. Every day Sabancaya Volcano spewed out thick plumes of ash. From my yard, I watched as the poison clouds emerged and became distorted, beautiful and grotesque, then gradually dispersed over the valley, plains, and peaks (Figure 5). Every day women swept their houses and patios, pushing the gritty cementlike ash aside, only to watch more fall the next day. Ash settled on the leaves and buds of growing plants as well; farmers could only hope that rain would wash it off. But no proper downpour ever came, just miserable sporadic drizzles that misted the plants, making the silica and other minerals in the ash into a natural cement that encased and suffocated the plants.

As we worked in the field, the ash coated us. My hands turned black as I separated *haba* pods from stalks. The fuzzy pods were ideal ash catchers; the leaves, also gray and chalky, released a charcoal haze. As we picked, we coughed and sneezed. I tried not to think of the harm to our lungs, and invisible sulphurous fumes made my eyes burn.[5]

At various spots around the field, shawls and ponchos spread on the ground were heaped with bean pods. Our backs bending, arms reaching, hands moving up the stalks from ground to waist height, we sought the last few elusive pods. One quick twist detached them; some were so dry they fell off at first touch and slid through my fingers onto the ground. I bent to retrieve them, put them in my pocket, and moved to the next plant.

Maxi wore a set of *bordados* (embroidered clothes) that included three ankle-length *polleras* (skirts). *Polleras* are well suited to handpicking, a daily task for most Caylloma farmwomen during harvest. The undermost layer works as a slip and the next one as a skirt. The top one is manipulated into a variety of forms and uses. Today it became an apron. To hold the beans as she picked, Maxi had tucked her top skirt into her waistband on two sides,

5 Sabancaya Volcano emits ash and vapor.

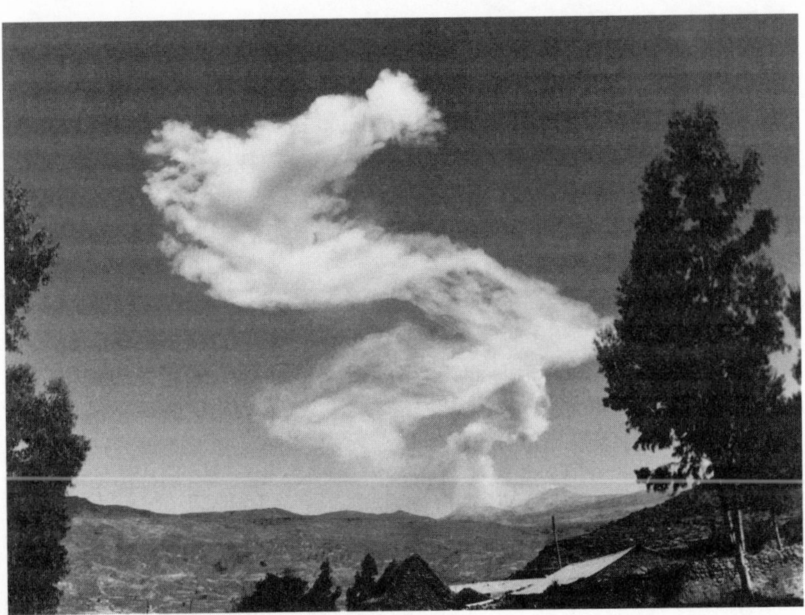

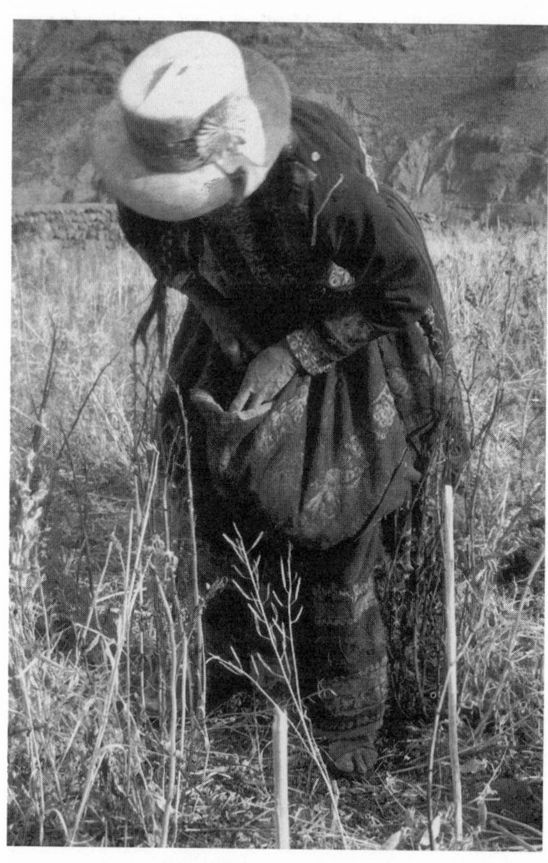

6 Maximiliana Terán picks dry beans.

creating a deep pocket reaching almost to her knees (Figure 6). When it got full, she stepped aside, untucked the edges from her waistband, and loosed all the beans onto a poncho.

Once again I regretted not being properly dressed. I lacked suitable skirts to make a giant pocket. My own set of *polleras* were not only packed away but brand-new. I reserved them for occasional use at fiestas because they seemed too grand for daily field wear. Today, as usual, I wore several layered shirts, but, over long johns, only one skirt—my long, full denim "uniform"—which did not lend itself to bunching up deeply. I stuffed beans into all my pockets but had to make many more trips than Maxi to empty them. I pulled up one long shirttail to use as a pocket of sorts, but this left me only one hand free for picking. How poorly equipped was I for agricultural enterprise!

With smooth and apparently tireless skill, Maxi carried out the deceptively simple task of picking beans. Her slender frame and delicate looks belied the strength acquired through decades of farming, her movements coordinated with a well-practiced grace. Bean picking is stoop labor, hardly a romantic occupation. Besides the volcanic ash and the usual dust, the body's motions are impeded by backaches and cut fingers and diverted to dart off and chase toddlers. Yet Maxi's gnarled hands had a hard-edged beauty as they tucked each pod into the tattered skirt, its once bright embroidery faded and loosened from years of daily use.

Working alongside Maxi, I kept my mind on the task at hand, lulled by the rhythmic monotony. I also thought of many other times we had spent together in kitchens, fields, parties, festivals, dances, and political meetings. In 1992, as president of the Coporaque Club de Madres (Mothers' Club), Maxi's many duties included coordinating projects with the village's male authorities and agents of the state, Catholic Church, and nongovernmental organizations (NGOs). The Club coordinated the distribution of food aid, cooked breakfast for young children, and established kitchen gardens and a soup kitchen (*comedor popular*).

On June 24 the previous year, I had gone to Chivay with her and the Club. For the Day of the Peasant, a national holiday, its members marched in a parade, and the Coporaque school team won the province-wide dance competition. On other days, we had sat together in meetings of the Peasant Women's Federation while delegates hammered out platform points. Maxi did me a million favors, from giving me fresh alpaca meat to taking me to her relatives' parties; all this hospitality indebted me and precluded any hope of full repayment for the ways she had welcomed me into her community and home. Today I was happy to have a chance to help, even if I might give her only an hour.

But my story has gotten ahead of itself. On my last day, I did take the walk I wanted.

Upon leaving Maxi's group, I continue toward Wayna Lama. Turning off the road, I follow a broad well-trodden path, cross a stream on a line of stepping stones, and skirt the *pampas.* A gradual climb up the low hills, less than a half-hour walk from the village center, brings me to a small knob of land where I sit and look back at Coporaque. Although the community's center sits in its protected corner, its lands are quite exposed. Many terraced fields (*andenes*) zigzag up the steep hillsides. More than half of the *chacras* lie below the road, however; those are a mix of *andenes* and *pampas.* My eyes follow the narrow Río Chilliwitira as it passes through Coporaque and these eastern fields. In town the river is a slender, lazy stream, then etches an ever deeper and wider cut, which becomes, at the edge of the *pampas,* a large impassable ravine opening into the Colca River far below.

Vast, distant mountain ranges flank both sides of the valley; closer at hand, smaller hills and mountains perch above the villages and create barriers between them. The valley's villages are arranged in pairs along opposite banks of the river. From my vantage point on the north bank, the neighboring towns of Chivay and Ichupampa, just a few miles away, remain invisible around the bends to the east and west respectively. I see two villages across the river. Straight across is Yanque, its huge colonial church gleaming white. Yanque and Coporaque are so close that people walk daily between them, through the river's shallowest part (there was no bridge until 1996); in fact, part of Yanque's fields lie on the Coporaque side. The next village is Achoma. Some five miles farther west and higher up the slopes, it registers as a pearl gray mass against the brown hills.

The Colca Valley villages have been in their present locations for more than four hundred years.[6] Today all the townspeople live in the village centers and walk several miles daily to their dispersed fields; a forty- to sixty-minute walk each way is standard. Before the Spanish conquest, the population was less concentrated. In and around the contemporary villages are remains of pre-Hispanic settlements perhaps a millennium older. Coporaque has an ample number. I spend a few minutes picking my way through ancient stone buildings in varying states of repair which are no longer residences but are roughly maintained for temporary shelter or storage. During harvest, people sometimes sleep in the *chacras,* protecting their crops from thieves and not wasting valuable daylight time trekking to and from town. This necessity is not only a hardship. My neighbor Dionisio recommended that I try it. The air in the fields, he said, was fresher than in town; sometimes it was good to wake up and see the land around you.

Having reached my destination, I am momentarily content but still distracted by thoughts of all the preparations that remain before I travel to Chivay tomorrow. Seeing an old woman slowly drive a herd of sheep up the path, I realize it is time to head back. I take the last few photographs, turn to walk toward town, and stop to join Maxi in the field. We work together the rest of the afternoon, finally packing the beans into huge woven sacks (*costales*) for the men to load onto burros and take into town.

The walk I took that day was both unique and typical. Joining friends to work in the fields was entirely routine. Long stretches of solitary observation were also part of learning, as I sharpened my visual perception of people, farms, and landscape. Part of every day I spent with friends, settling into a dense and fragile web of kin and community, sewing clothes and eating meals in their homes, farming in the fields, talking over recent events, and listening to their stories. Another part I spent alone writing notes, composing my own stories, and tending my household.

Taking a walk, an activity both habitual and new, generates "successive encounters and occasions that constantly alter it and make it the other's blazon . . . , it is like a peddler, carrying something surprising, transverse or attractive compared with the usual choice" (de Certeau 1984:101). The last walk I took in Coporaque was a combination of novel and familiar, of solitude and sociability. It became a blazon, a proclamation of how hard people worked to make their living there, and a jarring reminder that the valley's physical beauty masked that harsh reality. Because it was part of my fieldwork pattern, that walk was a repetition of the usual that gave an air of normality to an exceptional day. Because it happened on my last day in town, the novelty of the final walk with its surprising encounters made me think long and hard of what my stay in Coporaque had meant.

Coming and Going, Being and Belonging

In this chapter, I situate the reader "at home" in Coporaque, Chivay, and Arequipa, and lead her on a journey among those places. Because the reader did not actually travel with me—walk down country lanes, pick beans in the fields, sew skirts in workshops, or ride buses through the mountains—those endeavors still may seem exotic, part of a foreign land so far from home. Yet those mundane activities, the stuff of normal life, are necessary steps that make an unfamiliar place a home.

My discussion of the politics of belonging remains grounded in the material reality of Caylloma people's lives, which is also shaped by ideological concerns: the construction of place, of community, of home. This chapter provides more than "background" and a description of the "setting" for events narrated in subsequent chapters. Rather, as it juxtaposes and alternates between domains of home and travel, it highlights the themes of belonging, transition, and the formation and transformation of identities that carry through the book.

Traveling is far more than moving between places. To travel means to understand space conceptually and the individual's position in it; to cover long distances but also short ones; to learn a place by traversing it, by walking on the ground, by staying home, by leaving home again. The final day in Coporaque crystallized activities and emotions that characterized my daily life there. Leaving never came easy, no matter how often I did it. Departure propelled me into a new phase of understanding what those experiences meant, as present turned into past and memories of departure blurred with those of arrival. All the travelers who have become characters in this book create and experience their identities in diverse physical and social spaces. As farmers and herders, artisans and merchants, women and men, Caylloma people engage in a multifaceted politics of belonging. They negotiate local, regional, national, and global spaces in ways that are structured by differences in gender, race, ethnicity, and class. And as an ethnographer, a woman, an academic, a hyphenated Chilena-Latina, and an American *gringa,* such differences structured my experiences and the politics of my belonging as well.

Many of the people with whom I lived and worked during fieldwork in Caylloma and Arequipa became friends; a few of them became *comadres* and *compadres* when I became godmother to their children. Because so many Cayllominos welcomed me into their homes, the intimate world of rural family life created my most indelible impressions of Colca Valley lifeways. It was largely through knowing Caylloma society in this personal way that I came to understand issues of self-representation and identity negotiation. The ongoing construction of my personal relationships is intertwined with the long, complex history of all my visits to Caylloma.

I am a widow. During fieldwork I lived in the valley "alone," that is, without family. My husband, John, died suddenly a year before I began fieldwork. This made me reevaluate all my life plans. We had hoped to do research there together, so I had to decide whether I would continue my field studies and, if so, whether I would return to Coporaque.[7] In earlier years we had been there together, although my stays were all too brief. I arrived to "begin" fieldwork in Caylloma seven years after my first visit with John. Two years after that initial visit, he lived in Coporaque for a year doing geography fieldwork, and I spent two months there with him. During that year John became friends with Maxi's husband, Fernando.

A few days before Christmas, 1985, I first met Maximiliana in the gloomy corridors of Arequipa's public hospital. Fernando was being treated there for a head injury sustained in a truck accident. John and I visited while Maxi kept vigil for several days, frightened and often alone. Fernando recovered fully.

Five years later, it was John who died suddenly. After fifteen months of anguished deliberations and preparations, I moved from Wisconsin to Peru in 1991 to do my dissertation fieldwork. When I returned to Coporaque, Maxi and Fernando received me with open arms. My friendship with Maxi is among the oldest and most durable relationships I have there. Knowing how tenuous is our grasp on life and livelihood, our bond is twined from the threads of human frailty.

My experiences as an anthropologist are not completely separable from my experiences as a person. The issues that I stress in my work pertain to vision and perception as they involve the environment and the human form: I look through the lenses of gender and ethnicity at ways people represent themselves and are represented within their political and ecological settings. But by participating in Cayllomino practices, I not only learned about Caylloma, I also experienced changes in my own perceptions, sometimes because I deliberately sought experiences that would change my views, and sometimes because I was inadvertently led to a new way of looking.

Coporaque, the Caylloma community I know best, provides me with a sense of home. By describing this home base in detail, I aim to give a sense of place and to stabilize a potentially dizzying array of actions and experiences. The reader should be anchored by knowing Coporaque, as it anchored me. The community's physical space is also a conceptual space—the realm of the quotidian, which will become quite familiar to the reader.

Coporaque is just one of thousands of Peruvian rural communities whose complexity depends on unequal relations of power. Maximiliana's situation was far from unique as she juggled different social positions, roles, and responsibilities in her personal life and family, and within and beyond her community. Gender, ethnicity, and class are central distinctions coloring the position of Cayllominos, for they are also Arequipeños and Peruanos. They actively negotiate identities based on their knowledge of those complex relations of power and their intimate understanding of inequality. When I think of Maxi, I think of a farmer, a hard worker, and a kind and motherly woman, but I know that many urbanites do not see past the dress and appearance of an "Indian." Living in Caylloma and Arequipa, Maxi's children grow up learning these power relations.

Each brief journey brought its own cultural transitions. Traveling from Chivay to Arequipa, I found the journey through the mountains both mentally taxing and physically exhausting. The changes in altitude alone are quite severe: an ascent from the valley, about 3,600 meters above sea level, up through the highest mountain pass at 5,000 meters, across the slightly lower *puna*, and a sharp descent to Arequipa at about 2,300 meters. More important, traveling meant adjusting from country life to city life. For a long time I believed that the adjustments were difficult for me because I was a foreigner. Later I realized that I was not alone in these travels and transitions. Although we all traveled together on buses that gave new meaning to the word "full," in other ways our travel experiences were vastly different. Traveling entails intercommunity connections, regional transportation patterns, and political and economic positions that situate Caylloma people within the transnational arena.

Although many Colca Valley people felt at home in Arequipa, their ability to negotiate urban society was blocked by racial politics as much as by class differences. My outsider status provided different avenues of incorporation into Peruvian urban white society, because my North American foreignness automatically conferred the status of white (*blanca*). Yet because I am a *gringa*, my racial and ethnic position, paradoxically, remained largely outside the micro-calibrated racial scale with which Peruvians judge each other.

Being and belonging meant coming and going. Being at home meant taking trips. The way I lived, moving between three homes, I was torn between city and countryside, between houses and cornfields, between kitchen warmth and valley expansiveness. But I was not unusual in having several homes or in shuttling between rural and urban areas. Most Cayllominos travel occasionally to the city of Arequipa, but others make their homes there. Some take the bus to Chile, where they buy contraband to sell illegally in Arequipa's street fairs. A few individuals routinely fly to the United States, and some settle with relatives there. Even when they stay at home, they are part of the global system because they buy and sell labor and goods in the fields, markets, and mines of Caylloma.

"Home," of course, was far from idyllic. Cayllominos manage the daunting task of growing crops at high altitudes under a volcano emitting toxic fumes in a seismic zone where tremors level whole communities. Ecological inconveniences are compounded, and sometimes caused, by political and economic difficulties. The civil war's intensity in the early 1990s deeply affected everyone. Cayllominos often lived under a federally imposed "state of emergency" and army occupation.

The war put me in a paradoxical position. As an anthropologist, I wanted to stay safe and to work in safe places but also to understand the war's impact. I wanted to study art and creativity and to understand creativity as both luxury and necessity. Doing ethnography was a strange occupation, but not only because of the war. It is the nature of the beast. Ethnography is a strange genre, neither fish nor fowl, neither fact nor fiction, yet its unique values cannot be duplicated in any other scientific or literary genre. My perspectives clearly resonate with those of numerous anthropologists, some of them self-declared feminist ethnographers, who have addressed the complex intersection between representation and inscription, the relations of power between authors and subjects, and, ultimately, how method informs theory. Thus, this ethnography about gender and representation necessarily considers how I represent myself: as a woman who is also an ethnographer, as a traveler who makes herself at home.

Making Myself at Home: The Fieldwork Lifestyle

During fieldwork I lived in Arequipa, Chivay, and Coporaque—city, town, and village. Four previous trips over a seven-year period had familiarized me with several locales. By doing fieldwork in three different-size communities, I reckoned to understand better the scope of regional life. In Arequipa, I rented an apartment, where I kept most of my possessions, including books, notes, and computer. In both Coporaque and Chivay, I rented a room in a house, where I kept a bed and minimal provisions. When I stayed in the valley, I divided my time between those communities and occasionally visited others, especially Yanque and Cabanaconde.

Arriving in February 1991, I lived in my Arequipa apartment for several months, establishing a base for urban fieldwork. I next rented the room in Coporaque so I could spend longer periods of time there, establish a base in one valley community, and orient myself to the rhythms of rural life, including the uses of dress in its mundane context. When I made forays to Chivay to work with artisans in the market, sometimes I stayed in chilly hotels. Because of the limited bus service, I often had to walk the seven kilometers (four miles) between the towns, carrying sleeping bag, clothes, and cameras. To return to Coporaque safely before dark I had to leave Chivay by 4:30, then cook dinner by candlelight. This was not for me. For sustained study of clothing production and exchange in the Chivay market, I established a third home base in Chivay.

Living in Arequipa meant partaking of the luxuries and conveniences of a large city while enduring its hazards and disadvantages. When I arrived in Arequipa after a stint in the valley, I was always glad to take a shower, cook on a gas stove rather than a kerosene-fueled Primus, trade my sooty field clothes for crisp clean ones, eat at restaurants, and see movies with my friends. Street crime, electric blackouts, noise, and pollution tempered these urban amenities, though. Arequipa is culturally distinct from the United States, but many of my activities and relationships there resonated with my U.S. identities of academic researcher, student, and teacher. I made friends with university professors, artists, musicians, and other culture producers, and I learned to negotiate Arequipeño society. But after a day or two, it always seemed that something was missing.

I would even start to miss Chivay: the buzz of the market, the thermal baths, and the artisans who shared their art, work, and time with me. Despite a few conveniences, Chivay is cold; the temperature drops too far at night, and people are too impersonal. My opinion of Chivay improved somewhat, but I never got used to it; it remained chilly and alien.

Coporaque was another story. It was there that I felt most at home. The village had no electricity, the house had no bathroom, and the running water consisted of a tap out in the patio. But the location of the house in the village and of my room in the house made me feel correctly placed. In some respects, my choice among the valley's smaller villages was arbitrary. With about 1,100 residents, this farming village at 3,575 meters (about 11,000 feet) is an average-size community, or district (*distrito*).[8] In another sense, my choice was inevitable. Because I first went to Coporaque so long ago, knew it better than other communities, and had friends and *compadres* there, it seemed logical to work there. Yet my attachment to the place was far more than pragmatic. Whenever I returned from a stay in Arequipa, only after a night in Coporaque could I settle in and feel at home. Cozy. Harmonious. Breathing.

The valley's volcanic ash, thin high-altitude air, and below-freezing winter nights all conspired against my respiratory system, long pampered by such luxuries as central heating. But only in that valley have I ever felt that I was fully breathing, not gulping or gasping but being permeated by long, deep breaths of nourishing air. But it was only partly physical. The air itself nurtured me because I believed in the power of place. The physical surroundings were also a spiritual home, generating a sense of belonging to a place quite far—both distant and different—from where I grew up. But there it was. Coporaque was the place I felt at home.

In *The Desert Year,* Joseph Wood Krutch proposes that certain places exert rare power at certain times in one's life, as Arizona did on him.

> [I]f I never learn what it was that called out, what it was that was being offered, I shall feel all my life that I have missed something intended for me. If I do not, for a time at least, live here I shall not have lived as fully as I had the capacity to live. (Krutch 1985 [1952]:5)

Mine is an emotional materialism. I believe in the concreteness of sentiment. Actively settling into my three homes made me feel moored and countered my constant coming and going. I hated to feel that I was floating from place to place, pursuing Knowledge for the sake of my Work. A nester at heart, I quickly set up in ways that feel cozy, homey, and natural to me. In any new home I hang paintings, strew shawls and ponchos around, turn bottles into vases, and gather some furniture. So, too, in my Peruvian homes I repeated this process in strange houses in strange cities and towns, which forced me to confront what made each place into a home. What provided the emotional warmth that crept into my heart? What was the source of the welcome that Caylloma's people extended to me? What qualities won me over and made me feel that Coporaque is my home? Why did it matter so much whether a place was really mine or not? Perhaps the sense that I could belong was a delusion.

As professional strangers, anthropologists find comfort in discomfort. That paradoxical pleasure comes with immersion in a different culture. Yet a deep sense of comfort comes from the at-home-in-the-faraway, and it does not come only from within oneself. When I was sitting on the front steps of my friend Susana's house and her brother-in-law Gerardo grabbed my hand and dragged me to a fiesta in a neighbor's house, saying "*Vienes. Hamuy. ¡Tusunsunchis!*" (Come. Come. We'll dance!). . . . When I walked into my *comadre*'s patio and my godson threw his arms around my knees. . . . When I visited Maxi at her house, bringing little sweaters for her young sons, and left with her gift of freshly butchered alpaca meat. . . . When those things happened spontaneously, I knew that I did not create or will into being the situation that allowed me to feel welcome. People in Caylloma welcomed me because an ethos of hospitality pervaded social interactions. Not that no one ever slammed a door in my face, but rejection of that sort was rare. Those conditions also allowed me to be taken into, absorbed by, and contained within Colca Valley society—all this without ever fully being part of it. How such conditions arise are part of what I have to explain. "Have to" in the sense of "feel compelled to," "must" explain, but also "what is mine to" explain, because this experience was uniquely my own—what was being offered, what called out to me.

"My Godmother Is Another Big One": Creating Kinship in Coporaque

¡Madrina! ¡Comadre! In Coporaque when I passed through the streets or entered someone's patio, people called me with these words. Amidst the general uproar of children playing in the plaza, the distant braying of burros and lowing of cows, and other sounds, a few sounds were directed toward me. Godchildren shouted "*madrina*" (godmother); others yelled my name. Adults might beckon me with "*comadre*" (co-mother), but most exchanged nods and murmured "ma'am" (*tía* or *señora*),[9] and friends called me "sister" (*hermana, ñañay*). In turn, I called older men "sir" (*tío, señor*), and elderly women "mother" or "grandmother" (*mamay, abuela*). People commonly address each other by their relationship and qualify names by kin terms or possessives. Not "Nilda" but "*comadre*" or "*comadre* Nilda," I learned to say; not "Ani" but "my Ani," my godson Dante called his baby sister.

Madrina (godmother) and *comadre* (co-mother) are two of my many identities in Peru. For several years I had only one godson (*ahijado*); this relationship inserted me into Coporaque and channeled the economic and emotional support I owed to one family. When I returned to the community, I was hesitant to take on more godchildren, but as I stayed longer, I became a godmother again. Each new *compadrazgo* relationship required assuming new responsibilities and new identities; each linked me not only to three people—parents and child—but to their network as well. Sometimes perfect strangers called me *comadre,* and then I would learn we had a *comadre* in common.[10]

Now I have three "official" godchildren (*ahijados*) from Catholic baptism—Juan Dante, Enadi, and Lucía—and an "honorary" goddaughter, Luisa. Two of my *comadres* are sisters who live in Coporaque: Candelaria and Nilda Bernal Terán. Candelaria and her husband, Epifanio Condorhuilca, are the parents of Juan Dante. Nilda and her husband, Juan Condori Valera, are the parents of Enadi. My third *comadre,* Flora Cutipa, and her husband, Miguel Monroy, anthropologists who live in Arequipa, are the parents of Lucía.[11] But with Maximiliana and Fernando, the parents of Luisa, I did not complete a formal contract.

Candelaria was my first *comadre* (Figure 7). My husband became friends with Epifanio in 1984 and baptized Dante at age one. I agreed to be the *madrina* but was not in Coporaque for the baptism. After John's death, godparenting responsibilities became mine alone—for the boy, who was eight in 1991, and also for his sisters, Marisol, then ten, and Ana, three.

Soon after I arrived, Maxi and Fernando invited me to become godmother by baptism (*madrina de bautizo*) of their three-month-old baby. The friendship between our husbands spurred me to accept their invitation, for at that time I knew Maxi only slightly. I sealed the relationship informally by giving the baby some clothes, but they never arranged for baptism with the Catholic priest in Chivay. (No priest resides in Coporaque.) We have a tacit understanding that I treat Luisa as my godchild, but Maxi and I do not address each other as *comadre*.

In 1991, a few months after I met Nilda, she asked me to become godmother by baptism of her daughter Enadi, then almost four (effectively making me *madrina* to two-year-old Lorena as well). In September we baptized Enadi in the Coporaque church. The importance of this event was great, although the celebration was small. Nilda and Juan did not want,

7 Candelaria Bernal vaults over a wall carrying an orphaned lamb.

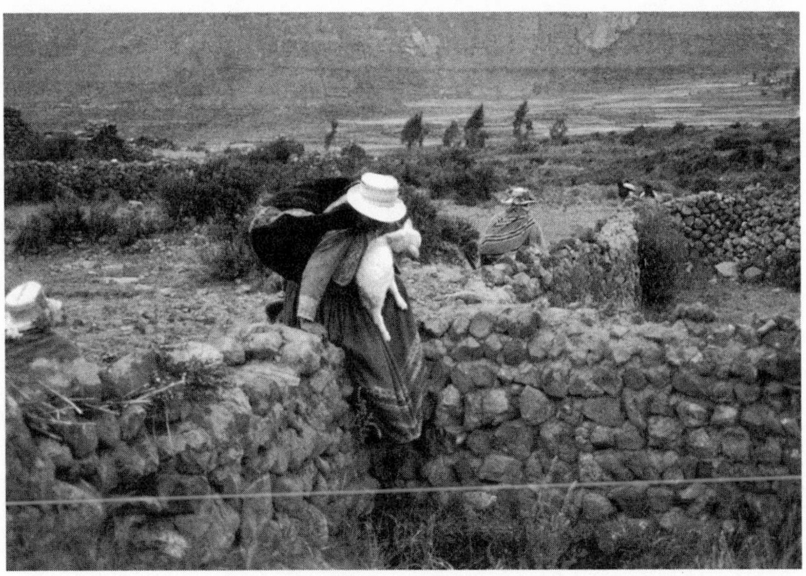

or could not afford, a lavish ceremony. This was the first baptism in which I took part (except my own), as well as the first official obligation that I took on alone in the community. Weeks before the ceremony, the priest held an instructional session in Chivay, which Nilda, Juan, the girls, and I attended.

The *madrina de bautizo* is expected to provide clothes. Although I wanted to encourage the girls to wear traditional clothes, I lacked the social resources to obtain an entire new set of girl's *bordados*. In addition, because Juan and Nilda are artisans themselves and Juan took particular pride in making the diminutive garments for his girl, I did not want to insult them by buying garments from other artisans. So I bought a commercial sweater, a type I had seen little girls wear, rather than a piece of *bordados*.

Utterly entranced with *polleras*, Enadi loved to dress up and dance and was constantly asking to wear the ones she had and wheedling her parents for new ones. Slender and light-skinned, she resembled her mother, but with much lighter hair, the tawny brown called "blond" (*rubio/a*) in the valley. The previous year, Juan and Nilda had been fiesta *mayordomos*.[12] Then Enadi got new *polleras* to dance in the plaza with her fellow Coporaqueños. For the baptism, Enadi insisted on dressing up in her *polleras*. At the church with the priest, her family, and me, she stood stiff and dignified, her immaculate braids poking from under her new white hat. But at home she danced exuberantly in the patio to cassette tapes of traditional Caylloma fiesta music, tickled to be the center of attention. Enadi was a vivid contrast to Lorena, stocky and with much darker skin and black hair (*moreno/a*), who was the spitting image of Juan's mother, Rosalía. Lorena had begun to wear Enadi's hand-me-down *polleras*. Even more than wanting to dance, the little sister wanted what her big sister had.

My social relationships in Caylloma were crucial in part because my own family and friends were far away. Only three Americans, my sister, Ramona, and two friends from Arequipa, Patricia Jurewicz and Catherine Sahley, ever traveled to Caylloma with me. Patricia is tall like me, 5'8", and we are both *gringas*, with light skin and brown hair. Several people in Coporaque thought we resembled each other and asked if she was my sister too.

Soon after arriving in Coporaque on the bus, Pati and I ran into Juan and his daughters on the plaza. Pati entertained the little girls by helping them blow soap bubbles. After a few minutes, we went our separate ways.

"I knew you were in town," Nilda said later when we visited their home. "The girls told me. Enadi said, 'My godmother has arrived,' and Lorena said, 'And my godmother too. She's another big one!' (*'Y mi madrina también. ¡Es otra grande!'*)."

A godmother was something every child should have, Lorena knew; Enadi had one, but she didn't yet. Since I stood a good six inches taller than any other woman in Coporaque, she identified me, in part, by my height. It seemed reasonable that she should have a big godmother, as her sister did. Lorena's analysis helped me understand how Cayllominos begin as children to create kinship and forge social bonds.

Visits, Homes, and Farewells

Visiting Nilda and Candelaria and their families at home was a regular feature of fieldwork life. For several weeks after I arrived in Coporaque in 1991, Candelaria and Epifanio's home was my principal, almost daily destination. Having been their *comadre* for several years accustomed them to my visits. Once Candelaria's sister became my *comadre,* I carefully balanced my visits to both homes, which soon felt equally familiar, as though I no longer was a guest. The sisters are similar in many ways: they look alike, although Nilda is thinner and Candelaria is taller; both are farmers; both are mothers with young children—Lorena and Ana are almost the same age. But Candelaria always wears *polleras,* and Nilda usually wears sweatpants (*buzo*), sometimes with a *pollera* over them. They are also different in personality, life experience, homes, and activities.

The two sisters live only two blocks apart, but their homes are different. Most houses in Caylloma villages are single-story adobe-brick structures, with either thatch or corrugated metal (*calamina*) roofs (Figure 8).[13] On the Coporaque plaza are several cement-block houses, some two stories high, all with *calamina* roofs. A number of old stone houses, some still occupied, also have thatch roofs. Thatch is labor intensive to maintain but makes the interior warmer. Metal, although easier to maintain, is expensive and does not retain heat well.

A typical rural Caylloma home is a compound. A stone wall surrounds four or five structures arranged in a rectangle around a central patio. One room commonly combines the living area and bedroom, and holds several metal beds and a metal-and-Formica table and chairs; a narrow adobe bench (*tiyana*) is built into the wall. As rooms lack closets and wardrobes, clothes are draped over a rope stretched diagonally across one corner (except for weavings stored away in ritual bundles). The rooms reserved

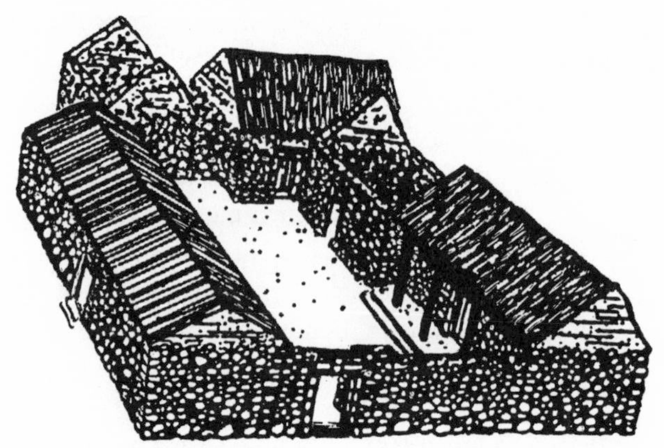

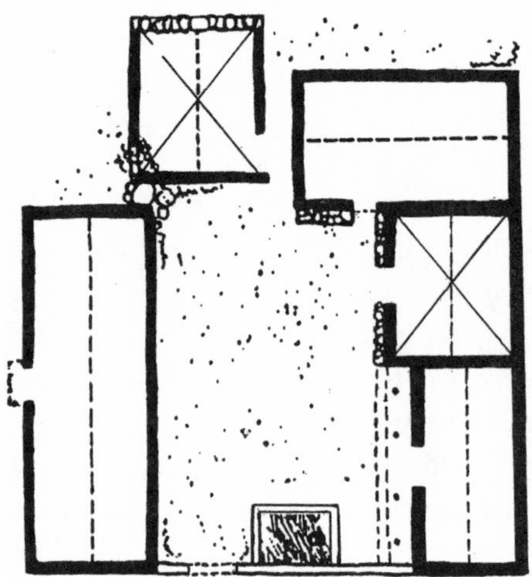

8 Layout of house compound, Colca Valley. Redrawn from Llosa and Benavides 1994:130, Figure 10.

for agricultural storage, although no different in shape and size from the living/bedroom, rarely contain furniture. In addition, a compound usually contains animal corrals or sheds. Run-down or ruined houses at the property's edge shelter trash heaps and makeshift latrines.

Because people are mainly farmers, much of their "domestic" space is dedicated to the current season's agricultural tasks. Processing and storing food requires considerable space and involves numerous stages. On visits to my *comadres*' homes, I witnessed, and occasionally assisted with, all kinds of products passing through various stages of transformation: being butchered, dismembered, peeled, plucked, severed, sorted, salted, chopped, sliced, and pounded flat.

Clothing production also requires space for working, equipment, and materials. Throughout the Colca Valley, with its tremendous amount and variety of textile craft specialization, embroidery and weaving production is unevenly distributed. In many families, at least one woman weaves some of her family's garments. In Coporaque, a handful of people occasionally embroider for their relatives, as Epifanio does. Only a few families in the villages are artisans who depend on embroidery for income, Nilda and Juan among them. Only Chivay and Cabanaconde have embroidery workshops.

Nilda and Juan have two homes in the village—one is considered hers, the other his. Juan's house is the nuclear family's main residence because it is only a block from the plaza and close to family. Nilda's parents live one block south, on the plaza; Juan's mother, sister, brother-in-law, and their children live one block north, farther from the center. After inheriting the plot from his late father, Juan raised the money for building materials and secured the labor for construction. The tiny property has only one building and a narrow patio. The house is one large room made of adobe bricks, stuccoed, with a metal roof. They sleep, cook, and eat in one end, which has two beds, a stove, and a table and chairs. The other end, set apart by plastic curtains, had been a store, but they no longer operate it. Shelves and a counter hold a few sundries and supplies for their embroidery business, and there are two sewing machines and another table.

Nilda's house, on the southwest side of town, was part of a large tract of residential land that belonged to her mother's father's family (Terán). Her mother gave her the property when she reached adulthood. Although the house has beds, Nilda prefers not to sleep there because it is farther from the village center, about five blocks away. She and Juan keep a few animals in the large patio and corral. Having two houses provides space for living, working, storage, and animals.

When I visited Nilda and Juan, we dissected the latest fashions emerging from their sewing machines. They are the only workers in their home embroidery business. We also spent hours catching up on daily occurrences. Enadi and Lorena would climb on me, demanding that I look at their toys and pets. Nilda was then in her late twenties. A champion conversationalist, bilingual in Spanish and Quechua, she had perfected her Spanish during four years working as a maid in Lima.[14] In her early twenties, she returned to Coporaque, married, and had children.

Candelaria lives down the street with her extended family: her husband, Epifanio, their three children, and his grandmother Donata, now in her nineties. The house belongs to Donata, who raised Epifanio after he was orphaned as a small boy, and it will pass to him when she dies. Candelaria has lived her whole life in Coporaque. She does not sew, embroider, or weave. Epifanio, also a Coporaque native, worked for several years in a Chivay embroidery workshop and lived in Lima.

I visited them almost daily to discuss events and make plans. Their house compound, like most, consists of four buildings around a patio. One enters through a gate between one long building and the corral, which have outside walls on the street. Burros often poked their noses over the wall of the corral they shared with the cows. Entering the patio, I would call hello and wait until the dog recognized me and stopped barking before I entered a room. Conversation usually revolved around family events, farming tasks, and food preparation. A few years older than Nilda, Candelaria is rather shy, and more comfortable speaking Quechua. Although I am five years older than Candelaria, I often felt like a little kid, pestering her with many questions in Spanish, which she answered patiently but succinctly. Epifanio enjoyed providing lengthy explanations and quizzing me about life in the United States. Sometimes he and I discussed embroidery, such as a skirt he made for his grandmother. Neighbors and relatives often dropped by to finalize arrangements for the next day's farming activities.

Differences between the sisters extend to their kitchens. Candelaria has the typical house-compound kitchen: a separate, windowless building with an opening in one corner of the roof serving as chimney. Candelaria uses the standard cooking fire of dried dung (*bosta*) and wood under a *q'oncha* (Quechua), a foot-high unglazed earthenware stand. In Chivay, many people use kerosene stoves, which are rare in other villages. Nilda is one of the few Coporaqueñas who usually cooks on a two-burner kerosene stove, set up in the single living/bedroom; she has no separate kitchen.

The kitchen is a focal point of warmth and companionship, and *q'oncha* is a synonym for "hearth" and the "warmth of home." (Other rooms are not heated.) In this primarily female domain, women cook almost all the food and serve male and female relatives and friends. Men do not cook and rarely serve food, except at ceremonial meals, but they eat in kitchens.

In Candelaria's kitchen, a dozen *cuyes* (guinea pigs) often run loose; their gurgles and squeals create an undercurrent of sound. At night the room is dark, lit only by the fire and a candle. The soups Cayllominos eat for lunch and dinner are creative combinations of crops produced in the valley, such as corn (as kernels, *mote,* or on the cob, *choclo*), fresh potatoes (*papas*), or dried potatoes (*chuño*); purchased foods, such as rice; and minuscule amounts of meat, usually alpaca or mutton. People eat *cuy* only on special occasions; Candelaria once prepared it for Abuela Donata's birthday. I loved to eat in kitchens like hers, where women cooked on a *q'oncha*. On winter nights, the temperature dips below freezing. The cooking fire and hot soup were the only things that truly warmed my toes. Even after I had established my own kitchen and made meals there, I ate in Candelaria's kitchen a couple of nights a week.

Breaking away from all of this was the saddest part of leaving. My return to the States ended the routine of daily visits and invitations extended and received. Hoping for short and sweet goodbyes, I deliberately downplayed my departure during my last few days in Coporaque. That way no one would throw me a party, a boisterous alcohol-laden affair that surely would delay my departure by several days. A quiet evening in my *comadres'* homes with their families seemed a more appropriate farewell.

On my last day in town, I bid farewell to many people. Bittersweet goodbyes occupy me from early morning, when Candelaria visits me, to late night, when I take leave of her. First thing in the morning, Candelaria brings her children and Nilda's children to my house. We assemble in groups and take several photographs. I put on my *polleras* for the occasion. Because the skirts are still brand-new, Candelaria has to coax the stiff fabric into the appropriate folds. Nolberto Delgado, my schoolteacher neighbor, takes some of the photographs so they will include me. Laughing, joking, and posing together, we create a small but festive event that helps mark our farewell.

Then I resume packing and take the walk to Wayna Lama. After I return, I assemble bags of supplies for my *compadres* and head for Juan's house. I visit Nilda for several hours, then eat dinner with Candelaria and her family.

Sitting in Nilda's house, we sigh to think how quickly the year has passed since we decided to become *comadres*. As we look over some *bordados* that she and Juan are making, I admire a lovely new design on a vest and commiserate because a customer has not paid for a beautiful skirt they spent weeks completing. Curious about my activities in the United States, Nilda asks if I will see the visitors she met. Reminiscing about Enadi's baptism and other times we have shared, Nilda—at least as sentimental as I am—once again gets out her photographs. I had taken a few for her, but many dated to her years in Lima and early married life in Coporaque. We pass the late afternoon reinforcing old memories and creating new ones.

Finally, Nilda has to finish cooking dinner. We say our goodbyes, and I go on to her sister's house.

For the night of my farewell, I have arranged to eat dinner at Candelaria and Epifanio's house as usual. When I arrive, everyone seems to be in the kitchen. Dante runs out to greet me with his reedy cry, "*¡Madrina!*" He pulls me into the kitchen, where the women are tending kettles of soup. This evening he and Marisol clamor to see their photographs. Because I sometimes shoot and give them Polaroids, they are disappointed that this morning I did not. I promise to bring today's photographs when I return in the spring.

As usual, the exuberant Ani causes a ruckus, then quiets down when food is served. We settle down to eat our soup and then chat quietly over tea. Epifanio is not there; he is playing cornet with his band at a fiesta in another town. I give Candelaria my remaining packages of spaghetti and other food, and we arrange for Epifanio to pick up the cot they lent me. We talk briefly about their upcoming activities here and mine in the States. But, thinking of the packing that remains, I do not linger. As the meal and our visit end, Ani dozes on her mother's lap; the older children assure me they will see me off at 6 A.M. tomorrow.

I step outside into the patio. How bright the firelit kitchen seems compared to the night sky. Streetlights on the plaza, powered by a diesel generator, are turned on only once or twice a year for fiestas. Navigating the three short blocks home is now routine, but I still recall the pride I felt the first time I walked across the little town without a flashlight, guided only by the scattered stars above and the piercing Coleman lanterns in stores on the plaza. Tonight, before setting forth, I pause to adjust my eyes to the moonless dark. Then I step into the inky blackness and make my way back home.

Journeys in the Mountain Lands

From Coporaque to Arequipa

I can't believe it's snowing. Now, in the middle of a drought, and the middle of winter at that, it precipitates with a vengeance. Never have I seen such weather in Chivay: thick fog, freezing rain, and sodden snowflakes more worthy of Wisconsin. From the doorway of the *colectivo* (long-distance taxi) ticket office on the Plaza de Armas, I scan the sky for some sign of relief. Thick gray clouds obscure the sky and mountaintops. Very little snow is actually falling in the valley, and since most crops are already harvested, there will be little damage. My concern this morning is the travel hazard, for we will leave for Arequipa at noon. I grimly contemplate the perilous journey. The *colectivo,* a 1969 Dodge Coronet with bald tires, is bound to skate all over the slick dirt roads and may bog down in the mud.

Another vehicle, another stage in the voyage home. Yesterday I came to Chivay from Coporaque on the bus, leaving one day to get everything done in Chivay and connect with the *colectivo* for today's journey to Arequipa. If I tried to complete the whole trip on the same day, experience had proven, the bus might bypass Coporaque, leaving me stranded there. But yesterday's leg of the trip went smoothly, and, once I got to Chivay, I was busy all day with more goodbyes and packing.

Now, with my luggage safely stowed in the *colectivo*'s trunk, I am eager to get moving again, although a few last-minute errands remain. Bundled up against this soggy nuisance, people scurry around bent over, head and shoulders hidden under a thick blanketlike shawl (*mantón*). I snap my down vest, zip my parka, and pull the hood tight around my face. Leaving the dry shelter of the office, I make a beeline for the market across the plaza.

Chivay's market building is the commercial heart of Caylloma Province. It is not just the only sizeable market in any community in Caylloma, but the largest commercial facility in the province and in the entire rural area northwest of Arequipa. Occupying one long city block, this squat green hulk has an adjoining fenced yard of outdoor kiosks. There are more than a hundred stands. The market is larger even than the church and most government buildings, although not as tall as the new two- and three-story hotels. Chivay is the Colca Valley crossroads because for centuries it was the only town with a bridge for vehicles. (Another bridge, between Yanque and Ichupampa, opened in 1996.) As the provincial capital, Chivay is home to much commercial and political activity and, with five bus companies, is the transportation hub for the valley and most of the province.

Skirting the makeshift plastic awnings draped over outside stands, I enter the market through the large main door and pause to scan for open stands. The market opens by 6:30 A.M., and most business is transacted before noon, even though it does not close until 4 P.M. My main goals are food and gifts. The trip normally takes four hours, but today the weather might delay us indefinitely so I need bread, cheese, and fruit. Most of my purchases, however, are craft items. Yesterday I bought heaps of belts and bags as gifts for friends in the States. What I still need are samples, as I promised several artisans that I would try to market their products or find materials.

This morning people are dribbling in. The weather is bad for commerce, so some vendors have not bothered to open, especially the outside kiosks. At the stands selling food and other essential goods and services, business seems average. Women buy food and prepare lunch no matter what the weather. People also have come from outlying villages to make purchases that they will not postpone because of mere weather. At one stand, a girl buys a liter of kerosene; at another, a man recharges a truck battery. Only Chivay has regular electricity; in the other villages, large batteries, which must be recharged in Chivay, power radios and televisions. Bad weather on top of the poor harvest means that many stands, such as those that sell embroidered clothes, have no customers. Furniture, housewares, and small appliances—never booming in the best of times—are doing little business.

Today my friend Susana Bernal's kiosk will be my last, quick stop. Yesterday, over dinner at her house, we determined which embroidered items I will take to the United States, said most of our goodbyes, and planned to meet at the kiosk this morning. Over the years, Susana and I have had many lengthy consultations about artisans' favorite topic: innovations and changes in embroidered items. She makes *bordados* with her husband, Leonardo Mejía, and sometimes with her brother Hilario Bernal. She needs to sell more. Most embroidery is used for Caylloma women's clothes, but that market is saturated. The national economic crisis means that local people have less money to spend on *bordados.* Therefore, the tiny tourist niche of the embroidery market has become increasingly important. How to make embroideries appeal to tourists has become a constant subject of discussion. How many hours have I spent scrutinizing her wares; designing my own *polleras;* watching her embroider; helping her sew; and swapping jokes, gossip, and favors? Between Chivay and Arequipa, I have also carried her onions, oral messages, and supplies such as zippers and Velcro.

This morning, as agreed, I greet Susana in her kiosk in the exterior yard. I press close against the counter, but the freezing rain still drips off the metal roof onto my back. Susana sits inside, bundled up but still sewing. I explain that the *colectivo* will depart forthwith. From a tall stack, I select a few purses and belts. Today Susana asks me to take a note to her sister Benita, the only one of her six siblings who lives in Arequipa. When

I hear the *colectivo*'s horn, I stuff the note and purses under my jacket, safe and dry.

"See you in six months," I promise.

"Safe journey," she replies, and I turn away toward the plaza.

Today's slack pace contrasts vividly with normal mornings. The market has many consumer products that are not available in the tiny stores in the villages, and it offers a wider selection of other goods, often at lower prices. Chivay is the main place where local farmers sell their produce, including corn, barley, and *habas*. Especially on Mondays and Thursdays, *feria* days, a bustling energy enlivens the scene. Traders flock into town not only from neighboring villages, but from provinces in distant departments such as Cusco. When trucks pull in with huge sacks of the dry, white corn of Cabanaconde, or llama caravans wend their way through the streets, each animal piled high with alpaca fleeces, then the market hums.

A massive shuffling of passengers and goods characterizes morning at Chivay market. The hardiest souls set up food and drink stands at dawn, musty smoke from their kerosene stoves filling the air. Around six o'clock the first bus horn blasts through the chilly calm. In the next few hours, seven or eight buses will pull into town. In Coporaque the bus pulls through the plaza around six. In the villages at the ends of the lines—Cabanaconde on the left (south) bank of the river and Madrigal on the right—travelers set out in predawn darkness to catch the bus by 4 A.M. Two hours, and fifty kilometers, later they alight in Chivay frozen, famished, and parched. Some passengers will return to the outlying villages the same day; others will continue to Arequipa.

The bus companies cluster their scheduled arrivals and departures. In theory, all Arequipa-bound buses leave around 8 A.M., but the decrepit, unreliable vehicles stagger in and out all morning. Last-minute trades, sales, and deliveries invariably create a crisis for at least one breathless passenger, who reaches the bus as it pulls away, pounds indignantly on the door, and demands that the *ayudante* (conductor) heft his oversized bundle onto the roof. Buses routinely pack in dozens of standees, sometimes so many the driver must crawl in through his window.

Besides the buses, there are few other vehicles: a handful of trucks, a *colectivo* or two, a few pickups owned by stores and NGOs, and two dump trucks owned by the municipalities of Coporaque and Chivay. With private vehicles so rare, men who drive their own trucks are well known, even infamous; they are identified by not only their vehicles but their personalities. One man usually agrees to give rides; another, notoriously cavalier about animal and even human life, was reputedly involved in a hit-and-run. Watching these vehicles careen around, I sometimes felt displaced, as if I were not in the Andes but in some other dry and dusty place like Wyoming, populated by men in cowboy hats and pickup trucks. But no gun racks. And then the army convoy trucks pull through, and I am reminded that the province is under military occupation.

For travel to Arequipa, the *colectivo* proved the best mode of "public" transportation; it breaks down much less often than buses, usually leaves on schedule, and, despite imperfect shock absorbers, offers a more comfortable ride. Señor Gómez, the driver, is invariably called by his nickname, "El Chileno" (The Chilean). He is experienced and careful, not reckless like many bus drivers. After twenty years, he knows every bump and boulder on his route.

This morning as I approach the car, El Chileno kids me that I am late and delaying them. In fact, only a *gringa* would believe that the first horn blast means the vehicle is actually leaving. I recognize several waiting passengers. Schoolteachers and bureaucrats, who travel often, are among the few Cayllominos who can afford the higher fare: $7.00 one way, double the bus fare, is almost a full week's wage for a laborer. After arranging our belongings, we pile into the car. I find myself alone in back but know this is temporary. El Chileno almost always travels full: four passengers in the backseat, three in the front.

As we pull away from the plaza, I feel a sense of exhilaration. This is short-lived, for several blocks later we stop to pick up three *mestizas,* two elderly ladies and a teenage girl. The women look so alike I think they must be sisters; the resemblance is compounded by their similar dress in dark straight skirts, short wool coats, cotton stockings, and chunky-heeled shoes. The girl, in jeans and a windbreaker, helps them settle into the backseat next to me. "*Abuelita*" (Grandma) she calls them both, a common term of respectful address; neither is necessarily her grandmother. After she tucks thick wool blankets over their legs and squeezes in beside them, finally we can go.

The Dodge pulls out of Chivay and starts to climb. As we gain altitude, I crane my neck for one last glimpse of Chivay. Below, the hundreds of metal roofs, which usually glint in the sun, are oddly obscured on this cloudy day. I am overcome with nostalgic affection for this cold, uncomfortable town. Even more, I yearn for Coporaque, now invisible around the bend. Pushing upward into the very clouds, we veer left, then right, as one horseshoe curve follows another. Now I see nothing as clouds blanket the car, intensifying my sense of disconnection.

I feel lost.

I am gone.

When will I return?

The long, slow ascent out of the valley allows ample time to brood. Over the next hour, we gain 1,300 meters in altitude above Chivay until we make our way through the high pass at Chucura, a desolate and sometimes icy spot some 5,000 meters high. Melancholy maintains its grip on me until the wispy cocoon begins to dissipate. The road levels off as the clouds break. I feel relief as I sit back, exhausted from many days hurrying about and far too many sad farewells. True snowflakes sparkle as they dust the rocky plain. El Chileno steers the Coronet straight across the eerie lunar land.

Two hours later we reach Viscachani, our only stop, the halfway point on the only road from Chivay to Arequipa. Here are crossroads to Callalli, up the Colca River from Chivay, and to Cusco. The rudimentary truck stop has no gas station, just two restaurant/shops to buy lunch or Coca-Cola. Today only two trucks are in transit; four or five is more typical. A young *mestiza* woman approaches us looking for a ride to Arequipa, and the driver decides to shoehorn her into the backseat.

A more congenial mood prevails when we set out again, amidst light flurries that do not threaten accumulation. Scattered conversation enlivens the trip for a few miles. The road remains dry, but the snowy veil enhances the desolation. From time to time, I see an alpaca herd grazing, but less often than usual; many herders have sought shelter. We cross the remaining miles of *puna,* then gradually descend through the high desert. Sumbay, a train station and military checkpost, then Pampa Arrieros, a herders' hamlet, contain the last houses we will see for two hours. Approaching Arequipa, we spend another hour making our way around Chachani, a long saw-toothed mountain northwest of the city, and passing through deep drifts of sand that remain bone dry. The cement factory at Yura is the beacon of civilization ten miles from the city. We pull into Arequipa in mid-afternoon, dusty but safe. The weather has slowed us slightly, extending the hundred-mile trip from four hours to five. The last few clouds are left behind, clinging to the tops of Misti, Chachani, and Pichu-Pichu, the city's guardian mountains. In Arequipa, the sky is as clear blue as ever.

After dropping off passengers in several neighborhoods, El Chileno deposits me at my house in Umacollo, a middle-class suburb. We say goodbye. I open the gate and haul my gear upstairs to my apartment. Home again in yet another home.

Getting over Green: Life in a Dry Climate

> *You have to get over the color green; you have to quit associating beauty with gardens and lawns; you have to get used to an inhuman scale; you have to understand geological time.* — WALLACE STEGNER (1992:54)

On my first journeys between Caylloma and Arequipa, the numbingly empty brown and gray expanses seemed a stretch of obstacles that metered hours of monotony to be gotten through enclosed in a vehicle crawling through the long dull distance that separated me from my destination. I had no name for it. What is the opposite of scenery? After a few trips, strange contours turned into landmarks as I recognized the larger features. Here we are on The Moon, I would think, when we reached one high plain that was desolate, rock-strewn, and devoid of visible vegetation. Its name, I learned, is Pata Pampa (Flat Plain), and the life-forms sheltered by its boulders are tiny ones adapted to 4,800 meters: *vizcachas* (squirrel-like rodents), lichens, and grasses. Although there are no other roads, faint trails crisscross the plains in all directions, worn by centuries of footsteps. Gradually I became attuned to seeing the land—looking not beyond the brown but into the amalgam of other hues within it. I sought spots I had spurned before, anticipating where the road-cut exposed a rock filled with delicate dove gray and lavender and coppery patina, a model of natural pointillism. Tawny clumps looking like bushes suddenly sprouted legs and walked away; these were vicuñas, wild camelids, roaming the Pampa Cañahuas nature preserve. Once the landscape was no longer monochrome, neither was it monotonous. Instead of wanting to rush past, now I wanted to know the land around me. Was this, too, part of feeling at home? Had I finally come to identify with another kind of place?

In "Thoughts in a Dry Land," Wallace Stegner ponders visual perceptions of the desert landscape. Why is an arid climate so difficult to portray? How can we respond appropriately to the desert's forms and colors? Stop depending on old perceptual habits, he recommends: undo them and acquire new ones. For those of us who did not grow up in a desert, this shift in perception has definite stages. First we learn all over again how to see; this he calls the hardest adaptation. Once we have learned to see "the new forms and colors and light and scale," then we must learn to like them (1992:52).

Stegner writes about the U.S. West, but his observations ring true for South America as well. "Perception, like art and literature, like history, is an artifact, a human creation, and it is not created overnight" (ibid.:54). Aesthetics, like visual perception in general, is rooted in ways of perceiving and appreciating the beauty *of* an environment as well as the beauty *in* it—both what it is and what it contains. The artifact of my perception was re-created during fieldwork as my ability to see changed. The perceptual shift occurred first on the largest scale, through appreciating the vastness of the highland setting. Observations of small-scale detail were more my bailiwick because of my life experience in the visual and performing arts. Bringing the great and small extremes together challenged my perceptions. Not only did the terrestrial textures change with the seasons, but I learned to see them anew each time I passed a spot. Distinctive shapes and colors, changes throughout a day, a year, a decade—all the visual characteristics of the physical and cultural landscape gained meaning in relationship to the dry high place.

Learning to see also involved learning to communicate. As I worked and lived in Caylloma, people explained to me how they see their landscape, and so I learned to value connections among vision, place, and action. Aesthetics is not only a realm of abstract thought, it also has practical and political value. People shaped a cultural landscape as they moved stones, making homes, walls, fields, and canals. They internalized that landscape, too, as they transformed visual images of its natural shapes into motifs on architecture, weavings, and embroideries. Landforms also have meaning as markers, indicating the presence of water, boundaries between communities, and historic struggles over land that shaped survival in the harsh desert clime. Of course, this is a political landscape as well.

As mountain dwellers and as farmers and herders, the people of Caylloma cope with a capricious environment. Their interactions are both demanding and respectful, and their social organization enables them to wrest a livelihood from this difficult land, with political networks to assert their demands and religious practices that include ritual propitiation of the mountains.[15]

The dramatic beauty of Caylloma's powerful mountain landscape astounds me. The exaggeratedly vertiginous aspect of highland life intimidates me. The scale seems, as Stegner suggests, inhuman. So much mountain towers over so few houses. At every turn, mighty snow-capped peaks (*apus*) hover over fragile villages and fields, dwarfing every human-made structure, from the herders' stone huts clinging to the ground to the whitewashed churches' bell towers probing the sky. Where is there room for people? There is too much landscape, it must surely crowd them out. Although the mountains limit human culture, they also enable it. They dominate an ecology in which other climatic and geographic factors also play vital roles.

For the two drought years I lived in Caylloma, the paradox troubled me. The area was so dry that I failed to grasp the impact of water shortage. How can a drought occur in a desert? Why should lack of rainfall matter in place where it almost never rains? Although the high western slopes of the Andes are a permanently dry environment, subtle fluctuations in aridity make the difference between life and death.

The entire department of Arequipa is extremely dry, encompassing regions of true desert, like La Joya, where barren sand dunes regularly engulf the road. Caylloma Province is a "semi-desert with a desert heart" in Stegner's words (1992:54). It rarely rains; in Chivay and the middle valley to the west, the average annual rainfall is less than 400 mm (Treacy 1989: 53–62; 1994a:53–58).

The native cacti and shrubs of the high desert thrive with little rain. Vast groves of cacti outnumber the small native shrubs like *t'ola,* used for firewood, and the few trees, mostly exotic eucalyptus.[16] Some cacti, like the *tuna* (prickly pear), provide thirst-quenching fruit.[17] *Chuna,* a larger cactus, is used in shampoo and its huge white blossoms are visited by the world's largest hummingbirds (Hughes 1987). With so few trees and thus so little shade, the sun burns your skin—even in winter, when the days rarely top 65°F and the nights dip below freezing.

My respect for the mountains' power increased as I knew them better, although I learned their habits only in the grossest dimension. Knowing the mountains requires a lifetime. The largest *apus* hover around 6,000 meters above sea level. On the south side of the river, Ampato, Sabancaya, and Hualca Hualca guard the valley; on the north side, Mismi. Their shapes and masses create barriers that can cause or halt precipitation. Local farmers taught me that, far from consistently benevolent, the *apus*' actions are capricious. For a few months, I believed the drought would break.

Standing in a cornfield, my *compadre* and I watched clouds overhead as rain fell on the river's opposite bank. "It has to come our way!" I cried, but Epifanio merely sighed and explained that probably it would never reach us but would settle on the high peaks as snow.

Mount Ampato and Mount Sabancaya are both volcanoes, but only Sabancaya presented a threat. It had emitted vapor for many years, but in 1990 this activity intensified. It belched thick, ashy plumes, sometimes only twice a day, sometimes hourly. The ash that settled on fields hampered agriculture. When hot ash coated Hualca Hualca's summit, it melted the snowpack and sent water careening down the slopes, causing landslides (*huaycos*), washing out the road, and cutting off several towns for days.[18]

These huge mountains are several kilometers from the valley, but many smaller mountains and land formations, each with its own shape and name, lie closer to the villages. Finaya, a flat-topped volcanic massif, protrudes between Coporaque and Chivay. Saylluta, a distinctive knob-shaped mountain, juts out over Chivay. Configurations of boulders and outcroppings, all of them named, correspond to sectors of fields and serve as boundaries between fields or communities.

A major geographical feature and a boundary of another sort is the Colca River itself.[19] Its central valley, a 50-kilometer-long oasis, and several similar ones lacerate the southwestern slopes of the Andes. The entire Colca River runs about 450 kilometers; its name changes to the Majes, and then to the Camaná, before it joins the Pacific Ocean. In the highlands, its waters are not used for irrigation, but it receives all the tributary rivers, streams, and canals that flow through and around the villages. The dominant presence of the river unites the villages along its course, although it lies far below them. The villages are set onto a series of broad fertile plains, and between Chivay and Lari is the largest expanse of flat lands.

The limited moisture, high altitude, and steep rocky slopes present impediments to agriculture, but local farmers centuries ago discovered how to farm successfully. They made the most of rich volcanic soils, sheltered warm microclimates, and irrigation water from springs and mountain runoff (Treacy 1989:69–71; 1994a:63–64). To manage the scarcity of water, farmers have created and maintained elaborate terrace systems that turn the vertical environment to their advantage. So little rain, unevenly distributed through the year, is not sufficient to water crops; irrigation is always imperative.

Aridity and drought are not just natural phenomena. The cultural endeavor and political organization of irrigated terrace agriculture are "channels of power" (Gelles 1990) that shape cooperation and conflict among communities. Recently, Colca River waters have also been a factor in intensifying contact between Caylloma farmers and the global economy. A huge irrigation tunnel parallels the road along the river; near Cabanaconde it becomes especially noticeable. At other points, new concrete-lined canals snake across the hills or elevated metal tubes pass over the road. They are the legacy of the Majes Irrigation Project (MACON, Majes Consortium) of the 1970s, which stole Colca River water, diverting it to the Majes plains downstream. From the planning stages, local farmers and environmental groups hotly contested the project and, once it was implemented, outright resisted this injustice. To Cabanaconde's farmers, the sight and sound of valuable water rushing past their heads to distant coastal alfalfa fields was intolerable. In 1983, with picks, axes, and dynamite, they fractured the concrete tube (Gelles 1990:146–153; 1994:243–246; 2000:46–47, 62–66). Later, the Cabaneños' rights were officially recognized and a permanent offtake valve was installed, after they petitioned the president of Peru, then Fernando Belaúnde (Gelles 1990:149; 2000:63).[20]

The drought years I lived in Caylloma radically changed my sense of place. Getting over green was essential for me; I forgot about lawns and got used to the inhuman scale. My perception of subtle changes in the natural landscape improved at much the same pace as my perception of them in the cultural landscape. But my understanding pales in comparison with the knowledge of those who have lived there for decades or generations.

I grew up in the Middle Atlantic region of the United States, with luxuriant rainfall and semitropical humidity. I came to Peru as an easterner with "eyes trained on universal chlorophyll . . . [for whom] the erosional forms of the dry country strike the attention without ringing the bells of appreciation" (Stegner 1992:53). So much dryness hurt and frustrated my eyes as they constantly sought but rarely found the precious green.

Traveling the hundred miles that separate Chivay from Arequipa, I felt cheated by the paucity of green. My radar was so tuned to green that each point of verdant punctuation was a joyful highlight in the tedious trip. But these spots mean more than occasional visual relief; they give crucial practical information: the location of a water source, even if tiny. Sometimes water splashes out and tumbles down bare rock. In other places, it oozes into the lush emerald velvet *bofedales,* spring-fed marshes with watering holes. Alpacas and llamas eat native grasses (e.g., *ichu*) well adapted to aridity, but during the drought the marshes were even more important. In the high *puna* as well as the valley, ash from Sabancaya Volcano covered pasture, killing the camelids who ate the poisoned grass. Sixty thousand alpacas, mostly babies and nursing mothers, are estimated to have perished in 1992 alone.

The Colca Valley is the star attraction of Caylloma Province. It is the most populated area and has impressive natural resources and extraordinary physical beauty. But the cultural ecology of this river valley is part of the saga of the province's political ecology. Violence, disenfranchisement, and resistance become apparent when we examine this place as social and political space, considering how the physical place is located historically within a nation-state. The farmers now channeling mountain streams to grow their corn have not simply chosen to inhabit this place; their ancestors were assigned to this land in order to feed colonial-period Spanish settlers and miners. Intimate knowledge of the land tells them where to get water and how to manage it, but it also sparks memories of many centuries of cooperation and conflict between *mestizos* and *indios,* especially fights over land and water, that characterize the valley's history.

A renewed aptitude for envisioning is essential for learning culture and learning *about* culture. Seeing is such a vital cultural feature that, paradoxically, it is often ignored, perhaps because we learn so quickly to normalize and rationalize as natural that which we take in through our eyes. "Getting over green," as I have used it here, means enriching a visual appreciation of Caylloma's landscape, but not just aestheticizing that landscape. It means recognizing that people also created beauty in the cultural landscape and rejecting depoliticized representations that omit humans from an ostensibly "natural" landscape. Getting over green reminds us that a symbolic economy goes hand in hand with a political economy. Together they have influenced the construction and representation of culture, gender, and ethnicity in Caylloma in ways that are distinct to this place, specifically forged in Peruvian history, and cannot be subsumed within a homogenizing notion of Andeanism.

Fieldwork, Homework, and Ethnography

Becoming an ethnographer is something that happened to me while I was doing things that ostensibly were distinct tasks: "doing fieldwork" and "writing up." The longer I was involved with both tasks, however, the more they seemed to overlap. Every day I spent in the field, I speculated about the ultimate result, The Ethnography; every day I wrote, I reflected on what Fieldwork had been. The differences between them, however, became more sharply defined as well. Fieldwork was more enjoyable, even joyful, though not always easy; writing was painful, mysterious, and rewarding in tiny doses. Writing comprised a constrained space where joy dared not enter. Despite, and from within, the pain of writing, rare moments of clarity emerged with powerful force.

Over the long course of producing this book, my ideas changed as the work jolted between leaps and setbacks and, all too rarely, progressed through stretches when the whole project made sense or I recognized one tiny detail as a key to the entire experience. The indelicate balance between fieldwork and writing generated many questions about gender and representation, about identity and experience, where personal and professional concerns nervously converged. To answer these questions, I could neither push away personal emotions nor address only personal issues.

During fieldwork, I developed strong emotional attachments to people and places in Peru. For a long time I believed those attachments were something I had to "get over" in order to write a scholarly monograph. Although I remained committed to a highly personal ethnography, with lots of detail and real people who came alive through dialogues and descriptions, even that sort of objectification made me ethically queasy because the one who represents acquires so much power. If only I could set aside "unprofessional" feelings—nostalgia for joyful days spent in the field, longing to return there, and outrage over the injustices, neglect, and abuses of the abominably wealthy few, which keep people I cared for mired in poverty. . . . If only I could get over my feelings, I reasoned, my writing would go faster, my goals would be clearer, and my ethnography would reveal itself. It took me two years of writing to realize one thing:

I could not get over my feelings.

Which then led me to realize:

I should not.

For me, ethnography had emotional shadings and nuances, moments of empathy when strangers became friends during a brief conversation, intense exchanges when I felt my identity shift as I acquired a name or a position in another person's conceptual scheme, and extremes of profound alienation when a sense of the futility of efforts to alleviate poverty seemed not momentary despair but acceptance of a grim social reality. Getting over emotional interaction with my experiences could only lead, for me, to giving up all hope for communication.

The ethnography depends closely on the identity of the ethnographer who creates it. But the primary value of questions about the relationship of action and experience does not lie in ruminations on the Self or in distinguishing the Self as subject from the Other as object. This ethnography is not a disguised journal of a spiritual voyage through the alien domains of Otherland into the discovery of Self. Such a document, no matter how effective, would not be an ethnography. This document contains my efforts to explain the place where I was a stranger yet at home.

Ethnography is undergoing a deep, thorough self-scrutiny unprecedented in the history of anthropology as a discipline. This has both thrilled and unsettled my generation of ethnographers—those who earned graduate degrees in the 1990s. The exclusionary tendencies of practitioners, the positivist scientific tone, and the master-narrative whole-cloth ethnography combined for more than a century to make a discipline that paradoxically produced a very narrow view of the cultures it intended to portray comprehensively. Critiques of these practices have generated other styles of "writing culture" and numerous countercritiques.[21]

Within highly diverse critiques, one common thread is an emphasis on positionality. "Every view is a view from somewhere," Lila Abu-Lughod (1991:141) puts it. Each author speaks from a position shaped by academic background and personal heritage. When the author tells the audience what he or she was in a position to know and not to know, it becomes clear that the observer is neither innocent nor omniscient (Rosaldo 1989:66). Admitting the falsity of innocence, we question whether detachment and neutrality should be our goals.

While some differences among ethnographic modes of representation lie in the way they are written, others inhere in the subject of representation. "Subject" encompasses broad issues of epistemology. In this book, I consider them largely in the relationship between gender and genre: how the ethnographic project is conceived, what is deemed important enough to be a subject of ethnography, who or what constitutes a gendered subject, and how the ethnographer represents her own subjectivity as she envisions the enterprise.

For feminists, the question of position is further complicated. All anthropologists must confront the fact that ethnography is a predominantly white male enterprise, designed and developed as a gender-biased genre, yet increasingly practiced by women. Because the assumed subjectivity of the anthropologist is still white male (Newton 1993:8), the author is not required to self-identify as such. A nonwhite, nonmale anthropologist, however, qualifies her identity and, along with it, her work.[22] As I put the label "feminist ethnography" on both my project and my product, I am conscious of the awkwardness in that characterization.[23] Personal experience and personal identity occupy professional space; as many authors have noted, they are intrinsic parts of the ethnographer's occupation.[24] "Personal" in one sense means that the author is responsible for the text. Although a certain inevitable amount of ethnographic authority (Clifford 1988) must be acknowledged, taking a personal stance also demands accounting for variations in lived experience and subjectivity among the people with whom the ethnographer has worked, and for the impact of their experiences on the ethnographer and, ultimately, on the kind of ethnography he or she writes. The default as white male remains important.

Characterizing subjectivity through the relationship between "field" and "home" shows us they need not be separate locations. Rather than a place, "the field" is a relationship "between oneself and others, involving a difficult combination of commitment and disengagement, relationship and separation" (Lederman 1990:88). In this sense, being in the field requires "simply a shifting of attention and of sociable connection within one's own habitual milieus" (ibid.; see also Clifford 1990, 1997 and Gupta and Ferguson, eds. 1997). So too, "home" is not an unproblematic geographic location but a concept requiring us to turn our gaze homeward and attend to its conflictual construction (Martin and Mohanty 1986:196; Frohlick 1999:90).

The "shifting of attention and . . . connection" that Lederman suggests, however, is far from simple. My analysis of that shift began when I faced the importance of home, both for me as I came to feel at home in my field site and for people in Caylloma as they experienced the contradictory sensations of belonging to community and being pulled away from it. "Getting over green" also meant, therefore, moving beyond the naïve belief that home could be so separate from field.

Feeling at home and understanding that feeling has made me attend more closely to every kind of lived experience as creative experience. As "home" stands for the sentiments and ideologies of community and placement—the "politics of belonging"—it embodies the bases of creative work, the security of cultural identity, the fabric walls that house our bodies, and, by extension, all creative experience. Ursula LeGuin commented that one can return home once one realizes that home can be "a place never before seen" (cited in Visweswaran 1994:109, 111). Although this means accepting the importance of constructing a safe "homeplace" in which to make a community of resistance (hooks 1990:42), it does not mean treating home only as a safe haven. Home confines as much as comforts, excludes as much as includes, and relies on "the repression of differences even within oneself" (Martin and Mohanty 1986:196), and thus renders safety illusory.

Where should ethnography take us? Is it a literal journey to an unknown land? Or is it a conceptual journey through ideas? As anthropologists, we must decide what kinds of ethnography have a future. One central issue is what kind of ethnography does or does not address feminist concerns. Feminist ethnography is not impossible, it is imperative. Despite the "awkward relationship" that Marilyn Strathern (1987) has probed, ethnography that omits feminist concerns is not just inherently androcentrically one-sided but also irresponsible. Rather than wonder if ethnography can ever be feminist (Abu-Lughod 1990; Stacey 1988), we must scrutinize all projects that claim to be ethnographic or holistic and yet omit half the world.

Diane Wolf claims that living in another culture does not fundamentally alter positionality; it "may create more sensitive researchers and ethnographies but cannot change where we come from and where we return to" (1995:10). But if we don't change, why go? If our experience of life in other cultures and away from the confines of classroom and library has no real impact on the work we do, why not stay at home? The product that emerged from my research is different from the project I envisioned before going to Peru. While my personality affected how I worked there, the experience of fieldwork also changed me as a person and my way of approaching this work.

The question of positionality is a real one for anyone doing research, whether close to the "home" where one grew up or at a greater distances as I chose to do. Questions about position are questions about power. Power relations between ethnographers and subjects are undeniably unequal, but we need to look beyond what seems obvious about the first or third world and into the constitution of power in different societies (Mohanty, Russo, and Torres, eds. 1991). In traveling to Peru and making the field a home, I had to ask myself many questions. What does it mean to be "Hispanic" or "Latina"? How does this differ in Latin America and the United States?

How do race, culture, and origin relate in the person of the ethnographer? How would I be perceived without my husband in a community where one of my identities had been his wife? What are my responsibilities as *madrina* to my godchildren? How do I, a white foreigner, fit into communities where power is so severely proscribed by race? This chapter only begins to answer these questions; they will surface again and again.

Conclusion

> *What does travel ultimately produce if it is not . . . "an exploration of the deserted places of my memory" . . . ? What this walking exile produces is precisely the body of legends that is currently lacking in one's own vicinity; it is a fiction, which moreover has the double characteristic, like dreams or pedestrian rhetoric, of being the effect of displacements and condensations. . . . These signifying practices . . . invent spaces.*
> — MICHEL DE CERTEAU (1984:106–107)

The people of Caylloma live in tiny hamlets, small villages, and market towns but also in a larger region; a sense of that broad regional scope is part and parcel of their daily lives. Not every valley resident travels to distant cities or countries, but all residents know such travel is possible. Their awareness of their positions as members of a region and a nation shapes their identity. My awareness of their positions as well as my own has also shaped my identity. Through these signifying practices, we have invented spaces, and explored the deserted places of our memories.

What de Certeau calls "the long poem of walking" does not merely follow established paths and recognize established sights but "manipulates spatial organizations, no matter how panoptic they may be. . . . It creates shadows and ambiguities within them. . . ." (de Certeau 1984:101). My way of knowing Coporaque—footstep by footstep—also meant covering a part of its territory each day. I came to enjoy the feeling of being planted in Coporaque, feet on the ground, learning this new hometown through sustained interaction with my social circle. The shadows and ambiguities were part of the fieldwork process and part of the lives Caylloma people made.

Ethnographers' work and life are joined so closely it often makes us squirm. Perhaps anthropologists really are strangers in their own land, wanderers and misfits who seek to extend that sensation in another strange land. Many have speculated on the discomfort, (dis)ease, and alienation that drive us to foreign lands and make us "walking exiles" on a pilgrim's quest through unspeakable conditions to find the self-abnegating mystic hero within. But this does not tell my story or the stories of many anthropologists, particularly women who have written movingly of intimacy and distance. Rather than professional strangers, anthropologists may be the opposite: beings with an intense need and, if we are lucky, some talent for fitting in quickly, developing friendships, and building a network of trust—in short, for making ourselves at home.

In my case, "home" came to equal "understanding" not only my own ideas and emotions about people and places but those they expressed about each other and outsiders. Home, then, is not a place but a whole constellation of feelings. People in Caylloma made me feel at home on their terms. They were able to do so, in part, because they know what home feels like. Many people deeply appreciated the sense of home, not because they had been born and raised in the same village, but because they had not. They, too, had come and gone and had been transformed by a deeper sense of what home meant. Their travels also opened spaces to something different; they had experienced the double characteristic of being affected by displacements and condensations that de Certeau calls "travel."

About his stays on an unpopulated island in Alaska, Richard Nelson wrote that attachment to place is a shapeless desire in which loneliness itself takes on qualities usually found in company. That elemental comfort may seem sweet and fantastic, or it may seem "entirely commonplace, filled with the ordinary but indispensable satisfactions that also strengthen the bonds between people. Perhaps this is the essence of connectedness with place and home: bringing nature and terrain within the circle of community . . ." (Nelson 1989:163).

At various times in our lives, we all do both fieldwork and homework, and we should not always distinguish between them. I began this chapter with a story of leaving, achieving closure, and contemplating the end of a fieldwork phase in my life. This episode seemed to mark clearly a border between fieldwork and writing as two separate spaces of ethnography. Yet after I returned to the United States and began to write, I realized how mistaken I had been, how false this border would prove to be. Like many anthropologists, I believed that I was finishing fieldwork when I was truly only beginning it. I finally managed to understand that fieldwork *is* homework.

2

Fabricating Ethnic Frontiers: Identity in a Region at the Crossroads

Of Canyons and Crossroads

"I am ashamed," confessed Florencia Huaracha. Her statement shocked me. After spending many hours interviewing Chivay market vendors like her, I was accustomed to hearing about their pride in the beauty of *polleras.* Huaracha, then in her seventies, had worn *polleras* since childhood and for twenty years had run an embroidery stand with her husband. "Have you ever stopped wearing *polleras*? Why?" I asked. "Shame" (*vergüenza*) was the reason Huaracha gave. She only changed out of her *polleras* to travel to Arequipa. The way urban people looked at Chivayeños was what made her ashamed. Even when Arequipeños said nothing, rather than endure their disapproving gaze, she left her *polleras* at home.

Analyses of contemporary ethnicity often paint rural Cayllominos as fundamentally different from outsiders. Inhabitants of rural communities are the people most often called Indians in Peru, and they are also often identified with "ethnic" dress, such as *polleras.* This difference, some claim, originated in pre-Columbian times. Others say that the Spanish invasion nearly five centuries ago created the categories of race and ethnicity, which contributed new conceptual boundaries that crosscut existing political and cultural frontiers. Within a region, however, internal distinctions may be more crucial in self-identification. Residents view the canyon that splits the Colca Valley as an ethnic boundary. It is the legendary frontier between two quadrants of the Inka Empire, Qollasuyu (home of the Aymara-speaking Collaguas) and Kuntisuyu (Quechua-speaking Cabanas). Today Chivay and Cabanaconde, the towns at opposite ends of the valley, ardently contest the superiority of their community's size, language, and dress.

Living and traveling in Caylloma and Arequipa, witnessing Cayllominos' frequent interactions with outsiders, and observing material reminders of pre-Columbian and European influences, I came to see Caylloma as a dynamic crossroads, a land of physical and conceptual frontiers. In the lengthy fame it achieved as a land of wealth and plenty, cloth has always played a part. As textile-related activities articulated with mining, herding, and agriculture, they shaped the southern Andean regional economy and the future of the Peruvian nation.

This conclusion, however, is not shared by all observers. Mario Vargas Llosa, Peru's best-known novelist and Arequipa's most famous son, sees "almost total isolation" in the Colca Valley's "startling landscape" (1987: 27). David Guillet, an anthropologist, maintains that the valley experienced "historic isolation" because of difficult terrain and distance from Arequipa (1992:14). Contrary to such claims that Caylloma was isolated, I maintain there was a high degree of articulation. What constitutes isolation? This chapter examines the rationale for applying a term whose referents are negatives: what it is not, where it is not, what it does not have, and who does not live there. Isolation is relative to one's perception of the importance of other places and the people in them. If Caylloma has been isolated, then from what? and from whom?

The canyon is an ethnic frontier with a physical manifestation in the landscape, but other frontiers are formed by more personal boundaries, especially dress. Huaracha experienced the boundary created by *polleras* as shame. Throughout this book I argue that after gender, ethnicity is the most important factor influencing use of *polleras*. This chapter analyzes the way ethnicity operates in Caylloma and in Peru, beginning with an analysis of regionalism. Numerous long-standing factors in Caylloma's political economy distinctively shaped ethnic identity as well as the region's unique role in Peru. In examining the racial and class components of Cayllomino identity, I compare local variants of Indianness with those in the rest of Peru and the Andes. Among visual markers detachable from the body that are often used to ascribe ethnicity and race, dress is primary. Like Huaracha, many women mentioned that dress identified them with their community. Not one person who wears *polleras* in Caylloma ever told me that she (or he) did so because she was an Indian. To understand this apparent repudiation, I review the two main kinds of women's ethnic dress, "*de vestido*" and "*de pollera*," and briefly assess them in relation to the characteristics of men's ethnic dress. In considering how dress forms ethnic frontiers, I was forced to attend to the ways that the political economy of representation has long been intertwined with the relationships between ethnicity and race.

The "Regional Problem," Caylloma, Arequipa, and the South

The "regional problem" is a key to understanding Peruvian society and culture. Peru is not merely characterized by extreme regional particularity. The provinces have struggled so constantly and intensely against the inordinate centralization of power in Lima that the nation has been defined by that tension (Flores 1988:147; Mariátegui 1971 [1928]; Orlove 1977; Femenías 2000a). Regions, though often demarcated by shared ecological characteristics and extensive economic and political interactions, also have "qualities shaped by ethnic, ideological, and emotional structures and associations" (Orlove 1977:64–65; Flores 1977) that may fragment as well as unite. Caylloma is part of Arequipa, but it is also part of the southern highlands (*sur andino, sierra sur*). This vast stretch of mountain ranges (sierra) and high plains (*puna*) extends from Peru into Bolivia and Chile. Likewise, Arequipa's location in the southern highlands renders it geographically and conceptually Andean, but its seacoast and large urban center link it to Lima. In exploring Caylloma's placement within Arequipa, the Andean south, and the nation, I also address the ethnic, ideological, and emotional associations of the regions.[1]

Caylloma has always meant cloth. Probably during pre-Hispanic times and certainly in the colonial period, wealth was derived from woven textiles and alpaca fiber, largely produced by indigenous labor. More recently, a wide variety of textile-related activities, from herding animals to marketing finished cloth, characterized Caylloma's economy and Arequipa's industrial development. These were so meaningful in the southern Andes that, along with mining and agriculture, they not only shaped the regional economy but also molded the national political landscape.

Today, as in the past, Caylloma's primary political-economic allegiance is to the city of Arequipa. The southern highlands circuit, however, draws Arequipa's highland provinces—Caylloma, Castilla, Condesuyos, and La Unión—toward Cusco and Puno to the north and east. Several of Cusco's provinces are closely connected to Caylloma: Canchis, Chumbivilcas, and Espinar. Common interests in sheep and alpaca, in particular, sustained links with Sicuani, the capital of Canchis, a major wool marketing center (Orlove 1977:65, 71, 77). Across the *puna* through mountain passes, traders have transported cargo, first by llama caravans, then mule trains, and now trucks and buses.[2]

The main railroad lines, extending from the interior to the coast, connect few interior cities with each other. The railroad does not link Arequipa to Lima, only to Cusco and Puno, and it does not reach Caylloma. The road conditions range from poor to abominable. The Arequipa–Cusco road is unpaved except near the cities. A few more kilometers were paved in 2002 before the local elections. Both railroad and road construction proceeded apace with economic expansion and market penetration. Two significant construction phases were the 1870s, when the railroad system was initiated, and the 1910s–1920s, when the wool trade expanded.[3] Only in the 1940s was a direct road built between Arequipa and Chivay; another spur soon extended from Chivay to the Madrigal mines (Guillet 1992:27–28; Manrique 1985). Widened in the 1970s for the MACON irrigation project, the road has since been neglected, rendering it impassable after heavy rains.

The city of Arequipa owes much of its dominance in the *sur andino* to its distance from Lima (today, twenty hours by bus) and proximity to Chile (the border is five hours by bus) and Bolivia (Puno, near the border, is twelve hours by train). With 1 million people, Arequipa is the only large industrial city between two national capitals, Lima (8 million) and La Paz (greater metropolitan, approx. 1.5 million), as well as Peru's second largest city. Because of its coast, the department of Arequipa gained advantage over neighboring landlocked departments. In the age of sail, much communication and transportation was by sea. Nineteenth-century British and American ships docked at two adjacent towns, Mollendo and Islay, then the most important ports in southern Peru. About 1900, Mollendo became the terminus of the railway from the interior. Soon, as larger steamers demanded deeper harbors, Lima eclipsed all other ports and trains stopped running to Mollendo. Today, the emotional importance Arequipeños invest in their coast outweighs its economic importance.

"Most of the political upheavals that shook our nation until recently originated in this land of poets, lawyers, and clerics. In fact, there seems to be no Arequipa intellectual who has not fomented a revolution" (Bermejo 1954:36). La Ciudad Blanca, "the White City," is famed as the city of poets and presidents, revolutions and earthquakes, ballads and bullfights (Chambers 1999; Love 1999). The revolutionary reputation began early: in 1836–1837, the department seceded from the newly independent nation and joined with Bolivia in a short-lived confederacy. Throughout Latin America, the so-called "Independent Republic of Arequipa" is legendarily arrogant.

Situated at 2,300 meters above sea level, the city is surrounded by mountains. Arequipeños also have a reputation for being volcanic—unpredictable like their guardian volcano Misti, and one of their nicknames is "Mistiano." A local saying, "*tienen su sierra nevada,*" literally, they "have their snowy mountain range," means they are as stubborn, capricious, and clouded over or melancholic as the mountains. Nevertheless, many city residents do not consider themselves "highlanders," *serranos.* "White City" refers not only to its ubiquitous pearly volcanic-stone (*sillar*) buildings but to its idealized racial composition and conceptual geography. Mistianos who consider themselves whites (*blancos*) may also call themselves *costeños,* "coastal people." The white, cosmopolitan association of "*costeño*" contrasts with the Indian rusticity of "*serrano.*" Limeños, especially elites, usually regard such claims as pretentious; to them, anyone who does not live in Lima is nonwhite. Arequipeños, therefore, cannot be white; they are provincial and live in the mountains. In most of Peru, highland residence and the farming and herding lifeways of rural communities (Spanish *comunidad,* Quechua *ayllu*) are usually associated with Indian identity. The people who live in Arequipa's highlands and other parts of the *sierra sur,* therefore, are the ones whom other Peruvians tend to call Indians. It is also true that many trace their heritage back to the people who lived there before the Spanish conquest. Arequipa is usually considered the antithesis of Indianness—a very "Spanish" city, meaning racially very white.

The political-economic development of Caylloma and Arequipa is intrinsically connected to ideas about racial and cultural heritage. By the fifteenth century, Caylloma was a well-established constituent of the Inka Empire, a primary reason why Spaniards settled there just after founding the city of Arequipa (1540). To the conquistador Gonzalo Pizarro, the Spanish Crown awarded an initial *encomienda* (labor-land grant). New settlements (*reducciones*) were soon consolidated into a province, then called Collaguas, in the Spanish viceroyalty of Peru; the province became a critical way station in the rapidly expanding global network of communication and exchange. Colonization, evangelization, and modernization proceeded apace with indigenous resistance to Spanish colonial abuses, culminating in the eighteenth-century rebellions (Femenías 1997a; Manrique 1985).

After Peru became independent in the 1820s, foreign concerns dramatically accelerated their role in extracting productive resources and introducing consumer goods. After the mid-nineteenth-century guano boom went bust, wool quickly became a major export and British cotton textile imports deluged the market. In the 1880s, British firms absorbed the Peruvian state's debt (incurred by losing a war with Chile); soon they penetrated all levels of commerce and finance. European immigrants became established in trade, invested in modernizing the physical infrastructure (especially railroad and factory construction), diversified into banking, and leveraged financial advantage into political clout (Flores 1977; Rippy 1959; Thorp and Bertram 1978).

The singular importance of the wool trade distinguishes this epoch from all others. During the heyday, 1890–1935, as Arequipa blossomed into the southern regional anchor, the wool trade uniquely shaped the region's racial and political economy. The city of Arequipa became the global epicenter of alpaca fiber commerce. Its wealthiest wool businesses were British owned: Ricketts, Gibbs, and Gibson. Caylloma's resources and strategic location facilitated regional growth, which in turn increased the province's national and transnational articulation. Simultaneously, racial and class boundaries were redrawn.

Rural Arequipa and the whole southern Andes were dominated by powerful chiefs called *gamonales,* who drew labor for their large *haciendas* (agricultural or ranching estates) from the many adjacent *ayllus* (Aguirre and Walker, eds. 1990; Kapsoli and Reátegui 1987; Manrique 1988; Poole, ed. 1994). Caylloma's *estancias* (grazing lands) yielded small amounts of alpaca fiber compared to Puno, where vast *haciendas* resembled self-contained chiefdoms.[4] But wool-related traffic through Caylloma increased indigenous producers' contacts with *mestizo* intermediaries and dependence on global markets. Consequently, "*misti,*" a new, derogatory term for *mestizo,* insinuated that *mestizos* asserted racial superiority over Indians and sometimes dominated through violence. The *mistis* ultimately gained sufficient political power to challenge the *gamonales*' iron-fisted rule.

Clearly, this is not a picture of isolation. Instead, the alternating waves of investment and withdrawal, conditioned primarily by global markets, periodically stranded Caylloma. Once wool declined, the province was again relegated to the hinterlands. The state's new modernization initiatives, supported by U.S. and multinational capital, were administered through regions. These included the Southern Regional Plan of 1959 (Carpio 1990; Flores 1977:14; Gallard and Vallier 1988; Love 1989) and a national Region system established in the 1980s by Alan García's APRA government.[5]

Conforming to the 1959 Plan, the city of Arequipa grew into an industrial hub. A huge Nestlé/Carnation dairy concern, Leche Gloria, was the centerpiece of an industrial park erected on the city's outskirts (Love 1989). This affected Caylloma in the 1970s through MACON (the Majes Consortium), a multinational effort that diverted Colca River waters. The alfalfa grown on the newly irrigated coastal plains fed cattle to provide milk to Leche Gloria. Intense commercialization accompanied the huge influx of personnel and money into the Colca Valley, enriching some enterprising and opportunistic Cayllominos and foreigners (Benavides 1983; Carpio 1990; Larico 1987; Swen 1986).

Industrialization also affected textile production. The urban textile industry expanded and modernized from the 1940s through the 1960s but continued to process alpaca. Two European-owned enterprises—Inca Tops and Condor Tips—helped shift the focus to luxury fabrics for the European market (Carpio 1990; Markowitz 1992). Rural producers were pressured to commit, in advance, ever increasing amounts of high-quality fleece and fiber to the Arequipa cartel; domestic and local crafts were left with inferior-grade alpaca.

The push-and-pull of underdevelopment meant prosperity for the urban bourgeoisie, but it also attracted more, and increasingly poorer, migrants to the city. Two major earthquakes devastated Arequipa in 1958 and 1960, but they did not impede development for long; the task of rebuilding the cathedral and other structures ultimately meant work for laborers (Quiroz 1990; Carpio 1990). But as development slowed, migrants who did not find jobs in industry were left adrift in a sea of unemployed ex-*serranos* like themselves. By the 1990s, not only did old-line Arequipeños express alarm at the ballooning "invasion," but the mayor's policies aimed to reduce the number of migrants or at least to remove them from view.

Race, Ethnicity, and Asymmetries of Power

The paradoxes of racial classification in Peru are manifold. On the one hand, many Peruvians deny there is racism because all are *mestizos,* but, on the other, some make extreme claims to economic and racial superiority. During a conversation in a private home, I was chilled when an upper-class woman proposed to "kill all the Indians." That, she said, would solve all the problems: those of Peru and, more important to her, of Arequipa, making the White City white once more (Femenías 2000a). "Ethnicity" became a prominent analytical term as part of attempts to understand race as other than a biological concept. Focusing only on ethnicity, however, cannot explain the persistence of racism (Harrison 1995:47). By contrasting terms and practices of self-identification to imposed labels in both local and regional variants of racial and ethnic identity, I expand our understanding of Andean race and ethnicity as social categories.[6]

In Peru, I mostly discussed race with people I knew well. During a visit to my neighbors Agripina Bernal and Dionisio Rosas in Coporaque, I noted that city people talk about "*indios*" but people in the valley do not. I asked if they knew any *indios.*

"There are no Indians anymore," Dionisio replied. "They are all dead. They lived in the time of the Inkas." Looking over the stone wall surrounding their patio, he waved expansively toward the houses and fields. "The *indios* built everything we see around us."

Agripina, his wife, took issue. She did not claim there were living Indians but was unsure about those contributions. "They built everything?" she asked. "What about the church? The Spaniards built that." Dionisio replied that the Spaniards told the Indians what to do, but the Indians built the church, the terraces, everything. They were the ones who knew how to build and how to work. For him, the "*indios*" were not only long dead but defined by their practices. In work lay their knowledge. Although more adamant in attributing this knowledge and skill to Indians, his respect for the achievements of those who went before and his emphasis on skilled knowledge and work were typical of most Cayllominos. So was the fact that he did not self-identify as Indian.

I have never met an Indian in Peru, yet everything that I read and heard in the United States prepared me to meet quite a few. The population of Peru, Bolivia, and Ecuador is widely reported to be about half Indian. In Peru, this "fact" even appears in schoolbooks (Fuenzalida 1970:16). But a more accurate rendering is that "Indian" is something people call others; those who are so called do not see it that way. If no one admits to being an Indian but all only use the term to label others who also refuse to identify as Indians, then what does this infinite, elaborate chain of finger-pointing mean? How does this universal "passing" work in practice? Is Indianness, in fact, such a crucial aspect of identity that it must be clandestine?

It is precisely because, as social scientists have long observed, "Indians" in Peru do not call themselves Indians that it becomes necessary to analyze the characteristics of this category. During the 1990s, the term "*indio*" was not a term of self-identification. Many wondered if it would be reclaimed as a positive term of pride, as "black" and "queer" were in the United States. The Quechua term "*runa*" was sometimes deliberately used in political oratory and published works, simultaneously reclaiming language and ethnicity, and "*runakuna*" (plural) was a badge of group identity. But the reasons for avoiding "*indio*" are not explained by substituting another term, which is ostensibly a euphemism but without negative connotations. Others commonly used are "*indígena*" and "*nativo.*"[7] In Peru, a person does self-identify as "*originario/a*" to indicate that he/she is from a certain place, and this term need not have racial overtones. No matter how they are labeled, "indigenous groups" in contemporary societies, regions, and nations are ill served by being conflated as peasants or as "Andean" (Starn 1991, 1995). Arguing that "culture" has replaced "race" as the primary label for Indianness, de la Cadena (2000) likewise notes that the substitution has not generated a positive gloss.[8]

I never asked a person if he or she was an Indian. Even in my own country, I would not presume to ask people if they identified themselves by many of the ethnic and racial labels that others apply. In Peru, I refrained from suggesting an identity to which people did not subscribe because I did not want to offend anyone, put myself in danger, or, if everyone "knew" the criteria except for me, seem exceptionally foolish. After all, I was a foreigner. Maybe I just didn't get it. So I listened. Keeping my ears open and my mouth shut aided my investigation. People told me about their own racial and ethnic identity as well as that of others. No one ever mentioned being an Indian. No one even casually slipped it into conversation, much less proudly claimed it. Even when I asked an individual if he or she knew any Indians or knew where they lived, Indian identity continued to go unclaimed by the speaker for him/herself and usually for family members. Perhaps the people down the street might be, but often Indians were those who lived higher in the mountains. And the people who insisted that Peru, especially the highlands but increasingly the cities as well, was full of Indians were not happy about their presence.

"Indian" occupies a place in a set of relational identities. No one is Indian in and of himself or to himself; rather, other people are Indian to him, or he is Indian to another. As in kinship, one cannot say "I am sister," only "I am her sister," that is, a sister to someone else. As a relational identity, "sister" only has meaning depending on the speaker's point of view. What then is a relationship of Indian? Contrasted to Ego, the self of the speaker, a person with less power, prestige, money, and value is Indian to him or her (Mayer 1970).

Race and ethnicity have long preoccupied scholars of the Andes, and the identities most commonly addressed are the trio of Indian, white, and *mestizo*. Growing attention to the constructedness of these categories attends to nonphenotypical markers, including dress. Nevertheless, in both popular parlance and much social scientific literature, the Indian category is usually presented as having a "biological race" component, encompassing phenotypical attributes like skin color, eye shape, and face shape associated with "Native American" heritage. Discrimination against dark-skinned people is only part of the dynamics of racism in Peru. People who "look Indian" are rarely called Indian if they are middle or upper class, if most other family members "look white," or both. The visual aspects of race matter in part because they have been used so often to support notions that race is based in biology. In addition, when phenotypic characteristics are used to determine group membership, ethnicity becomes a matter of visual position in social space. While not ignoring phenotype, I concentrate on visual markers detachable from the body that dominate in the ascription of ethnicity and race (see Poole 1997).

"*Mestizo*" indicates a mixture of white and Indian, but there is considerable disagreement about the extent to which it indicates race. Most *mestizaje* literature, treating the *mestizo* category as "in between," focuses on *mestizos*' liminality, building on the assumption that "racial mixing" inherently creates difficulties. As a nationalist project, however, an ideology of *mestizaje* homogenizes. To be Peruvians, *mestizos* must reject specific ethnic identities and subscribe to assimilation. The utopian aspiration to form a "*mestizo* nation" is impossible because the mixture simultaneously depends on the recognition of both heritages and demands rejection of them.[9]

No matter how asymmetrical, the power relations between categories are constructed. Some scholars, therefore, argue that they are completely malleable. This pluralist model asserts that ethnic groups can coexist on equal footing once the negative connotations of certain categories are effaced (e.g., van den Berghe and Primov 1977). This rationale contributed to the 1960s ban on using the term "*indio.*" Peru's experience has shown, however, that plural models cannot be implemented successfully in societies where racism is deeply ingrained.

In Peru, race and ethnicity also symbolize place. Accordingly, "Indian" is associated with a rural identity, "white" with an urban one. This framework posits that ruralness consists of an Indian hinterland with a nucleated white center, mediated through towns where *mestizos* dominate social relations. Thus, people who live in the mountains are "*serranos,*" meaning both "highlanders" and Indians. Again, the model misleads. Attachment to place and continuity of community are important, positive factors in identity formation and maintenance. Fragmentation, however, is the inevitable negative counterpart. Direct connections between communities have been limited under Spanish colonial and republican national control. Although the whole hinterland is characterized as Indian, political control is denied to Indians. Therefore, mediation with centers of power occurs in a system of vertical hierarchy through channels with an undeniably racial tone: power is concentrated in whites and urbanites.

Ethnicity in Peru is shaped outside Peru, especially by ideas applied to a larger area, "the Andes." Many characteristics and cultural traits of mountain dwellers probably diffused over spaces with similar terrain, but a cultural ecology model is of limited use; unless historically informed, it often lapses into economic determinism. All the "Andean nations" are not alike. In Peru, despite the use of similar terms, ethnic and racial realities are in many ways as different from those of Ecuador and Bolivia as they are similar because of each nation-state's individual pre-Hispanic, colonial, and national heritages (Albó 1987, 1994, 1999; Larson 1995; Radcliffe and Westwood 1996; Urban and Sherzer 1991).

The question of time, as applied to ethnicity, formerly implied permanence. More recently, it has meant examining historical particularity. Attention to time also demands examining how ethnic groups were categorized on an evolutionary scale of modernization and progress. In this scenario, Indians have been linked to the past (de la Cadena 2000; Femenías 2000a; Flores 1987). In Peruvian political ideology, racist rhetoric blaming Indians for impeding national progress has gone hand in hand with the exaltation of past achievements that have bolstered cultural pride. Nevertheless, because contemporary culture has been so closely associated with the past, indigenous people have been rendered as relics, not as active agents. Such an abstracted "Other," in fact, "exists not across time, but at no time" (Abercrombie 1991:120; see also Larson 1995; Starn 1991, 1994).

In addition, "ethnicity" has been treated as a synonym for "class," and "indigenous people" have been termed "peasants" as analysts renounce the timeless Other and highlight contemporary aspects of conflictual identities and actions. In explorations of connections between different sectors of Peruvian society—and with other nations—indigenous people emerge as actors who have resisted outsiders' expropriation of their lands and lifeways. Sentimental uses become instrumental when ethnicity serves as a symbolic umbrella for political mobilization (Urban and Sherzer 1991; van Cott, ed. 1994). In Latin America in the 1990s, democratization and ethnic activism were nearly synonymous—a phenomenon that Hale (1997) calls "re-Indianization." The indigenist political wave seemed to sweep the Americas.[10]

In Ecuador and Bolivia, indigenous activism often takes center stage on the national level (Albó 2002; Radcliffe and Westwood 1996; Zamosc 1994). In Peru, however, perhaps the most bitter political irony is that in a country ostensibly full of Indians, groups which self-identify as indigenous have not united into an effective popular resistance front drawing on indigenous heritage (García 2000b:6, 10–11 n. 14; also Basombrío 1999; Marzal 1995; Remy 1994; Stern, ed. 1998; Yashar 1998).

Cayllomino Ethnicity

Hearing politically charged discourses about race and ethnicity in Caylloma and Arequipa, I was repeatedly surprised, on the one hand, by the vehemence of racism and racist rhetoric and, on the other, by the detachment of phenotypical features from cultural ethnicity. People frequently comment on the physical appearance of other people's faces and bodies, including skin color. Their awareness of race and ethnicity extends to the clothes with which they represent ethnic and gender identities and political loyalties.

In this section, I contrast my observations with published comments about ethnicity in Caylloma; some authors describe multiple ethnic groups, and others maintain that ethnicity is not an important factor. Each Caylloma community has its own distinctions, and the larger communities, especially Chivay, feature greater class differentiation. Nevertheless, these authors show such vast interpretive differences—stemming from ideology and the subject of the author's research—that it seems they were not even in the same region.

Today, while some "natives" of Caylloma often discuss their contemporary identity in terms of pre-Hispanic ethnic origins, others sometimes boast of their Spanish "blood." Even in acknowledging that "mixing" has occurred, people rarely self-identify as "*mestizo*"; like "Indian," it is usually a label for others. Racial labels overlap with class distinctions. "White" commonly implies elite status, not only skin color. For example, one elderly man said his family, now one of Caylloma's wealthiest, was among the "few white people" when they arrived in Chivay around 1910. People in all communities, highly aware that sharp distinctions exist, also use understatement to make ideological points about self-worth and collective worth. By saying "we are as good as they are," individuals may assert their equality to urban people or local *mestizos* and communicate their awareness that others deny it.[11]

At least since the Spanish arrived, the history of ethnicity in Caylloma has been characterized by the lengthy, complex process that is *mestizaje*. During the colonial period, two main ethnic categories were "Spaniards" (*españoles*) and "Indians" (*indios*), but "blacks" were also recorded as Colca Valley residents (Cook 1982; Gelles 2000:32 n. 8). Race factored into economic status because of Indians' heavy obligations for tribute and service as *mitayos* (conscripted laborers) in mines, noted in 1549 in Cabanaconde (Cook 1982:4); church baptismal records also indicated the race of parents and child (Gelles 1994). By the seventeenth century, ethnicity was linked to occupation. Spaniards settling in the Colca Valley worked in cloth production and exchange, and as *arrieros* (mule-train drivers) and innkeepers.

Later in the century, Caylloma's ethnic composition changed again. Newly arrived Spaniards entered areas beyond the Colca Valley, especially the town of Caylloma; a new mine sparked gold fever (but produced mostly silver).

One oft-employed category, "*español,*" is problematic. Although at first "*español*" applied only to a Spaniard—someone born in Spain—the term became synonymous with white. In addition, to avoid the demands of tribute and the *mita,* many "*indios*" fled their home communities; elsewhere they passed as white, representing themselves as "*españoles*" (Spalding 1984; Szeminski 1987). Today "*español,*" like "*blanco,*" usually means social superiority or dominance, not necessarily light skin.

To mean "race," the term "*raza*" was used more frequently during the nineteenth century, when it assumed a nationalist connotation that carried into the twentieth century. "Whites" were called both the "*raza española*" and "*raza blanca.*" *Mestizaje* became so closely linked to nationhood that "*raza peruana*" sometimes appeared. For example, in the civil registry for the 1890s–1930s in the Coporaque municipal archive, on birth registrations the race of parents and child was listed as "*peruano/a,*" as well as "*indio/a,*" "*indígena,*" and "*mestizo/a.*" By 1940, race was a sufficient national preoccupation to be a census category (Cook 1982).

Contemporary anthropological analyses of Cayllomino ethnicity begin with William Hurley (1978). In Yanque and Maca, where he studied MACON, people are known as "Indians" and "*mistis*" or "*mestizos,*" but "there are no precise criteria . . . to distinguish the Indian from the *mestizo*" (1978:126). Using cultural indices such as clothing and coca chewing is of limited use in interpreting "racial composition" (ibid.:129). Hurley argues that assimilation fundamentally shapes racial views, as the primary goal is to "whiten" away from traits associated with Indianness and low status.

> But as they increase in status, they are assumed to become less Indian. It follows, therefore, that . . . we cannot have a rich or high status Indian, because the Indian, by definition, is associated with cultural traits of the poor. Thus as the Indian increases in wealth, he also acquires a new race, that of *mestizo.* (Ibid.:128–129)

Because "changing race" has limited possibilities, Hurley posits, differentiation is a matter of class. Meaning a rich, influential person, the term "*misti*" is often "used in a derogatory sense because, traditionally, it has been the *mistis* who have exploited the 'Indians' (*indios*)" (ibid.:129). *Mistis* have more land and cattle and more education than Indians or *campesinos;* they are often priests and teachers. If a *campesino* becomes comparatively wealthy and then treats "his former peasant colleagues" disrespectfully, this snob "become[s] a *misti* despite his racial 'handicap'" (ibid.:130). He who was once Indian compared to the *mistis* leaves his fellow Indians and becomes *misti* to them.[12]

Bradley Stoner (1989), discussing ethnicity and class as related to health in Yanque, likewise contrasts *mistis* to *campesinos.* He notes that wealth and resources are often concentrated among *mistis,* "who despite their small numbers exert significant economic and political influence and power. . . . *Mistis* are generally lighter-skinned, more Western or European in dress and appearance, and economically more well-to-do than other peasants" (1989:55). Calling *mistis* a class which cannot accurately be identified "on 'racial' grounds," he uses the term in describing politico-economic problems associated with ethnicity and identity. Besides *misti* dominance, many generations of *mestizaje* have fostered Cayllominos' pride in their "'Andean' or pre-Incan and Incan heritage," so that a "cultural sense of . . . Andean or Indian identity is widely apparent in [their] . . . beliefs, attitudes, activities and behavior" (ibid.:56).

My own studies revealed that Cayllominos understand Indianness as more than "Andean" identity. Whether or not they have internalized its negative connotations as thoroughly as Hurley claims, they both acknowledge its relational qualities and avoid using the term. They often characterize Indians as those who live at higher altitudes and visit town to trade. Clorinda Maqui identified such people as Indians, but qualified her response: "We don't treat them as Indian" (*No los tratamos de indio*), meaning they did not address them as such and did not exploit them (interview, Cabanaconde, 1993). Paul Gelles (1992; 2000:42–43) identified local euphemisms, including "*caballerito,*" which patronizingly means "little fellow" rather than "gentleman" (*caballero*), for those higher highlanders whom valley dwellers believe are poorer.

Stoner's approach links ethnicity as a system of beliefs to practices and their outcomes that are related to health and the body, and thus resonates with my concerns regarding the body and dress. By showing the consequences of ethnic identifications and actions, he avoids essentializing indigenous identity. Such examination of practices as distinguishing ethnic characteristics helps us better understand how Cayllominos themselves form their identities. This approach is consistent with G. Carter Bentley's (1987) call to link practices to ethnicity. Likewise, irrigation practices, which Gelles (2000) analyzes in Cabanaconde, are based on "enduring cultural frameworks which underwrite ethnic identity" (Gelles 1992: 14). Stressing the specifically Andean quality and highly localized variants of Cabaneño practices, including dress, weaving, rituals, and language, Gelles also shows historical changes, which are ultimately linked to broader conceptions of class and race.

Class alliances in Caylloma have shifted along with its political-economic position. Differential power, status, and wealth are more easily observed in Chivay, where some merchants seem quite well-to-do, but even small communities evidence differences in land tenure, labor relations, and capital (Gelles 1992:20; Markowitz 1992; Stoner 1989; Swen 1986). In the province as a whole, and the Colca Valley in particular, most villages have territory in several ecological zones, usually contiguous, which often extends far into the *puna*. Even in the valley itself, a few large tracts have been held by the church and several private landowners (Benavides 1990; Manrique 1985:202–213). As the nineteenth-century spread of *haciendas* accelerated competition over land and increased peasant debt to *hacendados*, it contributed overall to social inequality and injustice. With the wool trade, the penetration of merchant capital exacerbated existing differences and generated new ones, charting the course that globalization would follow. MACON contributed substantially to reshaping class boundaries as more people, goods, and money entered the valley. Although this phase coincided with the reassignment of racial and class labels from *indio* to *campesino,* that change did more to obscure than to illuminate the workings of race. Class differences in Caylloma are also obscured because community members have dispersed residences and large landholdings are concentrated among a few absentees. In addition, much of *comuneros*' income is derived from outside sources, ranging from seasonal wage labor to urban real estate.

Political, economic, and historical specificities are crucial in analyzing ethnicity together with race because the recent "focus on ethnicity euphemized if not denied race by not specifying the conditions under which those social categories and groups historically subordinated as 'racially' distinct emerge and persist," as Harrison (1995:48) has cautioned. Specifying conditions means attending not only to underlying causes but also to "structural consequences of race—forced exclusions and stigmatized labor—[and the ways they] differ from those generally associated with ethnicity . . ." (ibid.).

Ethnic identity in Caylloma is distinguished by a series of markers.

Showing how ethnicity intersects with economic status, these emblems connect class to race. If I was shy about asking who was an Indian, I was bold in pursuing other issues. I constantly asked people in Caylloma why women wear *polleras*. Cayllominos never said that they wear *polleras* because they are Indians. In discussing their unique embroidered clothes, Cayllominos did speak openly and eloquently about community, custom, and tradition, as well as beauty, pride, and shame.

Dressing the Ethnic Body

"Una Cosa de Polleras"

Previous visitors and researchers, commenting on Colca Valley embroidered clothes, have noted gendered differences in ethnic style. Proposing that dress is an ethnic marker, Hurley remarks that "women continue to dress in a far more traditional way than do men" (1978:127–128). Contrasting gender and ethnicity, Stoner claims that "women . . . dress in a much more traditional fashion" than men and that "the avoidance of traditional modes of dress . . . helps emphasize and reinforce . . . *misti* identity . . ." (1989:55, 58–59). In a coffee-table book, photograph captions point to tradition, contrasting it with the modern: "women and girls, descendents of the Collaguas, with their traditional dresses" and "note the use of certain modern elements such as slippers and trousers in the peasants' dress" (de Romaña, Blassi, and Blassi 1987:94, 95). In analyzing contemporary usage, however, the contrast between tradition and modernity is unsatisfactory in explaining relations among dress, gender, and ethnicity.

There are two basic styles of women's dress: *de pollera* and *de vestido* (literally, "in a skirt" versus "in a dress"); they are almost mutually exclusive. Understanding why women wear *polleras* requires isolating specific reasons that they do not wear the "*de vestido*" style or sometimes change to it—the ways that relationships among race, ethnicity, and class are manifested through dress. Among the many names for Caylloma women's clothes, some pertain to individual garments and others to the whole ensemble. People in Caylloma refer to their embroidered clothes generally as *polleras* (Spanish, "skirts") or *bordados* (Spanish, "embroideries"). I follow their practice, which means that for the most part I use both terms interchangeably but differentiate meaningful connotations of each term. A sizeable sector of Caylloma women dress "*de vestido*." They do not wear *polleras*—not daily, rarely for fiestas, or never. How does ethnic identification correlate with those customs? What are the attitudes of those who dress "*de pollera*" toward those who dress "*de vestido*"? What happens when women shift from one style to the other? The two categories of dress complexly crosscut and overlap with, rather than neatly correspond to, the categories "Indian" and "non-Indian." There is a multiplicity of varieties of clothes: they may be handmade, factory made and purchased, locally made and purchased but modified, and more; from these overlapping sets of categories, people characterized as "indigenous" choose their attire, as Zorn (1997b, 2003a, 2003b) has noted for Bolivia; (on Ecuador, see Rowe, ed. 1998; Tolen 1995).

Although "*pollera*" literally means "skirt," and "*vestido*," "dress," these terms are used far more broadly than literal translations can convey. Dressing "*de pollera*" means wearing an ensemble of clothing, such as Caylloma *bordados*, that is usually associated with rural peasant or urbanized popular ("*cholo*") classes (Figure 9). "*De pollera*" may be identified with "Indian" by outsiders. "*De vestido*," in contrast, connotes "modern," "western," "commercial," industrially produced clothes. These are not limited to a dress (*vestido*) but include a blouse with a short, straight skirt and even pants, especially nylon running pants or sweatpants (both called *buzo*) or jeans (*blujín*). For the mass-produced clothes encompassed by "*de vestido*," English has no single inclusive term that is a satisfactory translation. Factors of race, culture, geography, gender, and forms of production all figure into the meaning of "*de vestido.*"

Many Caylloma women commonly live outside the province, which influences their choice of dress. Most women with whom I spoke had lived elsewhere for part of their life, especially in Arequipa or Lima. As travelers whose kinship and social networks include members in Arequipa, almost everyone has made numerous trips there for reasons ranging from daily travel for commerce to long-term residence for work and/or school. Almost all women who had lived outside Caylloma told me that in those times and places they gave up their *polleras.* Changing to "*de vestido*" includes adjusting other related practices of personal adornment; in particular, women cut off their long braids.

When "*polleras*" and "*bordados*" are used to mean the whole embroidered outfit, they act as synecdoche for ethnic dress and more broadly for ethnicity. Each term also connotes certain aspects of that style of dress. "*Polleras*" means the skirts, which are one part of the ensemble; "*bordados*" means the embroidery, which is decoration applied to the garments. "*Las*

9 Margarita Sullca at her stand in Chivay market

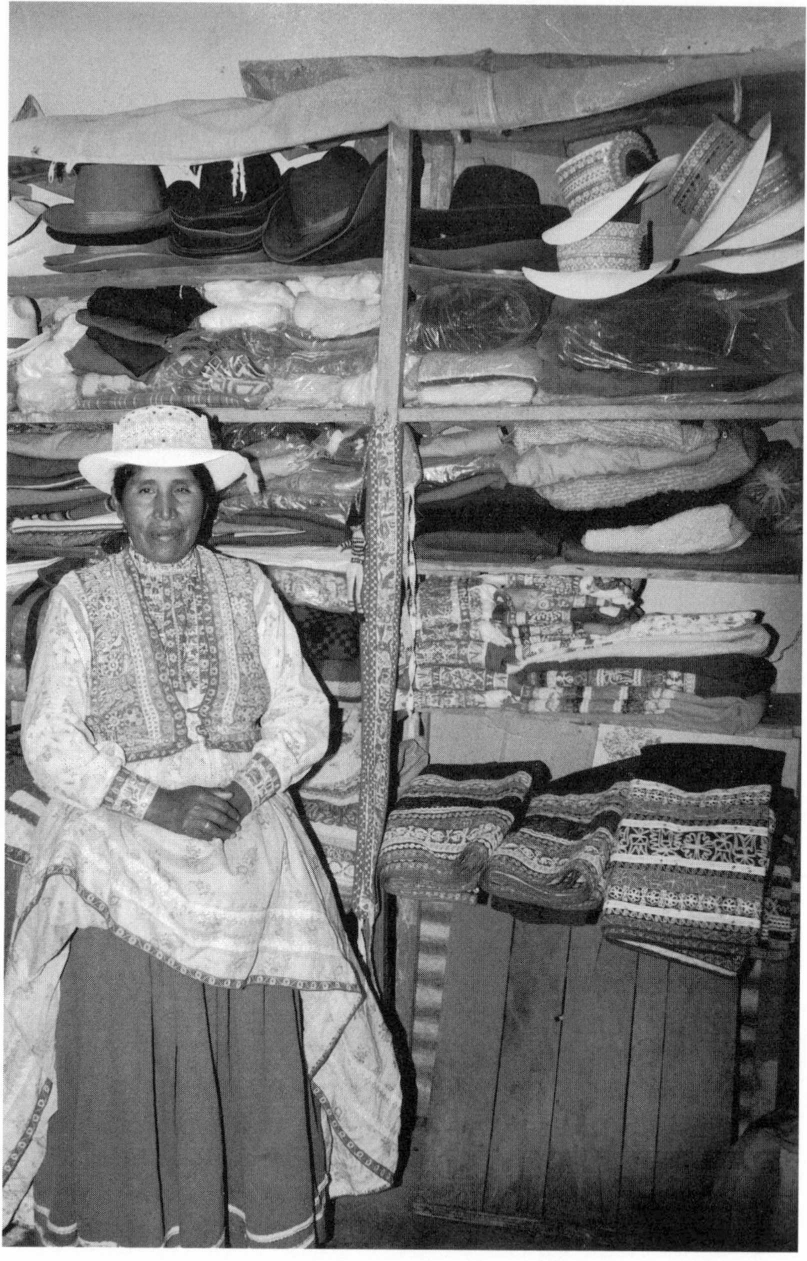

polleras bordadas" that women wear in Caylloma are highly complex, featuring intricate designs, meters of shiny trims and laces, and other lavish decoration. Among all Andean *polleras,* they are some of the most elaborate garments in terms of amount and kinds of embellishment and material. These features are not characteristic of all *polleras,* however. Throughout the Andean nations, market vendors and poor rural women wear less ornate *polleras.* Even in Caylloma Province, women from the town of Caylloma and environs wear *polleras* without embroidery, which are hemmed below the knees and feature rows of horizontal tucks. These *polleras* resemble a style worn in Puno and Bolivia; some Puneña migrants living in Chivay continue to use it. Still other styles are worn in Cusco, in Moquegua, and elsewhere in Bolivia (Barragán 1992; Stephenson 1999; Weismantel 2001).

The meanings that whites assign to *polleras* rarely take into account the variation, embellishment, or expense. Lumping them together, whites use "*de polleras*" as an epithet. With its derogatory overtones, this strident racist insult alludes to negative characteristics that whites attribute to Indians and rural women, and connotes poor, dirty, worthless, or common. When applied specifically to women, it means sexually unrestrained, slutty. The phrase is also applied metaphorically to arenas detached from dress and bodies. To call something other than clothes "*una cosa de polleras*" is to dismiss it as worthless.

Schoolteachers, medical professionals, and other outsiders who live in Colca Valley villages freely told me that *polleras,* as garments, are bad. *Polleras* lead, they claimed, to lack of cleanliness. *Polleras* drag on the ground and get caked with dirt in muddy fields. People also said that women blow their noses on the hem and that they do not wash their clothes. The frequent claim that women do not wear underwear beneath them seems related to myths of sexual availability as well as poor hygiene.

The phrase "*de polleras,*" especially the negative use of it, perplexed me for a long time. I racked my brain but failed to think of an epithet that similarly links ethnicity, gender, and dress in the United States, and that has equal negative impact. But no such equivalence exists. I believe that is part of what makes *polleras* unique to the Andes, or makes the Andes unique in terms of how race is characterized. "*De polleras*" condenses racism precisely in the relationships among dress, ethnicity, and gender.

If "*de polleras*" is such a filthy insult, why do women wear *polleras*? The negative stereotypes are light years away from the fancy *polleras* that Cayllominas proudly flaunt at fiestas. "*Polleras*" is a vast category; the class and status distinctions within it are often as important as the distinctions between "Indians" and "*mistis.*" Because of these positive connotations, *mestizas* occasionally wear *polleras,* especially on ceremonial occasions when fancy *polleras* serve as markers of both high status and community membership. For most Cayllominas, like Florencia Huaracha, the pride they feel in dressing well, usually within their community, is challenged by the shame of being mistreated, usually outside it. As they appreciate the positive value of *polleras* but routinely face discrimination against using them, pride and shame dog their steps.

Condensing Ethnicity in Men's Dress

During the 1993 municipal election campaign, an image of two man's caps appeared in posters all over Arequipa. "*¡Marca los dos chullitos!*" (Check the two little caps!) was the slogan of Frenatraca (Frente Nacional de Trabajadores y Campesinos, National Front of Workers and Peasants). Mayor Luis Cáceres founded this political party in Juliaca when he was its mayor. Because illiteracy is so high, all Peruvian parties use icons for campaigning and on the ballot. In adopting the cap (Quechua *ch'ullu;* Hispanicized *chullo*) worn by male farmers and herders, Frenatraca referred to the party's Andean roots. Cáceres symbolically deployed the *ch'ullu* to attract the support of migrants—the people who once wore those caps—by relying on its ethnic allusion; the symbolism contrasted vividly with his treatment of the migrants. In addition, as a male symbol, the *ch'ullu* enforced the association of politics and masculinity.

If *polleras* are the primary emblems of ethnicity and they are explicitly women's dress, then how do men represent their ethnic identity? My decision to focus on *bordados* was guided by their predominance in women's clothes. This meant that my gaze turned away from men's attire. Men's dress seems less obviously "ethnic." Although Caylloma men use a few unique garments, for the most part, they display distinctive garments on a daily basis far less frequently than women. They rarely wear embroidered garments. One thin band with a simple embroidered design sometimes graces the neckline of a poncho. This rarity makes it highly significant that in ritual contexts men wear and dance in women's *polleras.*

Several male garments most concisely display ethnic affiliation: poncho, *ch'ullu,* and hat. In Caylloma, the poncho that most men wear is heavy, striped, and handwoven of alpaca (Figure 10). Tan with blue border stripes and dark pink with green are typical colors. Other styles of poncho, some of which are industrially woven and commercially sold, are less commonly worn. The poncho is generally considered a rural garment. During the course of the day, men usually remove ponchos, which makes them the clothes of early morning and night. In the city, even on cold nights, men seldom wear ponchos.[13]

Men, even more than women, consistently wear hats outside and inside buildings. Straw and wool felt hats, similar to U.S. "cowboy hats," are typical in Caylloma. A few men affect hats of other areas and ethnic groups because they hail from there or have adopted them as their own. Notable among these are a heavy handmade white wool felt hat with brown designs, made and worn in Chumbivilcas, Cusco, and an oversize straw hat favored by *chacareros,* farmers of the *campiña,* the agricultural zone surrounding the city of Arequipa. Instead of a hat or underneath it, men and boys wear a *ch'ullu.* This hand-knitted cap with earflaps, distinctive to the Andes, is worn in most of highland Peru and Bolivia. The *ch'ullus* worn in Caylloma come from several areas, including Cusco. In the upper Caylloma communities, an undyed alpaca *ch'ullu* is knitted and sold com-

10 LEONARDO MEJÍA SHAKES OUT A PONCHO.

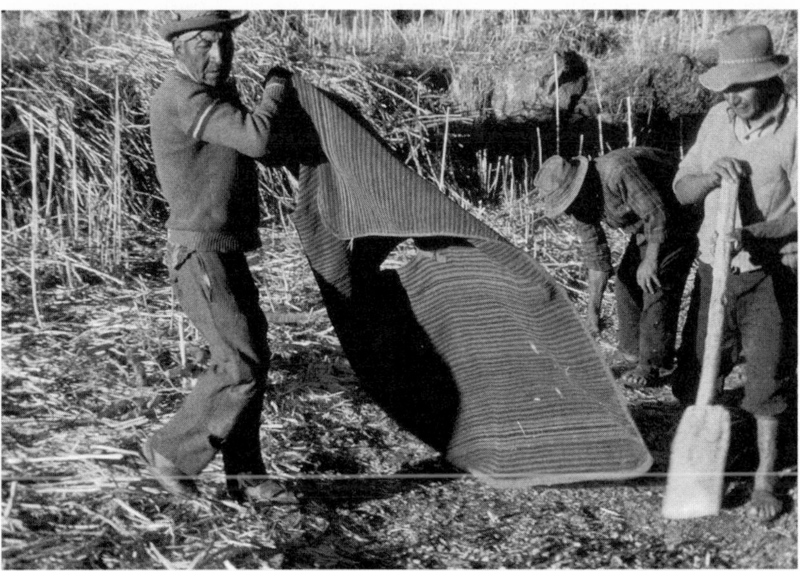

mercially through cooperatives, but less than half of local men wear this style.

Aside from the local variants of these three garments, there is little about Caylloma men's appearance to distinguish them from farmers of other parts of Peru. In this sense, men seem to have been more thoroughly de-Indianized than their female compatriots. Caylloma-style men's clothes have potency as ethnic representations, but it is generally diluted in comparison to women's *bordados.* Because items like the poncho and the *ch'ullu* are more routinely detached, their efficacy operates at a greater remove than women's garments. Once an event is under way, men usually take off the poncho. In contrast, women's *polleras* constitute an ensemble, containing garments that reach the skin, and women remove only the top layer, the shawl. Nevertheless, the significance of men's garments can be disproportionate to their number. In a specific context, one garment can be a potent, multivocal symbol of ethnicity. In addition, the condensed significance of a few items to indicate masculinity has not gone unnoticed by politicians who seek to maximize the instrumentality of dress. Cáceres was not alone in using an ethnic symbol connected with males. The use of *ch'ullus,* hats, and ponchos, as well as Amazonian headdresses, was a notable feature in the presidential campaigns and administration of Fujimori and, most recently, of Toledo, who makes a point of stressing his indigenous ancestry.

Conclusion: Articulation and the Politics of Isolation

As precious metals, a vast granary, and lustrous alpaca fiber, wealth has long been painted as a characteristic of Caylloma. The region caught the Spaniards' attention because it was known as a land of vast resources. Wealth simultaneously generated poverty, structured by ethnic relations in which indigenous and foreign interests clashed. Current racial, ethnic, and class distinctions are rooted in historic trends related to Caylloma's place in the region. Although indigenous leaders resisted Spanish plunder, Cayllominos have endeavored not to cut themselves off from modern society but to secure their rights as citizens of the nation-state.

How can we explain the "isolation" of Caylloma? Undeniably, the mountains are high and the roads are poor. The ambiance in the rural areas of Arequipa is different from the big-city feel of the department capital. These facts do not explain the "isolation," which is always politically constructed. Spanish colonial policies and practices laid the groundwork for political economic developments in the republican period, including British and U.S. neocolonial investment and resource extraction, which had a heavy impact on Cayllominos. "Isolation" did not deter the Casa Ricketts from extracting tons of alpaca fleeces. "Isolation" did not prevent MACON from tunneling through rock to reroute the river. The illusion of isolation results from isolationist policies (Markowitz 1992:67). Largely ignoring the rural areas, the state intervenes only in areas deemed central to national interest. Rather than isolation, in truth this is neglect (ibid.:32; see also Stoner 1989).

A road connects Caylloma to the White City of Arequipa, the Pacific Coast, Puno, Cusco, and Lima—all the destinations travelers from Caylloma have reached for thousands of years. A road of ruts, potholes, landslides, and sandtraps, always crumbling and always in disrepair. Like other aspects of rural infrastructure, the road is sometimes upgraded, but rarely in order to bring the benefits of modernity to Caylloma. Rather, the principal motivation for such investment has always been extraction: to take out precious goods—metals, grain, wool, and water—and an equally precious resource—human labor. For many centuries, Cayllominos have labored to build the physical infrastructure: *indios* built the terraces locally, and *serranos* built the churches and mansions of Arequipa. They have always been part of larger political units and incorporated into regional exchange systems: at the crossroads of two Inka *suyus,* in the *encomiendas* of conquistadores, as *mitayos* and *arrieros* for silver mines, and as artisans and merchants in workshops, markets, and fairs.

In a country where mountains are seen as racial and cultural barriers, and all who live in the sierra are *serranos* as well as *indios* and denied a place in national society, "isolation" also means racism. Ethnic identity in Caylloma is marked by dress and other symbols, but these boundaries are subject to interpretation. My analysis of the ways in which these emblems show how ethnicity and economic status intersect, and how both connect to class and race, is linked to the broader analytical move I suggest: a move away from bounded ethnic groups to politically related dominant and subordinate groups. This requires paying more attention to the practices through which domination was established. The visual and corporeal characteristics of ethnicity have related to clothes and their production in crucial ways at different historical junctures. Structural placement within the region and nation often has greater power to shape identity than have the internal distinctions that Cayllominos find potent. No matter how wealthy a *campesino* may be compared to others in his village, outsiders lump them together as peasants and malign them as Indians. Yet for all the shame she experienced in Arequipa, Florencia Huaracha was proud to wear her *polleras* at home. Understanding race and ethnicity in Caylloma, Arequipa, and Peru demands that we examine internal differentiation within a community and a region, and that we recognize that it is practices—what people do—that create what others see as essences—who they are.

3

Clothing the Body: Visual Domain and Cultural Process

Changing Clothes

When the summer sun warms the February days, the fiesta season nears its end. Carnival in Caylloma! Then we will see some fancy *polleras.* From December through February, embroidery artisans are busiest, providing women with elaborate outfits. This week, I am spending a few days in Chivay, where the artisans' workshops are concentrated, and looking forward to celebrating Carnival in Coporaque.

Leonardo Mejía and his wife, Susana Bernal, live with their four children and make *bordados* in their home workshop in Chivay. Since 1985, I have spent hundreds of hours in their homes and workshops, often dining there and discussing *bordados* as an art and business (Figure 11).

Tonight in their kitchen, Susana and I talk over the upcoming fiestas while Leonardo embroiders designs on a vest and their children dash in and out. The conversation turns to two *polleras* (skirts) that Susana has agreed to make for me. Two months ago, encouraged by several friends, I wore *polleras* for the first time. For that fiesta in December I had improvised with borrowed skirts; now, for Carnival in February, I want *polleras* of my own.

Leonardo is sewing on a machine, as he and Susana often do in the evening, taking advantage of the few hours of irregular electricity. A single huge bulb, intended for a streetlight, alternates erratically between blinding glare and dim obscurity. We often converse invisible to each other beyond the glare, or I watch Leonardo sew, but we cannot talk over the noise of the electric machine. Their others are treadle operated; it would be futile to depend on electricity to get the sewing done. The sewing machine, table, chairs, and stove—all old but still functional—leave little floor space in the tiny room. The stove and light bulb help create a warm, energetic atmosphere. When the machine stops humming, the stillness is palpable.

We settle down to our *bordado* business. Already I own several gar-

11 Susana Bernal and Leonardo Mejía in their workshop

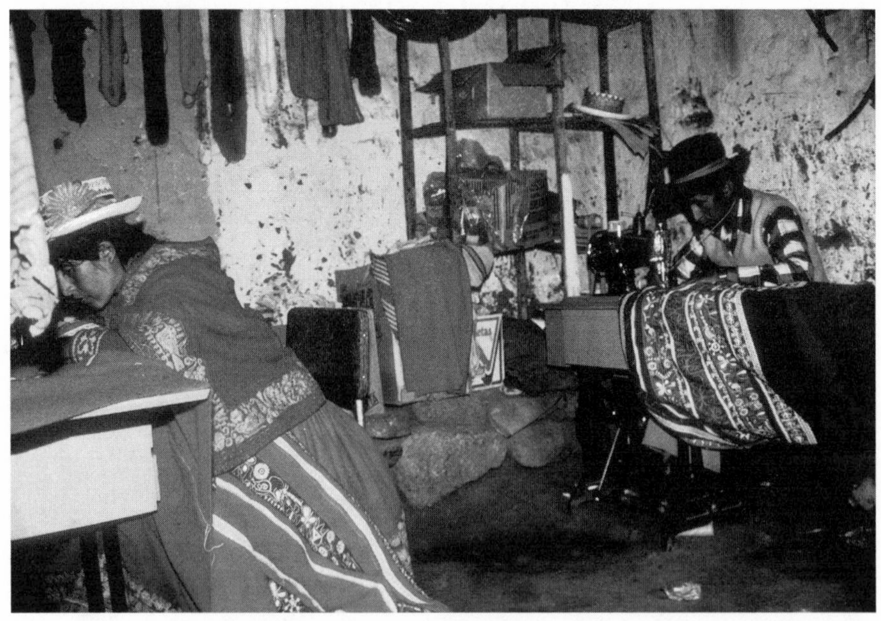

ments. My first step was to buy a vest ready-made from Susana. To go with it, she made me a blouse. Pleased with its design and fit, I have asked her to make my *polleras.* My vest is plaid flannel—turquoise, black, and white—with a fuchsia band and multicolor embroidery. The blouse is pale pink printed with small red flowers; a central band of embroidery adorns the breast. As we review materials, Susana spreads out bright bolts of fabric, including some that a vendor recently brought from Arequipa, and miles of ribbon and lace. She patiently explains some options: number of *polleras,* colors, fabrics, braids, trims, laces. . . . Soon my head is swimming. She tells me which colors go with the garments I own, but I am not convinced. Self-conscious in this enterprise, I am surprised that my aesthetic opinions veer toward more subdued combinations, which she tactfully considers before rejecting.

"If the vest is blue, shouldn't the skirt be blue?" I venture, clinging bravely to the concept of "matching."

"Perhaps. But that would be very dark," Susana asserts.

"What about lilac?" Leonardo adds his two bits. "Lots of ladies are wearing lilac this year."

"What ladies? Old ladies," Susana dismisses. "Lilac is for old ladies."

"What do I know? These are women's things." With a sigh and a shrug, he turns back to his sewing.

The children join in. Erika and Marleni, the two oldest girls, ages ten and eleven, already know some basic *pollera*-construction steps. They stand me up straight to measure the correct skirt length, from waist to ankle bone.

"One meter! How can you be one meter? Nobody is more than eighty, maybe eighty-five." They reduce my height to my legs' length in centimeters.

The details of *pollera* design occupy us for more than an hour. Finally we settle on the kinds of *polleras,* a schedule for completion, price, and arrangements for payment. By making one decision, to wear *polleras,* I enter a complex chain of corollary decisions and social interactions. I sigh to think how little I know about Cayllomino fashion and taste! What kinds of embroideries suit me? Which fabrics, styles, and designs correspond to this stage of my life? How do my selections relate to the choices Caylloma women make? What do they choose for different life stages?

Susana's knowledge of such matters was obviously superior to mine. At age thirty-eight, she had been sewing for almost thirty years and wearing *bordados* for longer than that. To wear *polleras,* I had to entrust my self-image to her expertise, which signaled another dimension in our relationship. Placing myself in another person's sartorial custody challenged my self-perception. Wearing *polleras* allowed me to try a new identity, with new visual and kinesthetic elements. While deciding how to represent myself as an adult woman in Caylloma, I also acknowledged my immaturity and need for guidance in learning culture.

The body-clothing process builds on the sense of visual appropriateness developed through life, the conception of physical self, and the expectation that others will recognize him or her. Yet the process is not separable from the objects involved. Each garment has a life of its own, beginning with a shared understanding between creator and wearer. The artisan, as the garments' creator, actively mediates the relationship between gendered body and collectivity. The garments' wearer composes them into a unified, often elegant ensemble. The social life of *bordados* unites individuals even as it transcends the individual to create a collective presence among all women who choose to don this dress.[1]

The Colca Valley is the most clothes-conscious place I have ever lived. Everybody is an expert on *bordados,* and nobody hesitates to share his or her opinions. Their experience with embroidered clothes involved wearing, making, buying, selling, or at least seeing them. Wearing similar clothes helps constitute a "community of practice" among women. If some ten thousand females in more than twenty Caylloma communities are wearing an average of eight garments at a time, then eighty thousand garments are displayed throughout the province on a given day. The visual appreciation of clothes goes beyond involvement in production per se; it is a standard part of cultural currency. Seeing clothes presumes cultural knowledge. Caylloma people's awareness is not just "fashion sense"; rather, the clothing domain is both a kind of cultural good that is "owned" by everyone and an individual statement. As a form of symbolic capital, *bordados* "belong" not only to the person who actually owns them, but to all members of her community of practice—those who see her and with whom she interacts.

Friends and acquaintances frequently pressed me to wear the finest garments. For the December fiesta, Susana made herself a new jacket of luxurious red stamped velvet (*chinchilla*). Elsa Mejía, Leonardo's sister, encouraged me to get a similar jacket. "That would be *chévere*!" she enthused. (*Chévere* is Spanish slang for "excellent, far out, awesome.") I thought not.

Better to be underdressed. . . . Give me some middle-of-the-road *polleras,* nothing fancy. Maybe I would wear them every day, I rationalized, after the fiesta; maybe I would make a permanent change. All *bordados* were plenty flashy for me.

For the skirts, I chose two synthetic fabrics of different weights and colors. Both *polleras* can be made of the same fabric, but I opted for an under-*pollera* of blue *diolén,* a heavy knitted fabric, and an upper one of pink *tela poliseda,* a lighter-weight polyester. The *diolén* skirt would be embroidered in "second-quality" (*de segunda*) style. Susana approved my having two blue garments only if I would wear the blue *pollera* under the pink one so it would be separated from the blue vest. Contrast between colors—those I knew as warm and cool—was the operative principle of combination. To make my *pollera de segunda,* she would sew on the correct number of bands, each using the correct quality of materials and appropriate designs, and then embroider them, as well as apply trim, lace, and yarn between the bands.

"As easy as changing one's clothes" we say about changing one's identity. But literally changing my clothes was not easy. Clothing the body is a lifelong process. I decided to stake a claim in that process by clothing my body in Caylloma style, even though my stay in that community of practice would be temporary. Bringing embroidered clothes into my lifestyle went beyond method, beyond aesthetics, and beyond narcissism. Commissioning *bordados,* I envisioned a new concept of the physical gendered person. Wearing the *polleras,* feeling their shape and weight on my body, I learned how these clothes incorporate experience. Wearing *polleras* altered my sense of belonging to a community; I shared a mundane experience with other women and, at times, with men. But it also accentuated the gulf that separated me from Caylloma women, and made me aware of the limits of incorporation.

In this chapter, my discussion of the meanings of Caylloma *bordados* which unfold through the process of clothing the body is centered in modes of visual representation, beginning with the clothing itself and extending to the gendered bodies that clothes conceal and reveal. The visual and formal aspects of clothes include their configuration as art forms, objects, and means of communication. In Caylloma, beauty is linked to skill, and person to place, but how does the visual domain of representation through clothes work in practice? How is this system of communication embedded in single garments? And in the total repertoire? In Chapter 2,

I discussed the association of gender with ethnic identity; here I focus on specific visual criteria and narrower distinctions. How do particular features of clothes identify persons of different races, places of origin, and economic statuses in Caylloma?

I began the chapter in Susana's and Leonardo's workshop to acquaint the reader with the process of obtaining *bordados* and to emphasize the role of the artisans in it. About 150 embroidery artisans make clothes for some ten thousand consumers. Representation through dress ultimately depends on the power relations between wearer and audience and on their forms of mediation, in which the artisans play prominent, complex roles. As businesspeople with vested interests, artisans encourage women to wear the clothes. As "spin doctors," they are brokers who link making clothes to wearing them. I pay special attention to these men and women because of their power to shape images and bodies. My analysis draws heavily on artisan surveys, in which they articulated their insights about the place of *bordados* in life and art.

Each of the constituent garments in a set of *polleras* is a unique exemplar of a standardized style that Cayllominos recognize. Community, quality, designs, techniques, and the artisan's status contribute to making *bordados* so costly in both social and monetary terms. Cayllominas' experiences of clothing the body are as diverse as their reasons for wearing *bordados* or not. Over a Caylloma woman's life course, changing into *polleras* always requires changing out of something else. For the artists, however, sharp aesthetic sensibilities prompt them to create embroidered landscapes, not just lovely fashions, as *polleras* connect them to the places they call home.

Finally, I discuss how dressing served as a research method. Buying a vest here, borrowing a skirt there—obtaining an ensemble of *bordados* became a central strategy through most of my fieldwork period. Situating my involvement in this ethnographic experience, I explore the idea of changing clothes literally and extend it metaphorically to the anthropologist's enterprise.

Characteristics of Women's Embroidered Garments

There are no generic *polleras*. All have specific characteristics—in terms of appearance, materials, and, of course, cost—that are appropriate to their intended use. The latter ranges from the most mundane activities such as agricultural labor to benchmark events such as sponsoring a fiesta.

Through such specificity, their creation and acquisition mark key points in a woman's life course. Juggling cost, status, and class distinctions, people make choices—between clothes and animals, between spending money and exchanging other goods. A top-quality set of *bordados* will set the buyer back $400–$500—about the price of a bull; a set of "western" clothes will rarely cost even $50—the price of a fine alpaca. The wide range of styles and qualities of *polleras* also prompts a wide range of opinions about them, depending on people's class, ethnic, and generational backgrounds.

Garments, both as individual objects and as elements in sets, have varied effects on the gendered body. As a specific element, each garment is a unit of embodiment, with physical and emotional impact on the body of the wearer. Each unit relates not only to the other units, but also to the whole, the larger ensemble. Each garment uniquely imposes sensation and meaning on the body. Its impact has to do with its position on the body—for example, skirts weigh on the waist and surround the legs—and its position beyond the body—for example, a first-quality blouse should be worn with first-quality skirts. In another respect, however, all parts are equal; because all should be worn together, the absence of even one garment, such as a hat, can distort the whole ensemble and render it inappropriate. Certain objects condense meaning, especially skirts, hats, and shoes.

To be correctly clothed in proper Caylloma style, a woman wears at least eight different garments at once, most of which are embroidered: blouse, vest, two (or more) skirts, jacket, belt, hat, shoes. Most women have a full set of daily-wear and one of festive-wear *bordados,* and a few additional blouses and underskirts. At any one time, the average woman owns about twenty-five garments; throughout her lifetime, she will probably acquire and wear several hundred.

Women's embroidered garments:

- *camisa,* blouse
- *corpiño,* sleeveless vest
- *saco* or *jubón,* long-sleeved jacket
- *pollera,* skirt (two or three are worn together)

These terms largely originate in archaic Spanish. There are no original Quechua terms for these garments, and some Spanish terms have merged into Quechua vocabulary. The jacket, *saco* (Figure 12), in Cabanaconde is called *jubón,* a term used for "doublet" in sixteenth-century Spain (Anderson 1980); throughout Peru, the term for most other kinds of jacket is *chaqueta* (Spanish). Likewise, the short fitted vest (Figure 13) is called *corpiño,* rather than the usual term for vest, *chaleco* (Spanish). Adrián Zavala, a man in his seventies from Maca, insisted that "*corpiño*" is a Quechua term and "*chaleco,*" Spanish. Because the pronunciation is markedly Quechuized, variant spellings occur, such as *kuropino* (Markowitz 1992:91).

We cannot pinpoint when these items entered the Peruvian repertoire or became associated with Indians. Similar garments, documented in sixteenth-century Spain (Anderson 1980; see also Femenías 1996 [1991]), may have been introduced as early as 1532. Spanish garments may have been imposed in the 1780s, as edicts forbade the wearing of Indian garments after Túpac Amaru's rebellion and other uprisings. Yet Caylloma garments also resemble nineteenth-century European folk costume, so they may have originated as recently as two hundred years ago. The use of embroidery probably began only in the mid-twentieth century.

Garments usually embroidered:

- *sombrero* or *montera,* hat
- *faja* or *chumpi,* belt

Several different types of hat, both men's and women's, are called *sombrero* or *montera*. One common type is made of white straw, and another is of wool embroidered all over. A handwoven belt called *chumpi* (Quechua) may have an embroidered border.

Garments possibly embroidered:

- *phullu,* small shawl
- *lliklla,* carrying cloth
- *ch'uspa,* small bag

These garments are known by Quechua terms and are probably pre-Columbian in origin.[2] The *phullu* (Quechua; Spanish *manta*), a small shawl, is generally handwoven and usually has an embroidered border. The *lliklla* (Quechua; there is no Spanish term), carrying cloth, may be handwoven or industrially woven. Made of two equal-size pieces sewn together, it occasionally has a strip of embroidery covering, or two strips parallel to, the seam. A small bag, whether embroidered, or handwoven, or both, is a *ch'uspa* (Quechua; Spanish *bolsa*).

Most women wear *ujutas* (Quechua), rubber sandals made from tires, but sneakers are almost as commonplace now.

The significant differences among *polleras* fall into five categories: com-

12 Woman's embroidered jacket by Tiburcio Ocsa and Vilma Mejía

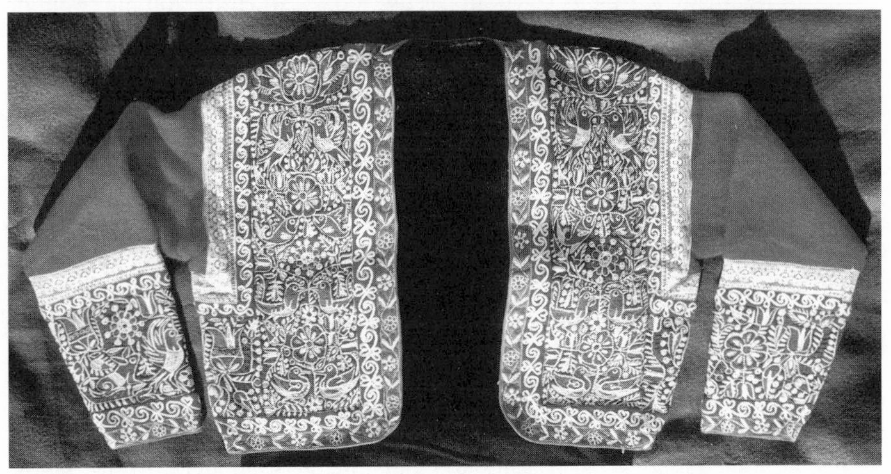

13 Woman's embroidered vest by Susana Bernal

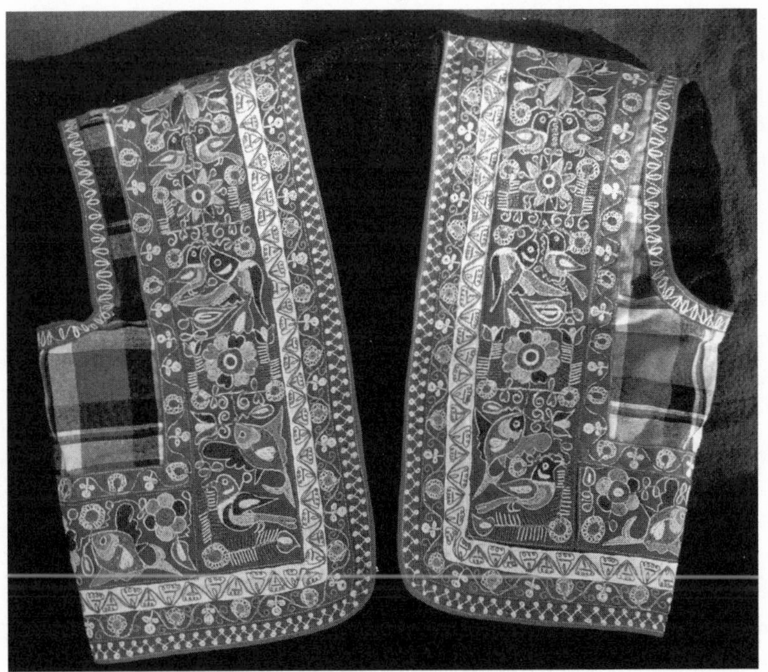

munity, type, quality, materials, and artist. I can only briefly describe a few of the many garments Cayllominas use today. An entire volume could be dedicated just to illustrating variations on *polleras.*

Community: Even quotidian *polleras* are distinguished according to the Colca Valley community where they are made and/or worn. "There have always been differences between above and below" the Canyon, explained Marcial Villavicencio (interview, Cabanaconde, March 1993). His assessment of the upper- and lower-valley styles was common not only among embroiderers but among valley residents in general. This cultural knowledge is far from esoteric; even small children could point out basic differences, especially in hat style and decoration, designs on skirts, and techniques.

Caylliominos draw many distinctions among *polleras.* Women in the upper valley and higher-altitude herding areas, around and above Callalli, wear a *pollera* that features appliqué in large solid areas. In the middle and lower valley, from Chivay to west of Cabanaconde, they use *polleras* with wide bands of sewing-thread embroidery and narrow applied trims. Around Callalli and Chivay, another type of trim is done with yarn (*lana;* Figure 14). Around Cabanaconde, secondary trim is usually rickrack (*trencilla;* Figure 15). Other differences pertain to the amount of embroidery, width of bands, organization of designs within bands, and motifs.

Hats in several styles are primary means of distinguishing between communities. In Callalli and Chivay, white straw or canvas hats are most common. In Cabanaconde and the lower valley, embroidered wool felt hats are standard (Figures 16 and 17). Near Lari, heavy wool felt hats, trimmed with a narrow band, are sometimes used.

Pollera type: Caylloma skirts feature horizontal rows of trim. There are two basic types used in the Colca Valley. The first is "embroidered" (*bordado*). The second, "with ribbon" (*con cinta*), is often called "of fabric" (*de tela*).

Quality: Embroidered garments come in different grades or qualities (*calidades*). Within the Chivay style, there are first, second, and third quality (*primera, segunda,* and *tercera calidad*). A garment *de primera* is made and worn only for fiestas and other ceremonial and official occasions. Made of velvet, with wide bands of polychrome embroidery, its execution and material should be first-rate. Such a *pollera* costs about $125 (prices range from $80 to $150); a jacket of that quality, about $40 (range: $35–$60). Second- and third-quality garments should be well made, following clearly

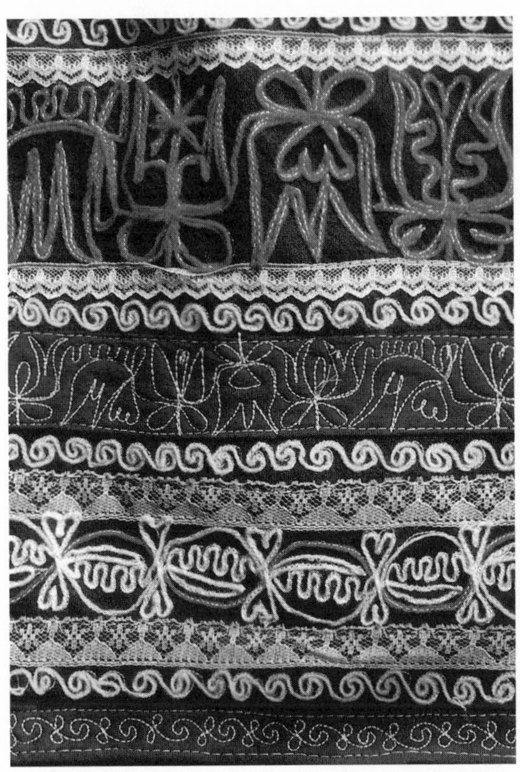

14 Chivay-style embroidered *pollera* by Susana Bernal, detail

15 Cabanaconde-style embroidered *pollera* by Hugo Vilcape, detail

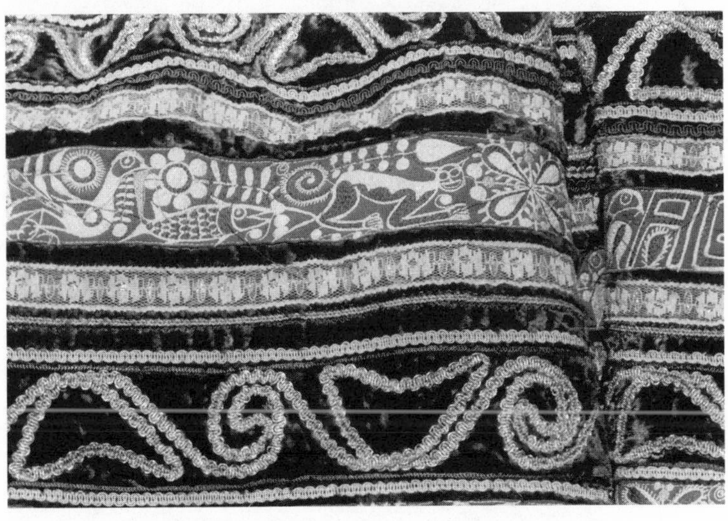

16 Cabanaconde-style embroidered hat by Leonardo Mejía

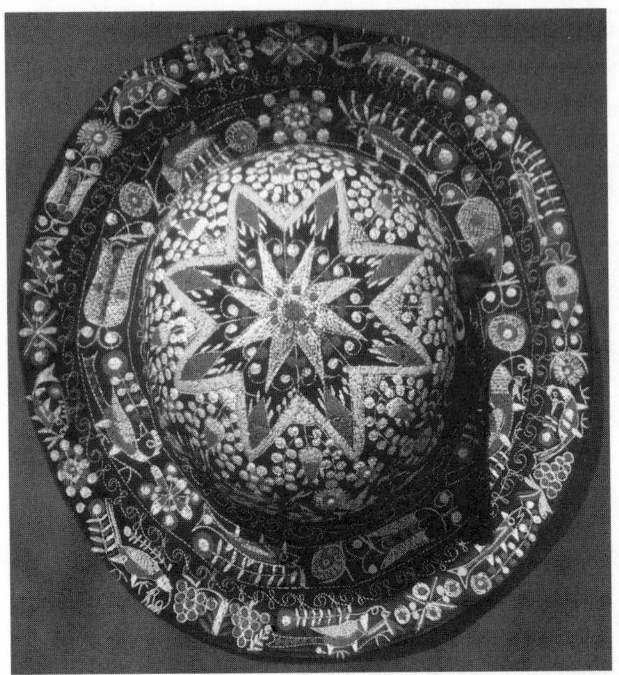

17 Cabanaconde-style embroidered hat by Hugo Vilcape

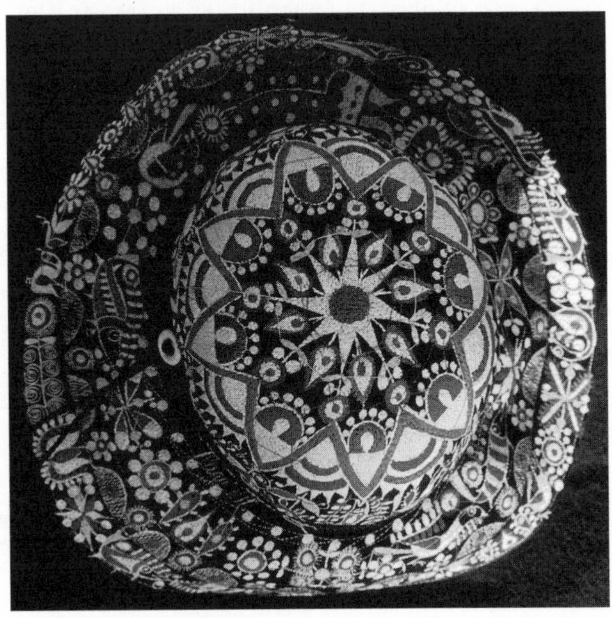

established norms of style; they are not poorly executed versions of a first-quality garment. A second-quality (*de segunda*) *pollera* is made of synthetic or industrially woven wool fabrics. The embroidered bands have only two colors of thread, and the other trims are also fewer and may be less costly. Most women use this *pollera* as daily wear; they often own several. The embroidered *pollera* I commissioned was second quality (see Figure 14); that type costs about $30, and a jacket of similar quality, about $20. Third quality (*de tercera*), often the only kind very poor women can afford, is also used as an extra skirt, underskirt, or for warmth. Usually made of *bayeta* (handwoven wool), this type has embroidery sparingly done in one color, plain cloth applied trims, and little additional decoration. The cost is $10–$15.

Materials: The ever changing array of materials in *polleras* also factors into their categorization. A single garment typically employs fifteen or twenty different materials. The quantity and quality are intertwined with community, artistic choice, and overall quality. For example, a first-quality *pollera* must be made of velvet, never *bayeta*. Likewise, narrow glossy braid (*cola de rata,* "rat-tail") is used on a first- or second-quality garment, and shiny lace is appropriately teamed with *diolén* (heavy polyester) or velvet.

Artistry: While Cayllominos agree that *bordados* are beautiful, "art" (*arte*) is the most ephemeral attribute of their beauty. There is tremendous variation in embroiderers' style and skill. An artisan develops a personal style and a reputation as an artist as he or she uniquely combines his/her understanding of contemporary fashions and established conventions. Caylloma embroidery is a riot of color, a dense conglomeration of threads where five or six colors negotiate a tiny space in every motif. The artisan's goal in creating exceptional design is not so much to challenge aesthetic norms as to exaggerate them or to innovate embroidered motifs. Considerable technical proficiency is needed to control the machine and create the precise motif outlines and color combinations that are pivotal aspects of aesthetic merit.

Different artisans aim for different market niches. Only a few artisans claim to be artists and pride themselves on creating the finest work. Others are yeoman workers who stay in business by producing low-priced, second- and third-quality garments for regular customers. Personal artistic style, therefore, can never be completely divorced from customer preferences, which in turn depend on her ideas about *polleras*' place in her life.

Clothing the Body as Lived Experience

In these clothes we were born. In these clothes we will die.
— FERMINA ROJAS (Arequipa, October 1991)

A dozen girls rush up the bleacher steps and crowd around a duffel bag overflowing with rainbow-hued garments. A middle-aged woman attempts to control chaos of the sort only teenagers can create. Her graying hair comes undone from its ponytail, and her plain brown cotton dress twists awry as she pulls out skirts, blouses, and hats, doling them out to the demanding throng.

"Do you have a jacket for me?"

"Is this skirt long enough?"

"The waist is too biiiiig!"

They push and screech and preen, giggling as they trade *bordados* around. Volleyball uniforms disappear under long-sleeved blouses and ankle-length skirts; sweatpants, shorts, and T-shirts are engulfed as the girls try *polleras* on for size.

"Hurry, hurry!" shouts Señora Fermina, the director of the girls' dance troupe. The stadium of Arequipa's Universidad Nacional de San Agustín (UNSA) is filled with Cayllominos. I have come with anthropologist colleagues, Flora Cutipa and Miguel Monroy, to talk with urban migrants. Today's ceremonies and games will launch another season of social events and sports for the Provincial Association of Caylloma (APC, Asociación Provincial de Caylloma) in the city of Arequipa.[3]

The day begins with a parade in which all the Caylloma villages are represented. Soccer and volleyball tournaments fill the rest of the afternoon. The outcome of abbreviated matches will decide this season's sequence of competition for the league's twenty-some teams. Teenage girls play volleyball, while the teenage boys and men play soccer. For the moment, however, they are dancers fixed on preparing to perform.

Village team dance groups of twelve to twenty members carrying flags and banners emerge from beneath the bleachers and line up at one end of the stadium. First comes Chivay, setting the pace as capital of the province. As Sra. Fermina leads the fifteen dancers around the track, the girls and a few boys twist and dip and whirl in the dance called Witite. Some of the boys are dancing in *polleras,* as is customary in the Witite dance. Of the many Caylloma festival dances, Witite is most closely associated with being

Cayllomino. Tall, proud, erect, Fermina seems a different person from the nondescript woman I just met. Now she is in her element, dressed in *polleras,* graceful in costume. Her energetic motions reveal the skill accumulated in years of dancing, as she turns in place, skirts flying out.

The Chivay group finishes its turn around the track and steps to the sidelines. Fermina is grinning proudly but looks tired. Her group has trained and performed well, I think, although some young girls are obviously uncomfortable in their borrowed finery. I expect her to climb up and join her associates in the bleachers, but she does not. My attention returns to the parade.

"There she is again!" cries Flora. Now Fermina is dancing with the group from Madrigal. After their turn ends and the parade finishes, she appears beside us, glowing. While she collects the *polleras* from the girls, I ask her why she danced twice.

"Chivay is our capital. As head of the troupe I have to dance with them. But Madrigal! That's my hometown! I have to dance with them, too."

"Do the girls like wearing the *polleras*?" I want to know.

"The girls love their *polleras.* We have to wear these clothes," she asserts emphatically. "In these clothes we were born. In these clothes we will die." (*En esta ropa hemos nacido. En esta ropa vamos a morir.*)

What did Fermina mean by saying "we were born and will die" in Caylloma clothes? What do *polleras* represent for Cayllominas in their home communities? How does that differ for those who live, work, play, and dance in Arequipa?

Fermina was "born in these clothes" in Madrigal, wearing *polleras* from early childhood, but she moved to Arequipa when she was twelve years old. Over time she restricted her use of *polleras* to dances and fiestas. When I first met her, she was not wearing *polleras* but a plain commercial dress, indistinguishable from the daily wear of any poor Arequipa woman. Her own daughters wear *polleras* only at fiestas and to dance in the troupe. Last-minute adjustments and preparations were necessary because the teenage girls were *not* born in these clothes. Most of them were born and raised in Arequipa, children of migrants from rural Caylloma. They may travel to their parents' home communities only once or twice a year.

"Born and die in these clothes" came to seem an appropriate summary of the Caylloma body-clothing experience. Fermina's forceful statement spurred my reflection on the lifelong meaning of dress. But the scene I witnessed contradicted her assertion, as did many conversations I had with other Caylloma women. Women insisted on their right to wear *polleras.* "We have to wear these clothes," said Fermina. "I have always worn *polleras,*" said many others. Asserting Caylloma identity by wearing *polleras* in the city is a vital part of survival, connecting women with each other and with their native villages, re-forming community. Fermina phrased the experience more tidily and emphatically than others, but she was not alone in this opinion. Still, no matter how firmly they believed it, their view was riddled with contradictions.

For the rest of the afternoon, Flora, Miguel, and I talked with dozens of Caylloma migrants who constitute the APC. They come from different walks of life, and in the city they work at different jobs. One man is a teacher at Flora's son's school. Another runs a printing business.

The *polleras* the girls wore that afternoon had varied sources. Parents had brought some from their hometowns. Workshop artisans had brought others on regular visits to Arequipa a few days before fiestas. Some *polleras* were produced in city workshops, especially those of Leandro Suni, known as the "Chivay Chino," a spectator with whom I spoke that day.[4]

The APC events are folkloric spectacles that coalesce the sociality of urban migrant life, including the places of *polleras* in it. The APC transforms Cayllomino life into urban folklore, challenging our ideas of what cultural authenticity means in an urban context. At the same time, because so many Cayllominos' experience of "home" is limited to visits, APC membership and performances help keep alive the idea of a cultural home. Costumed events like the APC's sports matches and dances extend beyond their frames because preparations for them are ongoing activities.

Clothing and the Life Course

Women cannot expect to begin wearing *bordados* at an early age and continue to do so straight through adulthood. They must continuously negotiate their clothed identities because they are participants in Peruvian society and because the state enforces nationalized norms of clothedness on their bodies. Giving up their long full skirts for a short plain dress, cutting off their long braids for a frizzy perm, and trading rubber *ujutas* (sandals) for sneakers or heels—all these are elements of change that females repeatedly undergo. Their choice is free only to a certain point. Parents may encourage daughters to wear *polleras* for special occasions, but national society prevents girls from wearing *polleras* daily. Women claiming to have "always" (*siempre*) worn *polleras* have usually worn *them* at various points in their life, but with numerous interruptions. My survey inquired about significant events or phases that coincided with changes. When did you start wearing *polleras*? Did you ever stop wearing them? When and why? The wearing process, it became clear, was not one long seamless segue between phases, but a stop-and-start pattern. Changing back and forth is a habituating process as well. Disrupted habituation is the rule, rather than the exception, for females of Caylloma.

The embodiment of Caylloma culture on gendered bodies begins at birth, as Sra. Fermina claimed. Women wear *polleras* while giving birth, and the baby emerges into the world enveloped by the voluminous skirts. At birth, new Cayllominas sometimes acquire and wear their first embroidered garment (Sara Kaithathera, personal communication, Yanque, 1992). All babies are swaddled with a long, narrow band (*cinta*); a girl's band, if embroidered, resembles a longer version of the adult woman's belt.

Many girls acquire their first set of *polleras* by age three, for their baptism or for a fiesta (Figure 18). Embroidering small garments for little girls is time-consuming for artisans, and buying them is expensive for parents. Younger daughters' first *polleras* are often hand-me-downs. Out-of-fashion adult women's *polleras,* if still serviceable, are sometimes cut down for older girls. Almost all girls have white hats, usually the sturdier, lower-priced canvas ones. In the lower valley, girls may wear embroidered hats, especially for fiestas.

Since most girls do not wear *polleras* every day, an outfit purchased for a fiesta usually lasts longer than a year. Although many families ideally would give each daughter a new set of *polleras* annually, few can afford to do so. Parents most often cite the high cost as the reason their girls do not regularly dress in *polleras.* Daughters of artisans are more likely to wear *polleras* because their parents make their outfits. Felícitas Bernal, Susana's sister, and her husband, Gerardo Vilcasán, both embroiderers, have seven daughters and one son. Although it was expensive to keep their daughters in *polleras* from age three, the parents felt strongly about the positive value. As long as their girls wanted to wear *polleras,* they would provide them. Felícitas still wears *polleras* daily, but her daughters reserve them for fiestas.

Girls cannot wear *polleras* all day every day. They must attend school, and so they must wear the school uniform. Public schools have become a central arena of Peruvian state sumptuary regulation. Plain uniforms of white shirts, gray sweaters, and gray trousers for boys or gray jumpers for girls are mandatory for all schoolchildren. This national legislation, im-

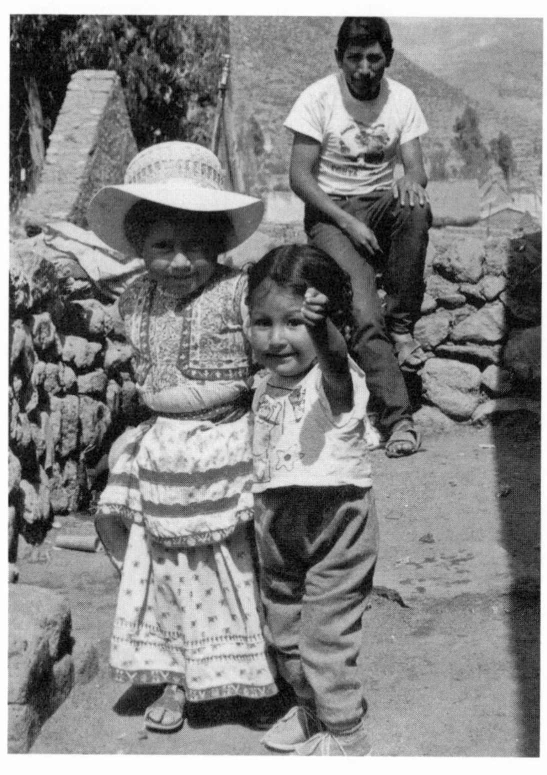

18 Enadi Condori Bernal in *polleras* after her baptism, with her sister Lorena and their father, Juan Condori

posed in the 1960s, was intended as a symbolic leveling mechanism, but it actually legitimized discrimination against indigenous children: wearing traditional clothes to school became a "crime." Another consequence was that such clothes came to be considered a costume available to children of all ages and ethnic groups. Not only in urban festivals but in rural school "folklore" celebrations, non-Cayllomino children assume "native" disguises.[5]

During adolescence, acquiring *polleras* and displaying oneself in them becomes more important. Girls take a greater interest in obtaining fancy *polleras* for fiestas, which, as social occasions that include courtship, are focal points in their lives. Most girls now migrate from Caylloma to Arequipa or Lima to work while in their teens. Because most small villages lack secondary schools, any child who wants to attend high school must travel at least to Chivay, Cabanaconde, Yanque, or Callalli. Parents often prefer that the child study in Arequipa, which has better schools, despite the additional expenses. Even children living with relatives in Arequipa usually work, pay rent, send money home, and financially help younger siblings attend school. Girls as young as eleven are employed as live-in maids, and employers regulate their clothed bodies, requiring that they don an apron or uniform.

As adults, women face new choices. When a young woman finishes or leaves high school, she may have a child and get married or, more frequently, enter a live-in partnership (*convivencia*) with a man. If she chooses to remain in the city, her use of *polleras* diminishes even further, to occasional festive attire. Only if she returns to Caylloma is she likely to wear *polleras* daily.

Young married women who wore *polleras* more often when they were single spoke nostalgically of their beautiful, luxurious fiesta *polleras.* Natalia Suyo, born in Maca, moved to Arequipa at age six. As a teenager, she loved to return home to dance. "By the time I was seventeen, I had seventeen *polleras,*" is how she phrased it. But then, soon after finishing high school, Natalia married a man from Cusco, had her first child, and remained in Arequipa. Traveling to Maca became more difficult and her reasons for dancing diminished once she no longer needed to attract a partner.

At the first wedding I attended in Coporaque, in 1989, the bride wore white—Juana's purchased white wedding gown with veil was borrowed from a teacher. The bridegroom, Elías Yajo, wore a plain tan suit and tie. After the church ceremony, the civil ceremony was held and celebrated with an hour of dancing and champagne-drinking in the town council building. Then the newlyweds walked home, accompanied by many celebrants. Within ten minutes, Juana had changed into *polleras*—not a brand-new outfit, but a first-quality ensemble. Wearing white has become the contemporary custom: the bride wears a borrowed or rented wedding gown, then changes to *polleras* for the party afterward, which usually lasts several days. Sometimes new *polleras* are provided by the bride's *madrina de matrimonio* (godmother who pays most wedding costs); other times they were acquired for a fiesta earlier that year. Weddings often occur on or near a fiesta date, providing a combined occasion for acquiring *polleras.*

Generation and age affect social custom and, consequently, *pollera* use. When women now in their fifties and sixties were young, girls rarely migrated for work or finished school. Thus, more older women wear *polleras* daily. Eufemia Feria, a Cabanaconde artisan married into the Tejada clan of artisans, told me that she had worn *polleras* "always, since birth" (interview, Cabanaconde, February 1993). In her midsixties, she dressed in good-quality Cabana-style *polleras* and embroidered hat. Because of her age, it seemed feasible that in her case "always" did mean she had worn them constantly, but then she told me of numerous interruptions. For more than ten years she and her husband lived outside Cabanaconde, her native community, on a Peruvian state-run estate. There, she dressed "*de vestido.*" Even now, when she travels to Arequipa, she does not wear *polleras.*

Today, by the time girls reach adulthood, the conflictive habituation has become so well established that state regulation is usually redundant. Normative sanctions are often as effective as workplace regulations in preventing women from using *polleras.* In both the private sector and state-run organizations, uniforms are required for professional and paraprofessional positions such as nurse, teacher, and secretary. Even the city street sweepers have a uniform: members of the unionized, largely female force wear a blue coat.

Taste and style in *polleras* vary by age. As noted above, when Leonardo recommended the color lilac for my *pollera,* Susana dismissed it as an old ladies' color. Women over sixty tend to wear dark colors: black, navy blue, burgundy, or brown.

"In these clothes we will die." Many, but not all, women will be wearing *polleras* at the time of death. Color is linked to the ways women commemorate the death of others in their community. Elderly women often wear black because of their status as widows. In mourning rituals, embroidered garments are used in specific colors, mostly black with white and blue. Fermina may have meant, as well, that she expects to be buried in those clothes.[6]

Love and Money: Community and Class in Pollera *Style and Use*

> *It's one's typical dress; it's from one's people/village* (pueblo).
> — MARGARITA SULLCA (Interview, Chivay, April 1992)

> *The better one dresses, the prouder one seems.*
> — SEBASTIÁN QUISPE TICONA
> (Interview, Cabanaconde, March 1993)

These statements were made by embroidery artisans. Sullca stresses community membership—what is typical of the people among whom and the place where one lives. Quispe mentions the quality of self-presentation, dressing better than others, and pride in appearance.

At her embroidery stand in Chivay market, Margarita Sullca has spent thirty years dressing Caylloma women. A native of Chivay who wears *polleras* daily, she reflected on commonalities and differences among Caylloma communities: *polleras* are the clothes "*de su pueblo,*" of one's people/village. While Cayllominas appreciate the positive value of *polleras* and feel pride in dressing well, usually within their community, they are equally aware that they may face discrimination whenever they wear *polleras.* Yet the fancy *polleras* women flaunt on ceremonial occasions mark high status as much as community membership. "Pride" is related to individual self-esteem and class standing within the community, valley, and province. Artisan Sebastián Quispe Ticona of Cabanaconde stated that "the better one dresses, the prouder one seems" (. . . *más orgulloso se ve*). Pride (*orgullo*), he believed, had to do with the quality of one's *polleras* and was directly linked to money: wearing *polleras* "depends on the money (*plata*) [he or] she has" (interview, Cabanaconde, March 1993).

Another artisan linked the high cost of *polleras* to vanity, the dark side of pride: "Women put on [*polleras*] for vanity. They want to show they have more money," said embroidery artisan Livia Sullca (interview, Chivay, February 1992). Her association of *polleras* with ostentation prompts questions of conspicuous consumption. Have *polleras* become fully commoditized? Can anyone consume and use them as signs of high status?

Polleras are expensive, as everyone in Caylloma knows. Their price is a significant factor in purchase decisions and a topic of daily discussion (as is the price of most commodities in a country suffering from hyperinflation). *Bordados* are a medium through which women show their prosperity, both in monetary wealth and prestige, because acquiring *polleras* requires social connections as well as money, and credit or obligation may substitute for cash. During the course of her lifetime, a woman can expect to spend thousands of dollars (or the equivalent in products and services) on the hundreds of *bordados* she will wear. Some garments, like blouses, must be replaced every year; others, like skirts, last a few years. Occasionally, sponsoring a fiesta demands significant expenditure on fine clothes.

Rosalía Valera, the mother of my compadre Juan Condori, has an embroidery business in Coporaque. In the 1960s, when she was young, she worked in the Majes Valley in commercial agriculture and abandoned her *polleras* for several years. Now, as she actively sells embroideries and travels frequently, Rosalía prefers to wear *polleras.* "I travel in *polleras* so people will think I don't have money. When you travel in *polleras,* the women love you, they share with you" (. . . *las señoras te quieren, te convidan*). This affectionate reception, she claimed, held sway not only in Caylloma and neighboring provinces, where women wear similar *polleras,* but as far away as Mollendo, on the Pacific coast, and Tacna, near the border with Chile, where this type of dress is rarely seen.

"To show they have more money" apparently contradicts "so people will think I don't have money." How could the same garment indicate two opposite conditions? This is possible because of the grades. A *pollera* of rustic, homespun *bayeta* is light years from one of shiny, high-priced velvet. Rosalía travels in older, shabbier *polleras* so people will not rob her. But her choice also expresses her sense of ethnic background and class; others recognize and welcome her as a sister highland peasant. Rosalía glosses this generous, positive reception as "love": "the women love you, they share with you."

Love merges with money in *polleras'* instrumental applications, for affection factors into commerce when women sell other Caylloma goods, such as fruit, corn, and cheese. They wear *polleras* on the hottest days to sell cactus fruit in Arequipa and beyond. One summer weekend I went to the beach at Mollendo. At the end of the sidewalk, 200 yards from the Pacific Ocean, sat two women from Maca with baskets of cactus fruit. On an 80°F day, thirsty beach-goers in bathing trunks and bikinis were glad to purchase the fruit from the Maqueñas covered from neck to ankles in *polleras.* The commercial advantage of identification with place superceded comfort.

There are times, however, when women say that *polleras* are not appropriate. Emotions, attitudes, and practical reasons intertwine in every decision to give them up. "I am ashamed," admitted Florencia Huaracha, who changed out of them for city travel (Chapter 2). As they become an item of conspicuous display, *polleras* also become less accessible financially. Women abandon the practice when they can no longer afford it. "I buy new *polleras* from time to time, for fiestas, but they are too expensive for everyday," was a frequent refrain. Replacing only worn or inexpensive items, mainly blouses and vests, is a stop-gap measure for those reluctant to abandon *polleras* completely.

For other women, practical matters of climate and comfort separate them from their *polleras.* Many women explained that *polleras* are warmer than *de vestido*–style clothes, and certain fabrics, especially *bayeta* (wool), are warmer than others. "It's too hot in Arequipa," some women claimed: the climate of Arequipa averages 10° warmer than Caylloma. But others spoke of emotional temperature. When they take off the long skirts that envelop and protect them, they feel "cold"—vulnerable and exposed.

Polleras "are very heavy" (*pesan mucho*), women say. The weight of many meters of fabric presses down on their waist and hips. Removing the physical weight of voluminous skirts, they feel lighter. Other kinds of weight, however, remain a burden. In analyzing their choices, I found it impossible to separate emotions from economy. All too often, the stigma that *polleras* carry as emblems of rural origins, poverty, or Indianness effectively counters pride in wearing luxurious *polleras.*

Juan Tejada, a senior artisan in Cabanaconde, equated clothes with custom, and both with return migration. Coming home meant wearing ethnic dress. "The Cabana women who return, they bring their fabrics, they change, they put on their customs from birth" (. . . *sus costumbres de su nacimiento se ponen;* interview, Cabanaconde, February 1993). Many migrant women who gave up *polleras* in the city were happy to put them on again. They associated *polleras* with returning to their native village, whether temporarily, to dance, or permanently, to settle down and raise a family. Despite many disruptions in the practice, wearing *polleras* and the possibility of returning to them shape women's bodies and lives. When women go home and exchange the physically hot and emotionally cold environment of Arequipa for the affectionate surroundings of home, they "put on their customs from birth." Thus, we can understand clothes as a kind of place. Sra. Fermina's phrase "in these clothes we were born" then comes to mean "in this place we were born": *polleras* are the clothes of our people and place, our *pueblo.*

"Embroidery Is a Lovely Thing": Aesthetics and Fashion

> *[Embroidery] is an art that should be highly esteemed. I think this way, but others think only about their business. It is an artistic matter and not an economic one.*
> — LEONARDO MEJÍA
> (Interview, Chivay, February 28, 1992)

Embroidery was not just a business, Leonardo Mejía liked to say. His observation was based on twelve years of experience working in a workshop with Susana; helping in several other workshops, including those of her brothers; and teaching other people to embroider. Because I had known them the longest, I tested the survey form with Leonardo and Susana before I surveyed the other artisans. Once he had completed all five pages, he chided me: "*¡El arte!* The art! You didn't ask enough questions about the art." He then made the above statement, and I modified the form. Many artisans share his pro-art attitudes, but Leonardo was the most adamant among those who claim embroidery is an art form. Artists recognize their creative role in expressing and shaping the aesthetics of valley residents. They are not only in it for the money.

"*Los bordados son bonitos,*" artisans stated: women wear them because "the embroideries are pretty." *Bonito,* "pretty," also implies "lovely," "suitable," "nice." "*El bordado es algo bonito,*" people say, "embroidery is a lovely thing." Almost half the respondents to my surveys used *bonito* to describe embroidery, making it the second most common term after *costumbre,* "custom." Yet there was no clear consensus about the most important quality that makes *bordados* pretty. Rather, numerous factors combine to create a harmonious whole, an ideal of beauty that looks right to those who wear them and those who gaze at them. Beauty, while embedded in the garment, is also embodied in the person of the wearer. The ideal defies consensus, and disagreement is par for the course.

Questions of aesthetics have meaning only in a larger realm of cultural and social process. Broad considerations of community and region come into play in choosing a garment, such as a type of hat. Even the tiniest technical feature, perhaps undetectable to an untrained eye, is often an arena of conflict where community variations and individual preferences become meaningful. As Caylloma people related their sentiments about beauty, I came to realize that aesthetic factors are fully integrated into the way they conceive of a garment as a whole. Considering recent changes is also important, as artists make innovations that both satisfy their creative urges and keep their work selling, and as customers compete in the arena of self-adornment. In a word, fashion.

Anne Hollander, a fashion historian, calls fashion "a compelling new system of Western elegance" that has arisen since the late Middle Ages (1994:14), rendering it distinct from all other modes of dress. Positing this modernist "fashion" against a traditionalist "non-fashion," she maintains that "Western fashion [has a] unique method of dealing with the human body, creating an eventful visual history quite separate from what I call non-fashion, the sum of other developments in dress and adornment . . . all over the globe" (ibid.). Fashion, Hollander maintains, is modern because if offers "fluid imagery for its own sake, to keep visually present the ideal of perpetual contingency. Meaning is properly detachable from form" (ibid.:17). "Traditional dress" is "non-fashion," she believes. Rooted in a different set of temporal and visual values, it creates "its visual project primarily to illustrate the confirmation of established custom, and to embody the desire for stable meaning even if custom changes—it is normative" (ibid.). Were we to focus on form, as Hollander suggests, we would be forced to label Caylloma dress "traditional." I reject this sharp division of clothing into two camps, however, because it obscures the very real connections between them, especially the influences of "other developments in dress" on constructing the fashion of the "West." Furthermore, Caylloma *bordados* are simultaneously "non-fashion" in their preoccupation with perpetuating form, and "fashion" in offering "fluid imagery" that presents an "ideal of perpetual contingency." Dichotomizing the West and the rest as fashion and non-fashion obscures the choices that all people must make about perpetuating or changing their clothes.

In calling attention to the fashion element in *bordados,* I do not intend to trivialize it or treat it as capricious or unsubstantial. Rather, I take issue with Hollander's polarization in order to emphasize that changes in appearance and representation occur constantly among indigenous peoples as well as among so-called modern societies. Caylloma *bordados* are not frozen survivals from ancient groups in isolated enclaves. They derive meaning from their flexibility and from appropriation. Caylloma artists appropriate national and international tastes according to local cultural preferences, which in turn contribute to developing and maintaining discrete ethnic identities among the women who wear *bordados.*

Among the most recent fashionable elements in embroidered clothes are synthetic materials and bright colors. By addressing such "foreign" elements, I aim to release them from their conceptual closet and to address how and why they became firmly established in the Caylloma clothing repertoire. The very brightness that is exalted as "lively" (*vivo*) by those who use it is all too often derided as "gaudy" by outsiders, even by textile scholars. This attitude inheres in outsiders' concepts of authenticity and identity, not in those of the people who make and wear the clothes.

Getting into Green

Caylloma people were far from shy in offering their opinions about appearance and style or in making personal comments and asking personal questions. I got used to being told how I should dress and to having frequent discussions about aesthetics, personal preferences, and taste in *pollera* fashion. One day in Coporaque, after obtaining my finished *polleras* from Susana Bernal, I set out to take them to my *comadre* Nilda Bernal so that she could show me how to sew the waistband properly.[7] On my way, I ran into Nilda's mother-in-law, Rosalía Valera, and a neighbor, Florencia, both regular *pollera* wearers. They asked what was in my bag.

I pulled out the brand-new skirts, never used, stiff and shiny. On the blue *pollera,* bands of trim and lace paraded up the lower half (see Figure 14); on the contrasting pink one printed with red flowers, a slender turquoise band trimmed the hem. I had already shown them to several people who praised their quality and beauty. Rosalía, however, heaped scorn on Susana's choices.

"That's already old-fashioned. Why did she use that outmoded design?" she railed, pointing to two rows of swirls executed in lime green yarn.

I was stunned. Having overcome my original reservations, I looked forward to dressing in Chivay style, wearing the latest *pollera* fashions executed flawlessly by my talented friend. Yet Rosalía put them down; my skirts were not fashionable enough!

Many North Americans have a phobia about bright colors. For a long time, I was among them. Lime green was the toughest; it is hard to love. Whenever artisans asked me what tourists want to buy, I never hesitated to point out that *gringos* abhor this color.[8] An internal struggle preceded my realization that Susana must embroider my skirt exactly as she saw fit. I chose only the background fabric—and that from among the options she offered. After all, she was the expert. I could not whine to her, "I don't want any lime green, any of that neon, acid, Gatorade green." So sure enough, lime green ended up in my skirt, just as in local women's skirts. Once I got used to it, I even came to like it. More important, I began to understand that it is now an established element of authentic Caylloma clothes.

Many artisans obtain their materials from a large fabric store in Chivay, where I once ran into Felícitas Bernal and Gerardo Vilcasán, who had come from Coporaque to stock up. Large colorful skeins of yarn were enticingly displayed through the openwork iron bars of the store's gate. Referring to a lime green skein, I used the Spanish for "light green," "*verde claro.*" Gerardo corrected me, "It's *q'achu verde*" (*q'achu,* "light" in Quechua; *verde,* "green" in Spanish; "green" in Quechua is *qomer*). He explained that *q'achu* means "light" only in certain contexts and in modifying certain colors. For "light blue," one cannot say *q'achu azul;* rather, the Spanish *celeste,* "sky blue," is used. *Q'achu* also means "new crops," "forage," and by extension, "freshness," ranging from green pasture to recently freeze-dried potatoes. The emergence of young crops in the naturally dry environment of the Colca Valley is precious. Contrasting with the gray and brown landscape, the green of new plants vibrates. Using *q'achu verde* affirms the importance of these green growing things.[9]

Bright colors—lime green, pink, and orange—are now used extensively in fabrics, threads, yarns, and trims. Yarn color seems to be a more serious fashion concern than changing hemlines. Bright colors claim an important place in Caylloma textiles, and they have done so for so long that, just as I began to warm to them, they were already beginning to be considered passé!

Rosalía's indictment of Susana's work also showed me how much opinion about embroidery aesthetics and fashions varies among artists and consumers. When it comes to judging each other's work, artists take no prisoners. When I discussed the incident with Susana, she defended her use of the green swirl and other design features and pointed them out on many *polleras* that she had not made. Furthermore, she educated me, my skirt's design was unique because I am tall, so it had to be longer. She modified the usual layout by adding another band of lace and yarn so that the trim would properly cover the area from the hem to knee height.

As I suspected, the aesthetic disagreement involved rivalry between workshops and individuals about fundamental issues of quality and professionalism. Susana was not just Rosalía's rival in another workshop but had worked for her. Years ago, from age ten to twelve, she had assisted Rosalía with sales and travels to the distant highland fairs. Susana also claimed that Rosalía did not know how to embroider at all and hired others to do her work. Realizing that the bad feelings between them ran deep, I did not press for details. In addition, I suspected that Rosalía was annoyed because I did not commission the *polleras* from her, her son, or her daughter-in-law, who were, after all, my *compadres.* Juan and Nilda were not troubled, however, because I purchased other embroidered objects from them.

Commissioning my own clothes forced me to come to terms with my own cultural biases about color. Displaying my garments put me on the line, exposing my taste (and budget) to scrutiny and judgment. My *polleras* became a proving ground. As it turned out, when I finally got to her house, Nilda was not home. Several weeks passed before we both found time for my sewing lesson. Although I did not accomplish what I set out to do that day, I gained insight into the social dynamics within the artisans' community of practice.

The Embroidered Landscape: Artists, Designs, and Style

> *[Embroidering] is like painting a landscape.*
> — MARCIAL VILLAVICENCIO CONDORI
> (Interview, Cabanaconde, March 25, 1993)

In proposing the embroidered landscape as an apt image for Caylloma *bordados,* I intend the phrase both literally and metaphorically. *Bordados* are a primary means of creative expression for hundreds of men and women. These objects are their representations of cultural and natural phenomena, not expressed the same way in any other medium. Locally meaningful, *bordados* also embody the appropriation and transformation of nonlocal designs, materials, and styles. Considering the embroidered landscape as a conceptual landscape enables us to understand how the ideas and products of distant places have found their way onto the bodies of Cayllominos.

Constantly composing his embroidered landscape, Marcial Villavicencio paints in thread. As we spoke in his home workshop in Cabanaconde, he explained that embroidery and painting were "similar in combining the little colors." The Colca Valley landscape around him inspired those designs and colors. As a schoolboy, Villavicencio began to draw on paper and then taught himself to embroider, at first by hand because his family had no sewing machine. When I interviewed him, he was thirty-seven, had been running his own embroidery workshop for eight years, and was well known for his hats. Devoted to the art in his work and persistent in preparing both quantity and quality *bordados,* Villavicencio took first place in a crafts competition at the 1991 Caylloma Provincial Fair. He later won a national award. Proud to be a representative of his community, he also regarded producing high-quality work with innovative designs as his individual achievement.

The ongoing interplay between inspiration and innovation is a dominant theme in artists' discourses. The natural environment of the countryside inspires Rodolfo Cayo, an artisan from Madrigal who maintains an embroidery kiosk in Chivay market. "I go out to the countryside; I figure out different things" (*cosas* [i.e., designs]). By embroidering, he makes sense of the natural world. The aspects he most enjoys are drawing the motifs and combining the colors.

Although there is considerable variation in individual style, each artist must master a standard repertoire of motifs (*figuras* or *dibujos; cocos* refer to geometric motifs). A single garment may feature fifty different complex figurative designs in the main bands, in addition to four or five simpler designs used for fillers, edgings, and borders. A star, the large, unifying feature on the crown of a hat (see Figures 16 and 17), also appears in bands. Motifs depicting animals and plants abound. Within a general category such as bird, numerous specific types are depicted, including dove, duck, rooster, and hummingbird (see Figure 19). There are more than a dozen varieties of flower, including that of the *chuna* cactus, rose, dahlia, and tulip; some appear in ornate flowerpots. Fish, usually called trout, are common, as are small rodents: *conejo,* although literally "rabbit," also refers to the wild, squirrel-like *vizcacha* and the domestic guinea pig (*cuy*).

Although most flora and fauna represented are local, others have never inhabited Caylloma. About two-thirds of the motifs are the same in the entire valley; others are exclusive to specific places. For example, the monkey, a tropical animal not seen in Caylloma, adorns Cabana garments (see Figure 15). Peru's national insignia (*escudo nacional*), a shield with a vicuña, a tree, and a cornucopia, is featured on the national flag and money; in Caylloma *bordados,* it is used only in Cabanaconde and the surrounding lower valley, often featured prominently on jackets.[10] The sky, which offers bright "stars" (including the planet Venus [Urton 1981]), is a nightly presence surrounding the valley.

In the cultural landscape, the primary source of design inspiration is other garments. Skilled artisans draw them with the sewing machine without looking at a model (see Chapter 7). A well-trained artist, therefore, need not directly copy others' work to be indirectly influenced by it or may draw from memory a design seen only once. The common currency of designs makes apparently minor variations significant and leads to conflicts as artists accuse each other of copying their original, unique motifs.

Artists also mentioned several kinds of mass-produced printed matter as sources. David Rodríguez, a Cabanaconde artisan who, at age twenty-three, had already been embroidering for eight years, said his drawings were his own creation but sometimes he copied images from a book (interview, Cabanaconde, March 25, 1993). Similarly, Mario Seyco, his brother-in-law, said he both created his own designs and got them from magazines (interview, Cabanaconde, March 25, 1993). Hugo Vilcape of Cabanaconde, ever on the lookout for inspiration, asked me to send him "an album with animal figures so I can try some new animals" (interview, Cabanaconde, February 1993).

Although not mentioned by artisans, other sources probably include weavings and architecture. Many embroidered motifs are also employed in locally woven textiles. Compare, for example, two contemporaneous hummingbirds: one embroidered on a *corpiño* (Figure 19), the other woven on a shawl (Figure 20). Both birds stand in profile with wings extended and their beak in a flower; stylistically, the embroidered motif is more curvilinear and the woven one, more rectilinear. Hand-weaving predates machine embroidery by several centuries, but in Caylloma both media have coexisted for fifty years, making it impossible to determine which one inspires the other. Similarly, carved motifs on colonial stone buildings resemble those on *bordados.* They are part of artisans' cultural visual landscape, thus a likely influence, but not one artisan mentioned "copying" colonial carvings.[11]

True artists must draw. They have talent, not just skill. Hugo Vilcape, famed in Cabanaconde as one of its best hat embroiderers, is highly conscious of the art in embroidery. "Embroidering is like drawing with a pencil," he claimed (interview, Cabanaconde, February 26, 1993). About forty when I interviewed him, he had been embroidering for fifteen years. Like Villavicencio, he acquired the drawing habit young, while still in school, which facilitated his mastery of embroidery.

Drawing combines creativity, command of the repertoire of motifs, and technical skill. "To draw" (*dibujar*) means to envision the figures and to use the sewing machine to outline them on cloth. All artisans draw directly on the fabric with needle and thread on the sewing machine. They learn to shape the designs by manipulating fabric under the machine's presser foot, which is kinesthetically different from moving a pencil over paper. The artisan who draws figures in pencil on paper is rare indeed, and some claim they cannot do so. None of the artisans I know collect their designs as drawings on paper.

After drawing with the machine, the next step is "to paint" (*pintar*): to apply colored threads inside the outlines, one color at a time, also called "to fill" (*rellenar*). Edgar Vargas, a Cabanaconde artisan aged twenty, said his older brother Cecilio, with fifteen years' experience embroidering, first

19 Hummingbirds and flower; detail of an embroidered vest by Susana Bernal

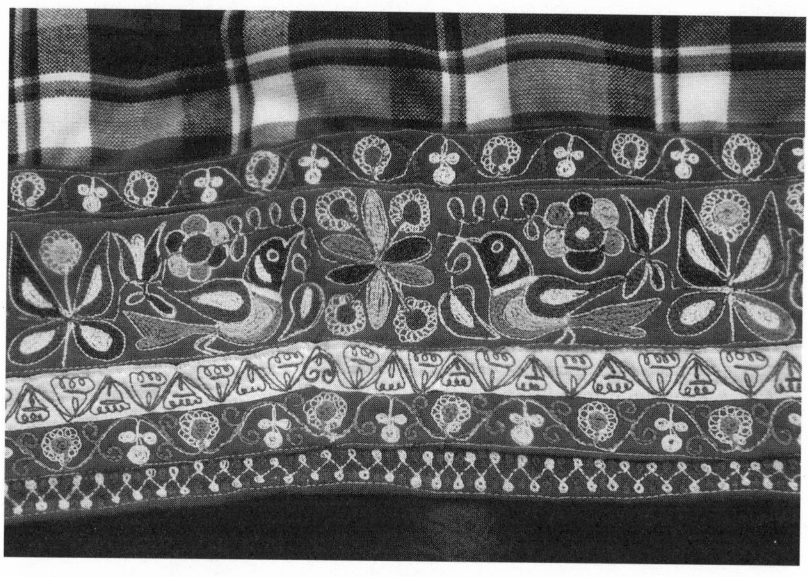

20 Rows of figures, including hummingbirds and flowers, on a woven shawl by Grimalda Vega

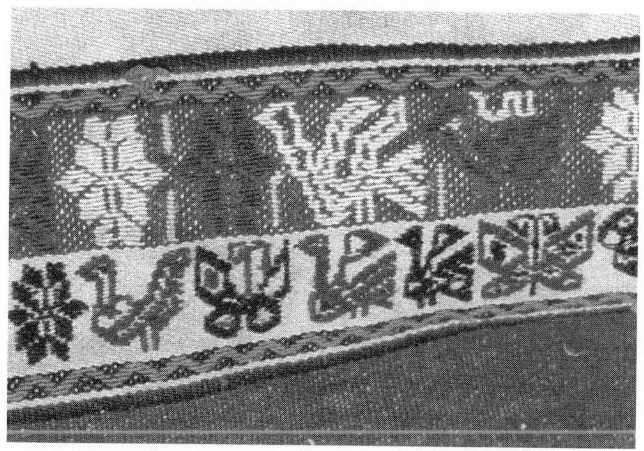

taught him how to paint and then to draw (interview, Cabanaconde, February 26, 1993). In painting, the artist follows the established outline; this familiarizes the apprentice artisan with the motifs and hones his or her color sense, providing a basis for learning to draw.

Men liked to talk about being artists. Almost all of the quotations about attitudes toward artistry presented here are from men. This apparent gender gap reflects gendered attitudes and a gendered division of labor in embroidery production (detailed in Chapter 7). In the Chivay shops, equal numbers of women and men work, and most do the same tasks. Cayllominos' perception of gender imbalance in specific roles is skewed. Although women artists do exist, most artists who speak of creativity in the work are men. Usually only one person, usually male, draws in each workshop. Because drawing is believed to be the line demarcating an artist, not everyone learns to draw. That line is so strongly gendered that most women do not draw. Attitudes, however, can change.

Susana Bernal, for example, began to draw after she had been sewing and painting for fifteen years. She taught some of her brothers, as well as many paid operators, to embroider. Nevertheless, for many years she thought she could not draw. In their workshop, Leonardo usually drew the designs. In 1991, he spent several months working as a teacher in a distant town. Then her brother Hilario drew until he got too busy preparing to sponsor a fiesta. She finally decided she had to draw. It proved not to be difficult, and perfecting her drawing satisfied her.

Rosalvina Cayo, a woman in her late twenties, operates a hat kiosk in Chivay market with her husband, Gerardo Alfaro. She is one of ten artisans who trim white hats with braids, laces, and ribbons. Three of her brothers embroider: Rodolfo and Rolando also have kiosks in Chivay market; Sergio lives in Arequipa, embroidering in his home and his parents' shop. Even though Rosalvina had often assembled garments for them, she claimed she did not embroider. Moreover, she believed she could not draw the figures: "*¡No puedo dibujar!*" (I can't draw!), she lamented one day. Susana ardently encouraged Rosalvina to believe she could.

"I used to think the same thing!" sympathized Susana. "But then I *had* to draw, and now I can draw. It's not hard. You can learn too!"

Embracing the role of artist was an empowering experience for Susana, and she wished the same for Rosalvina. Their conversation helped me understand the importance of drawing and the gendered aspects of artistic work. Susana's story is not unique, but women tend to describe themselves as sharing in a family enterprise and they rarely acknowledge a role in the creative side of their work.

Susana also consciously developed and fine-tuned her own personal style. After one year, she consistently drew slightly larger motifs, integrated the main motifs more smoothly with the background, and clearly defined each motif's outline and colors. Her husband, Leonardo Mejía, summed up style this way: "[N]o matter how much one teaches, the motifs don't come out the same. If there are twenty embroiderers, twenty different motifs come out although they have the same name. It's like, even if you're my brother, we're not the same" (interview, Chivay, February 28, 1992). Each artist's style of executing the complex embroidered designs distinguishes his or her work and accentuates the individual character of Caylloma clothes. Each garment bears the recognizable mark of the artist who made it, and the woman who wears it advertises his proficiency. Developing a personal style depends on individual flair and demands technical mastery of the sewing machine. Artisans constantly stressed the connections between the manner of embroidering motifs in each community and the skills, talent, and vision of the artists.

The Cabanaconde hat offers a good opportunity for analyzing two artisans' distinct approaches to design and for examining one recent stylistic change. One hat was made by Leonardo Mejía (Figure 16), the other by Hugo Vilcape (Figure 17). Mejía, originally from Coporaque and one of the few upper-valley artisans who made Cabana hats, now lives in Chivay. Vilcape is from Cabanaconde and still lives there. Both men were in their midthirties when they made the hats.

Cabana hats employ a standard layout: a central star, surrounded by floral, animal, and geometric motifs. Artisans use innumerable industrial cones of sewing thread. One month, no blue thread arrived in Chivay from Arequipa. Individual stocks were soon depleted and a shortage resulted. One day while I was at Leonardo's and Susana's kiosk, Marcial Villavicencio stopped to chat. Susana challenged me to pinpoint what was different about one hat, but I could not. The answer was, it had no blue. Leonardo had taken a bold step: he embroidered an entire hat without any blue thread and compensated with more yellow. Marcial did not contain his disapproval. In his view, Leonardo's attempt was an aberration. To be Cabana, he maintained, it had to have blue. But in Leonardo's view, the hat embodied his creative approach, as he made necessity the mother of invention.

Hugo Vilcape made a hat for me in March 1993 (Figure 17). Seated next to me one day at a party was the wife of Cabanaconde's mayor; she wore an elaborate set of *polleras.* Vilcape had embroidered her distinctive hat, which I so coveted that the next day I went straight to his house and commissioned him to embroider one for me, then watched it develop over several days. He signed the finished work with his embroidered name, which artists rarely do (see Figure 17, lower left center, on black band). Their iconic signature is sufficient identification. The central star, outlined in the traditional blue, has a distinct shape and texture. Its thick, raised surface is created by filling it with far more stitches and thread than others use. Vilcape's hats are pricey; he can charge more because of his reputation, but he justifies the expense because they take more time and thread.

Wearing my new Cabana hat around Cabanaconde confirmed how well Cayllominos know artists' styles. On the day I collected the finished hat, I wore it to another party. "Ah, Vilcape!" said one of the assistant mayors as I entered the parish hall. "Yes. How do you know?" I asked, removing the hat and handing it to him. He readily pointed out several distinctive Vilcape features, notably the double-filled star. Vilcape, in writing his signature, reinforced his self-identification as an artist.

Artists and consumers alike maintain that the quality of work is related to community and technique. "Thread" (*hilo*) is the technical feature that best illustrates Cayllominos' micro-level obsession with localized characteristics. Marcial Villavicencio was the first person to tell me that *hilo* matters: in the lower valley, artisans embroider with one thread, and in the upper valley, two (interview, Cabanaconde, March 1993). This refers to the number of threads that simultaneously run through the sewing machine needle. Embroidering with one thread makes for a finer outline and more precise designs. It also lengthens the time to execute a motif, especially to fill in the colors. The one- versus two-thread distinction, however obsessive, is not esoteric; consumers know their thread. In both Chivay and Cabanaconde, several artisans claimed they could embroider both ways and thus appeal to more customers and maximize their sales. Others would not cross the line, preferring to stay with their own community's styles and techniques.

"Ugly" (*feo*) is what Hugo Vilcape called Chivay *bordados.* He disliked the double thread, yarn, and large motifs. Only in recent years had Cabana embroidery become clearly superior; in the past, "it was poor work, not as well filled in; it didn't have a good image. [It had] deformed animals, like in Chivay, potbellied little birds (*pajaritos panzoncitos*), a few large drawings" (interview, Cabanaconde, February 26, 1993). Although Vilcape is an accomplished artist, in maligning Chivay designs, it was not his personal work that he claimed was superior, but that of his community.

The long-standing rivalry between the towns is played out in the domain of art. In my surveys, Cabana artisans not only spoke more often than Chivayeños of art and creativity in their work, they outright ridiculed Chivay-style embroidery.[12] Artisans in Chivay, while acknowledging differences between the styles, did not seem intent on asserting aesthetic superiority. Leonardo Mejía, Rodolfo Cayo, and others concerned with the creative aspect of their work spoke more about competition with other Chivay artisans than with Cabaneños. Their criticism centered on perfectionism: using one thread and being overly concerned with the art, Cabaneños worked too slowly to keep pace with demand.

To claim that one town stands for art and the other for commerce would be simplistic, but these ideas relate closely to the structure of production and exchange inherent in Chivay's historic position as Caylloma's market town. There are three times as many artisans in Chivay as in Cabanaconde (ninety versus thirty), they are more densely concentrated in one market building, and they rely more on volume sales. Because of increased competition and the larger market share, Chivay artisans have a wider repertoire. A few Chivay market artisans also embroider Cabana hats and other garments for the Cabana women who buy there. Some, including Rodolfo Cayo, apprenticed in Cabanaconde shops.[13]

The generation of the artist influences his or her work in ways that overlap with gender. Modernity and tradition coexist, however uneasily, in the *bordados* of embroiderers of all ages who are actively working today, and who often see art and style through different lenses. As women have become more involved in the creative aspects of the work, they also champion modern aspects of *bordado* fashion.

Alejandro Cáceres of Cabanaconde is one of Caylloma's most senior embroiderers. About sixty when I interviewed him, he had almost forty years' experience. Cáceres reflected on being a pioneer in the creative development of embroidery, especially the individual, inventive aspects of design. Originality, he said, was important in drawings. "Each person makes what comes out of his/her head, drawings that occur to one; they are inventions." Although the new *bordados* seemed crowded with motifs, he nevertheless admired the innovations of the younger artists. "[T]hey used to put on few new figures; now there are more. There were always flowers, little birds, and fish; now they have practiced more" (interview, Cabanaconde, February 26, 1993). The younger artists' chance to be creative, he suggested, builds on the foundation that he and his contemporaries laid.

Many younger embroiderers, however, claim innovation began in their generation, together with the shift to individual creativity and artistic achievement. At age twenty, Edgar Vargas had just begun to embroider. The motifs themselves were much the same, he said, but a significant change was the addition of "more art" (*más arte*). "Design depends on each person, it depends on his/her creativity. Before they didn't put much into this art. Now with more art, it's more fashionable to put more" (interview, Cabanaconde, February 26, 1993).

In discussing modern qualities of recent changes, artisans closely linked design and materials. They concurred that only a few motifs changed in any given year. Colors varied constantly, however, and within the last few years a large number of new materials had become fashionable. "To modernize" (*modernizarse*) was the term Marcial Villavicencio used for recent changes. In the times of his grandmother (*abuela* also means "ancestor"), he said, design was a simple thing—one just applied braid or rickrack to the fabric. Modernizing meant applying laces and metallic braids, and drawing neater, more precise motifs (interview, Cabanaconde, February 25, 1993). Livia Sullca likewise said today's "embroidery is more modern." Her large store in Chivay sells tourist-oriented embroideries. More was modern, in her vision: "we apply more materials, we put on plenty of decorations" (interview, Chivay, February 1992).

New materials are modern, claimed many artisans: contemporary fabrics and trims are both better and more varied than those available in the past. The superior yarns and trims include merino yarn,[14] *brillas* (metallic lace), and *grecas* (braids); the fabrics include velvet, chiffon, and *poliseda* ("polysilk"). During fieldwork, I collected eighty samples of fabrics and trims, mostly from four artisan workshops, which still underrepresents the variety available. The daunting array totaled more than one hundred. The artisans' lexicon, in addition to techniques and designs, is packed with a huge vocabulary of materials.

Lightweight polyester fabric, acrylic yarn, crushed velvet, and silvery lace are now elements of traditional Caylloma clothes. Some of these materials are found exclusively in *bordados,* but most are appropriated from the domain of national Peruvian society, where they may be found in an office-worker's blouse, a housewife's sweater, or a wedding gown. Fabrics are imported from Brazil, from Colombia, and (via Chile) from Asia. Very few materials are produced by Peru's textile industry, a moribund but still important branch of national enterprise (Cárdenas et al. 1988). Arequipa's alpaca textile factories are exceptionally dynamic; to supply the international luxury fiber market, they buy up almost all of Caylloma's alpaca fiber.

All the details of *bordado* design are overwhelming. I have highlighted a few key design elements that make Caylloma *bordados* unique, and a few differences among communities and among artists that local people said were important. This is just the tip of the iceberg. For every motif and fabric I analyzed, there are at least twenty I did not.

Past and present, continuity and change, modernity and tradition, fashion and non-fashion—these vexing dualisms are not supported by my analysis of Caylloma *bordados*. Rather, the modern embroideries of Caylloma continue to prove those borders false. The designs on the garments are clearly related to other domains, including printed matter and architecture, but they do not replicate any sources. Even as designs and materials shift with trends, *bordados* as a whole continue unchanged in essence. Although a few elderly artisans were downright curmudgeonly in dismissing the newfangled designs, most were glad that younger people were continuing the *bordado* tradition. Embroiderers develop their art so that it will excel over that which went before. "Since it now has regional, national, and—why not say so?—worldwide prestige," declared Fermín Huaypuna, "I believe that [our] embroidery will endure forever" (interview, Chivay, February 1992).

Other scholars writing about textiles have pointed out the falseness inherent in the traditional-versus-modern dichotomy, but often only in terms of iconography. Airplanes and televisions on Kuna molas and helicopters and machine guns on Hmong *pandau* have been touted as icons of modernity, derided as inauthentic, and lamented as emblems of the loss of traditional culture. Cayllomino artists do not draw airplanes, but their clothes are decidedly modern: the materials themselves are emblems of modernity. Studying woven clothes (*traje*) in Tecpán, Guatemala, Carol Hendrickson observed that "it might seem that a disproportionate number of the world's fiber manufacturers aim to supply Tecpanecos. . . . The map of the world is reflected in the . . . *traje* materials used in Tecpán" (1995:44, 50). In Caylloma as well, materials and fibers arrive from global sources.

The embroidered garments themselves are landscapes, not just interpretations of other landscapes. The garments contain the artisans' knowledge of local cultural and natural phenomena. The appropriation and transformation of local, national, and foreign designs, materials, and styles are ongoing processes. Designing and wearing Caylloma clothes crosses geographic borders to create, paradoxically, uniquely local traditions. Thus the embroidered landscape of Caylloma *bordados* is not only the local, natural, observable world. It is a conceptual landscape of global proportions.

Clothing the Body as a Research Strategy

> *Fussing with the complexities of clothing must not interfere with field work. . . . Frequently, the anthropologist does well to adopt the rule of dressing inconspicuously.*
> — PERTTI J. PELTO AND GRETEL H. PELTO (1970:191–192)

Skirts, hats, fabrics, colors, designs, artists—all these facets of Caylloma *bordados* weighed on my decision to wear them. I didn't want to commission a complete ensemble all at once. To obtain a complete new set of *polleras,* I decided to collect them piece by piece.

A set of *polleras* is not built in a day. It took more than a year to complete my basic outfit, and I still lack several items. In this outfit I invested many hours in consultation with Susana Bernal and other artisans, several hundred dollars, and some of my own labor. The gradual unfolding of this process enabled me to engage in the social process of obtaining garments, observe how garments are made, participate in making them, and spread out my expenditures.

I only wore a complete set of *bordados* to dance in one fiesta and to pose for farewell photographs. Getting used to wearing *polleras* on a daily basis would have been another project, one that would have required a commitment to fitting into a local identity and letting go of my "own" identity that was greater than I wanted to make. Yet only through such experiences could I have learned many lessons about the sociality in clothes and about wearing them as a bodily act. Clothing the body proved to be a sound research strategy.

In their manual *Anthropological Research,* Pertti Pelto and Gretel Pelto admit that "very little is known about the effects of anthropologists' clothing styles on their research" (1970:190). It is seldom advisable to dress "like everyone else in the village," they caution (ibid.:191); the anthropologist should not use dress to assume an insider status that he or she has not obtained, which might seem presumptuous or condescending.

How can the anthropologist be "inconspicuous"? She is likely to differ in race, class, ethnicity, education, and/or regional or national origin from the community members. She can scarcely be inconspicuous, so why do they give this advice? Some considerations are practical: "Fieldworkers must protect themselves from cold, heat, and other physical hazards, at the same time they must be able to carry certain minimal equipment—at least a notebook and a pencil—at all times . . ." (1970:191). Explaining how dress may be misunderstood, they recommend that the anthropologist cultivate an appearance that differs from "locally disliked types of persons," such as members of dominant society, "administrators, missionaries or rich merchants . . . , [or] 'people from the government' [who] wear shiny leather boots" (ibid.).

Despite the Peltos' sensitivity to issues of power and domination, they assume that research rests on dissociation from the subjects. I suggest a different approach: rather than assume that difference must be overcome, let us agree to transgress it, to cross cultural borders. By dressing like the people in the place where one studies, one can use clothing the body as a research strategy.[15]

My decision to acquire *polleras* was not a decision to select a primary research strategy. It seemed common sense; I had to obtain the clothes to understand how the body-clothing system worked. Wearing them was only one step in the process. As it turned out, it took a long time to finish my *polleras.* I couldn't wear them for Carnival. Although Susana Bernal's messenger delivered them from Chivay to my house in Coporaque on the first day of Carnival, I lacked the proper handwoven waistbands and the knowledge to attach them. That day, I could not finish or wear the *polleras,* so I created a compromise festive outfit—my white Chivay-style straw hat, my *corpiño* over my *gringa* shirt, and my regular denim skirt—and set off to dance. I finally finished the skirts several months later.

My *polleras* made their debut the day I left Coporaque to return to the United States (Figure 21). Still shiny and creased from being folded, they felt alien on my skin. Meters of fabric swirled around my legs and, tightly pleated into the waistband, weighed on my hips. I felt my person shrink inside the voluminous layers. My *comadre* Candelaria pulled up my overskirt and tucked it into my waistband, then arranged the sleeves of the hot pink wool jacket. Once I looked presentable, we took photographs with her children and Nilda's children; my neighbor shot several poses. Arranged in this new, luxurious finery, I was pleased to stand beside my *comadre,* and the sense of home crept into the fabric around me as the cloth warmed against my skin. But once the photography session ended, I felt so self-conscious that I took off my *polleras* and put on my "real clothes." Dressed once again like an anthropologist, I packed my skirts away.

Putting on a whole new set of clothes was more than a novel experience. In fact, my *polleras* are one of the fanciest outfits I have ever owned. In the field, my dress was casual in ways that suited my lifestyle. Although I tried to take some care with my appearance, style came after warmth and comfort. The kind of work I did, the climate, and my own sense of image all combined in my chosen rural wardrobe of T-shirt, turtleneck, long johns, flannel shirt, wool sweater, down vest, parka, hiking boots, and, almost always, a long full denim skirt. In Chivay, I often wore jeans, but in the countryside, I usually found the skirt practically and ideologically preferable. It became a badge of femaleness. Several times when I was wearing jeans, strangers called me "mister" or "*gringo*" from a distance.

21 Nilda and Candelaria Bernal's children, Marisol, Dante, and Ana Condorhuilca, and Enadi Condori, with Blenda Femenías

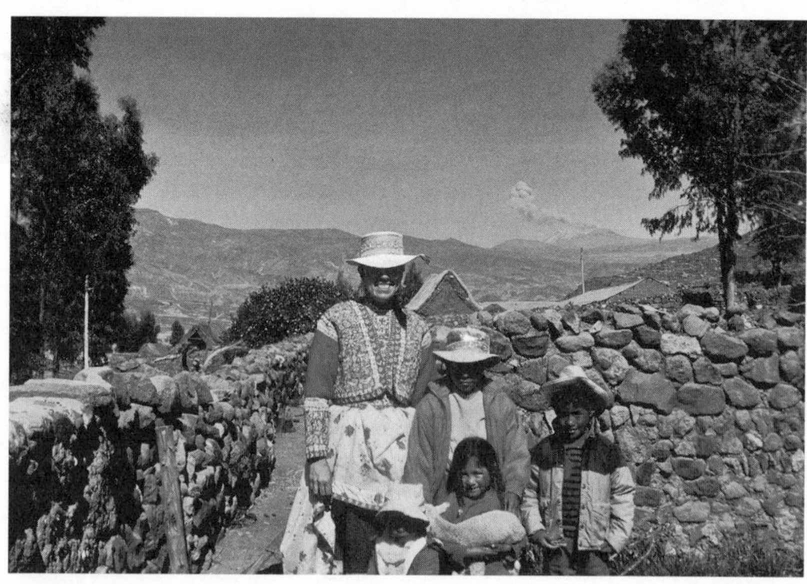

This never happened while I was wearing a skirt, and I preferred to avoid that gender confusion. The association of women with skirts, especially long full ones, connected me to indigenous women in the community and distanced me from *mestiza* women, who routinely dressed "*de vestido,*" in pants or short straight skirts. But that likeness was limited. My skirt was, in fact, like no other skirt in Coporaque and thus could not be placed in any locally familiar category.

Norma Vilcasán, daughter of Gerardo Vilcasán and Felícitas Bernal, is the fourth of their eight children. I have known the family since 1985 and often visit them in Coporaque. The sisters loved to wear *polleras* for fiestas. From age twelve, however, Norma's interest in clothes took a different path. Intrigued by other fashion currents, she and her sisters became staunch advocates of the miniskirt. One day Norma asked me why I wore "that skirt (*falda*)," pointing to my big old denim skirt. I explained several of its practical features. I could pull it up and put things in the pouch, it was comfortable, it made sitting on the ground easier, and so forth. You know, I told her, like a *pollera*.

"If it's like a *pollera,*" asked Norma, "why isn't it finished?"

"Finished?" I was puzzled.

"Why doesn't it have any embroidery?"

Embroidery, I realized, was not something extra added onto a Caylloma *pollera;* it was part of the definition of the garment. This is one reason that Caylloma women's clothes as a category are called both "*polleras*" and "*bordados.*" Norma's observation about my skirt's lack of embroidery crushed my naïve intuition that it was similar to other skirts worn in Caylloma. Substance merged with surface in ways I had ignored. In Caylloma, embroidery is substance, yet, despite my desire to see Caylloma garments "on their own terms," I had relegated it to surface.

Commissioning *polleras* helped me realize that clothing as a process, like learning culture itself, is never finished. Throughout this book I take clothing the body to be learning culture in literal as well as metaphoric terms. Thus, one task of ethnography is to cross cultural borders in another way. Metaphors about changing clothes as changing roles and culture abound in the English language: "putting on different hats," we say, "walk a mile in his shoes." We should sometimes take such phrases literally. For ethnographers, changing clothes inserts us into culture in ways that physically and mentally transform us and give us new familiarity with another way of life.

Fieldwork is cross-dressing. "Fussing with the complexities of clothing" *was* fieldwork. Far from "interfering with fieldwork," clothing in all its complexities became a central component of my methodology. I adopted "native dress" but only for specific occasions. And when I finally put on my *polleras,* I had to confront the self-consciousness that made me hurry back into my "real clothes." Clothing the body, as a set of interdependent practices, was a strategy that helped me understand all Caylloma social practices.

My body-clothing experience led to a paradox: I never felt completely at home in Caylloma clothes, but I never would have felt as much at home without them. I did become accustomed to my white Chivay-style hat, wearing it interchangeably with another straw hat from Arequipa; my embroidered hat felt too fancy. Everyone knew I was not a Chivayeña, especially me. Yet the close comfort of seeing myself dressed like others translated into feeling that others were dressed like me—the familiarity that makes us feel we belong to a group, that makes us feel at home.

Conclusion: Getting Dressed

In city and country, in festivals and cornfields, Caylloma women wear their lavish *bordados.* They devote time and energy, love and money to obtaining them. Through embroidered clothes they constitute an ethnic presence, representing themselves as members of a group—a community of practice—yet asserting distinct individual styles. Reviewing survey data and conversations, pondering why women wear *polleras,* I came to understand "the clothes of *mi pueblo*" as a literal and metaphoric reference to ethnic identity. Women put on their *polleras,* "their customs from birth," not once but hundreds of times in a lifetime. With each repetition, they affirm the importance of "changing clothes."

Because *polleras* are women's clothes, Cayllominas exemplify the intimate relationship between clothes and gendered bodies. Pride and shame, love and money, all figure into the ways women represent themselves. Moving through their daily lives, they are active subjects who choose to step forward in ethnic dress. Covered from neck to ankle with an elaborately embellished surface, women call attention to their bodies. Dressed in skirts, jackets, and hats—each having minute distinctions of design and meaning—women go about the business of "living and dying in these clothes." Dancing and parading in migrant associations, they perform a bit of Caylloma in the big city. Displaying the ultimate in festive dress, they flaunt their prosperity. But women are objectified when thus exposed to the gaze of others. Painfully conscious of their *polleras'* negative connotations and role in discrimination against them, some rural Chivayeñas choose not to dress "*de pollera,*" hoping to avoid being vilified by urbanites. For Florencia Huaracha, the gaze was unwanted; she felt *polleras* left her vulnerable to being the object of derision rather than of desire.

Embroidery is a lovely thing, most Cayllominos believe—both the women who wear them and the artists who make them. Hearing what the artists say about *bordado* aesthetics, we learn how women's right to self-representation intersects with the domain of fashion. *Pollera* fashions have cultural boundaries within which women make choices of taste, color, and materials. To understand Caylloma aesthetics, I had to recondition my tastes and "get into green," learn how to like the fresh, gaudy "*q'achu verde.*" Fashion also has monetary dimensions, and the cost of *bordados* depends on their grade or quality. But their cost includes social currency as well as money. The price of wearing *polleras* always depends on the social negotiations between consumers and artisans, workers and artists, and women and men.

Polleras are an embroidered landscape, drawn from all aspects of the cultural environments where Caylloma people live and travel. This landscape includes the garments themselves; the natural world of birds, fish, and flowers that artists see every day; and the local, national, and foreign designs, materials, and styles that Cayllominos appropriate. Situated in their landscape, the artists play out the gendered and community dynamics that relate art to ethnicity. As creative individuals, they serve as mediators between women's desires and their purses. Artists take pride in promoting women's decorative image as their product. They take equal pride in their skill and creativity in drawing each tiny, detailed motif. The elusive quality defining "art" and "artist," however, seems to be grounded in gender, as most self-identified artists are men. The exceptional case of Susana Bernal indicates, however, that gendered practices are flexible and have the potential to change.

In the fine-grained distinctions among garments from different parts of Caylloma, identity can literally hang by a thread, as both artisans and consumers enumerate the threads used to create designs. Counting threads may seem like splitting hairs, but the people of Caylloma are the ones doing the splitting. The fact that they emphasize such minutiae forces us to consider its significance. Through micro-details, artisans demonstrate their own virtuosity and actively foster pride in their own communities. Thus when discussing ethnicity, we must consider how artisans' competitive spirit, channeled through highly localized emblems, also mitigates against a more expansive collective identity. Examining the micro-distinctions in *polleras* shows how the "divide and conquer" ideology of colonialist domination impedes ethnic cohesion.

The landscape of Caylloma influences its people's actions whether they are in Caylloma or not. The clothes, like the villages, are homes to which Cayllominas can always return. Away from home, used for dancing in fiestas or to stimulate commercial transactions, *polleras* are part of women's survival strategy as they visually reinforce connections with "home." For merchants like Rosalía, the "love" that other peasant women showed her translated into good business sense. By insisting that they "have to" wear *polleras,* that they have "always" worn them, women insisted on their right to be Cayllominas.

For me, as an ethnographer, changing clothes was different. Instead of a "right," a way to claim identity, wearing *polleras* was a way to understand it. Bent on obtaining a complete ensemble of Caylloma embroidered garments, I initiated a research strategy that eventually forced me not only to envision a new concept of the physical person but to inhabit it, by assuming a physical burden. To analyze what changing into *polleras* meant, I had to consider what I was changing out of, to examine how I created and expressed my anthropologist role through my mode of dress. "Changing clothes" meant "changing identity" as a way to incorporate experience, but exploring the cultural boundaries of dress ultimately helped me be an anthropologist, not a Caylloma.

Choosing clothes is not always easy for Cayllominas because it means choosing an identity that conforms to the burden of racist stereotypes or submits to state authority, as in putting school uniforms on their daughters' bodies. But choice also helps them resist assimilation by wearing their *polleras* proudly and boldly on the streets of Arequipa. For the women of Caylloma, getting dressed means continually incorporating, considering, reclaiming, and rejecting a vast quantity of detailed information. Local connoisseurs of the Caylloma art called *bordados* become entangled in global capitalism as they partition and reassemble foreign materials into compositions meaningful to them. Getting dressed means being enmeshed in the conflicts inherent in unequal relations of power.

4

Addressing History: Representation and the Embodiment of Memory

"There Are No People, Only Indians"

In the center of Chivay, the plaza forms a perfect square. On its north side the church looms large, a quarter block wide, a full block deep. The *tambo* of Luis Salinas dominates the east side. This huge metal-roofed emporium is the commercial center of Caylloma Province. A narrow wooden balcony runs the length of its second story. From the main gate a train of llamas sallies forth, laden with sacks brimming with alpaca fiber. Each corner of the plaza boasts a stone arch. The llamas entered Chivay from the west, across the bridge that spans the Colca River. They will leave town heading east, under the arch to the road for Arequipa.

The center of the plaza holds a simple round fountain (*pileta*) of smooth hand-hewn stone. Free-wheeling commerce fills the open-air market (*feria*) around it. A woman ladles tall glasses of corn beer (*chicha*) from large ceramic vats for men in plaid homespun trousers. Here, a stack of brand-new hats tilts precariously. There, a woman haggles over the price of rubber sandals (*ujutas*).

Off to one side stand two tall men. They look aloof and out of place in stiff new hats and jackets. Beside them is a camera on a tripod. These North Americans have come to explore Chivay and to photograph this scene. The year is 1931.

I have never seen these arches, nor the *pileta,* nor the *feria,* except in the photographs and films the explorers took (Figures 22 and 23). The Shippee-Johnson Peruvian Expedition included these two men, Robert Shippee and Victor Van Keuren, as well as George Johnson and others.[1] I know their names, but not those of the other people pictured here. Today these people and places live on in the explorers' photographs (hereinafter, the "Shippee-Johnson photographs"), documents tucked away in local archives, and the memories verbalized by a few elderly Cayllominos when we talked of days gone by.

Now a more imposing fountain fills the central space. Star-shaped and crafted of cement, it boasts a chubby silver-painted cupid atop a lofty column. The *pileta,* for so many years the center of commercial activity, was modernized in the 1950s. Likewise, most buildings on the plaza were built within the last fifty years; almost all have stucco walls and metal roofs. This architectural modernization culminated in a hotel and monument built in the 1990s. The municipality owns the hotel, which has two stories and a balcony. The monument, designed by an Arequipa architect, is an imposing stone arch flanking the fountain. Although its form echoes the antique stone portals, it leads nowhere. The original arches are gone. Too narrow for trucks, they were torn down when the streets were paved. The *feria,* too, has been transformed—moved, regulated, and institutionalized. Now most commerce takes place in the market building a block from the plaza. In the street outside, traders at weekly *ferias* supplement the few regular vendors.

An air of antiquity remains in parts of the plaza. Rebuilt several times, the church was originally erected in the sixteenth century by Franciscans celebrating the advance of Christian faith.[2] The Salinas emporium has changed little since it was built in the 1910s. No longer a wool trade concern, it has housed many banks. But the clearest marker of antiquity is one

22 Vendors selling around fountain, Chivay

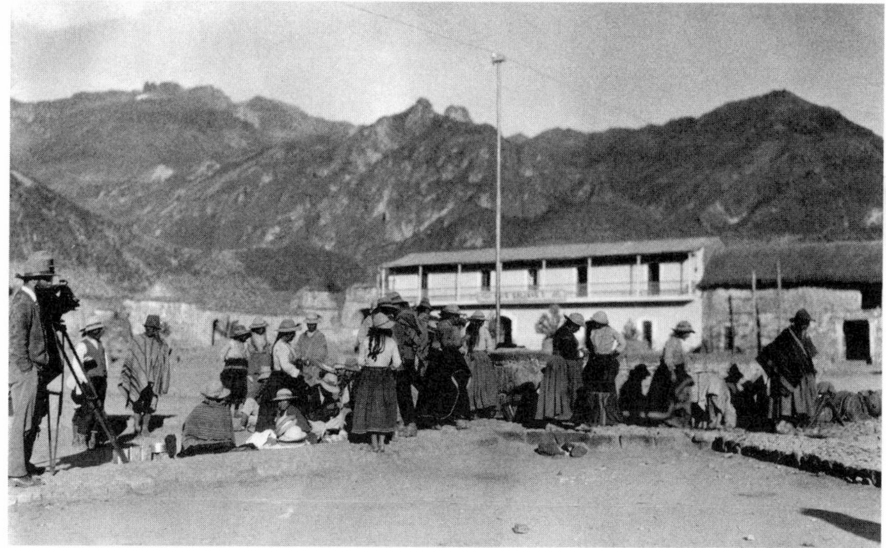

NEG./TRANSPARENCY NO. BB686 (PHOTO BY GEORGE R. JOHNSON), COURTESY THE LIBRARY, AMERICAN MUSEUM OF NATURAL HISTORY.

23 Llama train leaving Salinas emporium, Chivay

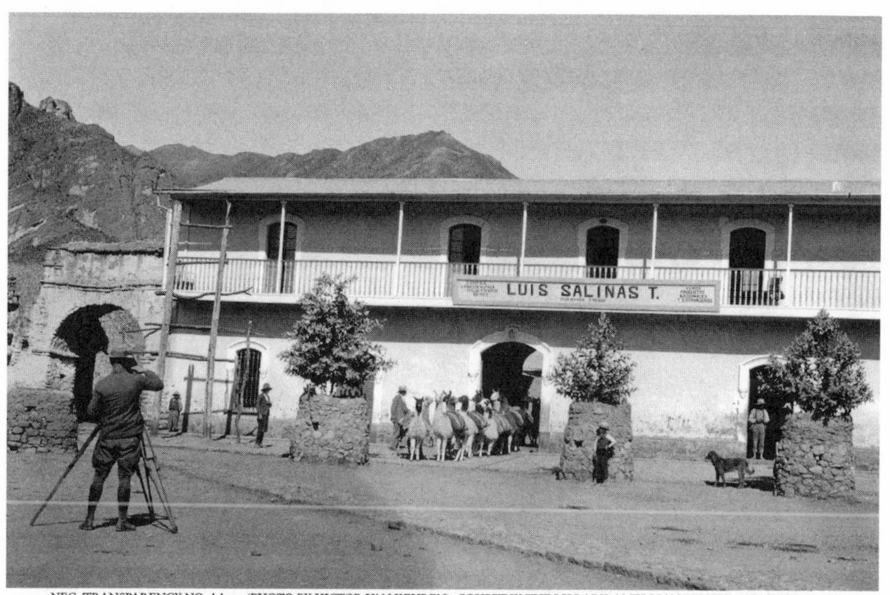

NEG./TRANSPARENCY NO. AA293 (PHOTO BY VICTOR VAN KEUREN), COURTESY THE LIBRARY, AMERICAN MUSEUM OF NATURAL HISTORY.

tiny "straw house" (*casa de paja*). The modest stone cottage with a thick thatch roof boasts a narrow front porch supported by rustic wooden posts. Few such houses, probably from the colonial period, remain in Chivay; their architectural style once dominated the entire Colca Valley. The last *casa de paja* on the plaza is owned by the senior member of the Cáceres family, a long line of merchants and landowners.

That house was my destination one sunny morning in 1993. A Peruvian anthropologist, Margarita Larico, and I went to talk with Eudumila Cáceres. The elderly Señorita Eudumila was still single and proud to be a Cáceres. A keen observer of daily life, she sat on a straight chair on her front porch, from which she surveyed the plaza. Her snow-white hair accented her regal bearing. A neat wool skirt was tucked around her knees, and as always, she wore a blouse, cardigan sweater, stockings, and low-heeled shoes. Though her clothes were good when purchased long ago, she could not afford to replace worn garments. A grande dame of Chivay's decayed society, she was preoccupied with multiple lawsuits to secure her hold on the last bits of family property. Most Cáceres of recent generations have moved away, and she followed their exploits while she secured the home front. As we began to converse, she was more interested in my *gringa* status than in Chivay, reeling off the names of her professional relatives in Arequipa and elsewhere. Surely I knew her nephew, a doctor in the United States. I tried to direct her attention to her hometown.

"Everyone has told me, Señorita, that you know more than anyone about the history of Chivay." I anticipated a rewarding interview. While viewing the Shippee-Johnson photographs, what stories would she tell about her childhood in Caylloma? What memories would surface from sixty years ago? But when we opened the album, she skimmed and quickly dismissed the photographs.

"Yes, that's the way Chivay was. But there are no people" (. . . *no hay gente*), she said disdainfully.

"Do you need a magnifying glass?" Perhaps the elderly woman's eyesight was failing, I thought. I pointed out the dozen people in a photograph of the *feria*.

"There are no people," she repeated, "only Indians, all of them."

If the "Indians" (*indígenas*) were not "people" (*gente*), who was *gente* to Eudumila? As we talked, I realized she hoped to see "gentlemen" (*caballeros*). What she and I sought in the photographs was not the same. Expecting her family or similar people, she was disappointed to see Indians, who were not, she believed, like them. Her father once was *gobernador*[3] of Chivay, and for years her uncle was mayor (*alcalde*); both had been active businessmen in the wool trade. Those men were *caballeros.* Because I hoped to learn more about every aspect of old Chivay, her narrow range of interest disappointed me.

The closer Eudumila looked, however, the more she was captured by the images of her past. She identified a few families of *gente* by their clothes and by buildings where they had lived and worked. From her ancient house, she gestured across the plaza toward a tall stone building which had been her uncle Juan's home. The arches caught her fancy too, and she pointed around the plaza to their former locations. Eudumila reminisced about the beauties and dangers of life in decades past. She brought to life the sights and sounds of a phantom Chivay, through which traders and pack trains had passed regularly. From Chuquibamba men walked for a week across high plains and through mountain passes. As they approached the town, she would hear them on the bridge. "*Chirilín, chirilín,*" tinkled the tiny llama bells; "*tolorón, tolorón,*" the larger mule bells rang.

I had limited success, however, in prompting her to say much about the people who were not "people." Their identification in the photographs was clear; one could not mistake "*gente*" for "*indígenas.*" "*Gente criolla*" and "*caballeros*" wore fine clothes, like Borsalino hats and high leather boots, purchased in Arequipa or imported from abroad. A native of Chivay, convinced of her racial and class superiority, Eudumila Cáceres refused to acknowledge any likeness to the hundreds of indigenous people wearing rough homespun clothes shown in the photographs.

Clothing, History, and Sentiment: Images and Discourses of the Past

In this chapter, clothing the body serves as a subject of history and a means to elicit history. Eudumila's memories, colored by her sense of superiority, illustrate how thoroughly status shapes perceptions of history, identity, and even who or what one sees in a photograph. Her judgments, elicited by visual representations of clothed bodies, helped me see how visual and verbal representations mingle as people construct a new past. I viewed photographs with dozens of Cayllominos, especially elderly people. Clothes prompted a disproportionate number of verbal reminiscences. Their mnemonic qualities, relating both to the objects and the processes of making and obtaining them, provided keys to understanding what the past means in the present—expressions that were often saturated with sentiment.

The history of Caylloma, moreover, is a history of cloth. It is in large part the history of *bordados,* the unique local art form thoroughly entangled with the regional and national politics of belonging. The clothes depicted in the 1931 photographs, worn by the people who were not "*gente,*" show no embroidery. No matter how much I speculate on the origin of embroidery, I cannot pinpoint the date. Nonetheless, I am confident that it was firmly established by the 1950s. Although many other traditional clothes antedate embroidery, for many Cayllominos I interviewed, today's embroidered *polleras* conjured up the past. Understanding this puzzling contradiction requires close attention to the depictions of the objects, as well as to the multiple and conflicting discourses in the interviews.

Because Cayllominos create and represent their histories through arts, the objects matter in particular ways. Garments are representations of history in and of themselves; they are heirlooms as well as mnemonic devices. After a person's death, his or her clothes usually pass to the heirs and continue to be used.[4] The fact that few embroidered garments survive several generations frustrated my efforts to document their history but also forced me to attend closely to why people endow absent objects with such importance. When I asked why women wear *polleras* today, many survey respondents referred to the past: they claimed "tradition" and/or "custom" (*tradición, costumbre*) as explanations for contemporary use. These concepts were both necessary and sufficient reasons for continuity and for innovation. In everyday conversations, *bordados* figured prominently in the stories Cayllominos frequently offered about their families: parents (*padres*), grandparents (*abuelos*), and more distant ancestors (*abuelos, antepasados*). History insistently intrudes in daily life because traditions play active roles in structuring society.

How, exactly, does the clothing experience color Cayllominos' views of the past? How does seeing women wear *bordados* influence the views of those who wear them, compared to those who do not? Why are *bordados* connected to the past? Women's bodies today, enveloped in dazzling baroque confections, have become armatures for adornment; this representation is always expressed in ethnic terms. In connecting the use of *bordados* to the past, gender assumes a large share of ethnic identification. Was this always the case? How and when did the symbolic use of women's bodies become connected with ethnicity?

I suggest that the symbolic legitimation of ethnic identity is closely tied to Cayllominos' ongoing efforts to establish, maintain, or challenge the power structure. This legitimation became more crucial each time outsiders decided to settle in Caylloma. In the twentieth century, they substantiated their claims to remain in numerous ways, and the clothes now called *bordados* came to symbolize belonging in the community. *Mestizaje* and the consolidation of patriarchal control proceeded simultaneously. Over several generations, gender and power were joined in patriarchy through intimate, personal control and through broader social control and political processes. Incorporation through clothes became increasingly important.

Cayllomino histories include experiences of violence, sexuality, poverty, work, family, and celebration—powerful experiences that generated powerful memories. Discourses were structured by age and generation through memories spanning about eighty years. Those who lived through the same times have some memories in common. Other identities and allegiances, however, shape memories as well. For elderly members of the same generation, memories of decades-old ethnic violence and gender-based conflict often remained vivid.

This chapter does not present the textbook history of presidents and coups. Perhaps because Cayllominos know how much impact national politics has on their lives, they rarely discuss it. It is the shadow and not the substance of their daily discourse. Nevertheless, power and representation emerge as central issues structuring discourses of history. Generated within Caylloma society, these discourses still involved me, the ethnographer. No matter how peripheral my presence, the people who constructed and performed these histories chose to involve me in them. They created ethnographic narratives.

My methods and sources of discourse elicitation included oral history with and without photographs, survey instruments, and conversations. Initially I expected a fairly direct link between one method and one result: oral history, for example, should produce a linear, chronological narrative. But quite the opposite occurred; oral history proved rich beyond my expectations in eliciting multiple discourses. The more I tried to direct and structure oral history interviews, the more perfunctory the responses became. The less I intervened, the more I heard other people's ideas, memories, and narratives. People talked openly about issues they cared about, even when I dared not ask. In recounting their stories, I respect their concerns and the individuality of the distinct voices they projected.

Written materials, especially documents from municipal council archives and newspaper accounts, have also been useful. Although small in quantity, the written documentation reminds us, first, that Caylloma peoples have written their own history and, second, that individual, personal stories relate to broader regional, national, and international events. Yet because I focus on historical changes that are often ignored in such sources, documents alone could not compose a solid body of evidence. Objects and oral sources provided decisive insights not contained in the written forms.

In the sections that follow, I rely once again on embroidery artisans. What role do they claim for themselves and their families in innovating and continuing *bordados*? Tradition and custom, the keys to unlocking these puzzles, are revealed in scrutiny of the ever changing fabrics as well as the embroidered decoration. The histories of family workshops reveal conflicting stories about the invention of embroidery. Finally, links between *bordados* and the radically accelerated, early-twentieth-century penetration of merchant capital prove significant.

A new ethnic economy developed as exchange relations in the 1920s and 1930s were divided along racial lines and restructured, influenced especially by arriviste *mestizos.* Through *mestizaje* and intermarriage, patriarchal control simultaneously extended over women's bodies and indigenous lands. Addressing the racial, ethnic, and gendered dimensions of patriarchy encourages us to understand Caylloma's political economy as a politics of belonging, in which an individual's status is intimately connected to his or her ostensible place of origin. Contemporary Cayllominos' ideas about the past are expressed through objects construed as ancient. *Bordados,* even with their new techniques, materials, and designs, have increasingly come to stand for old times and old ways.

Cayllominos' discussions of tradition and custom were full of sentiment, but not prettified. The commemoration of struggle and resistance is part of Caylloma's tradition as well. *Bordados,* the pretty clothes with an ugly past, are contemporary representations of tradition and custom that reflect on conflict-ridden times. The embodiment of memory in women and their dress uneasily expresses, but never resolves, history.

Contested Histories of Embroidery

Who Invented Embroidery?

> *Since I was little, my father was always embroidering. He was the first. Emilio Tejada Riveros was his name. He traveled all over the province with his machine, embroidering for people.*
> — JUAN TEJADA
> (Interview, Cabanaconde, February 26, 1993)

> *I was the first. The first works I made were for my wife. When I had just begun [to embroider], the women liked it and it became a custom.* — MELITÓN PICHA
> (Interview, Cabanaconde, February 25, 1993)

Floral embroidery on *polleras,* most people agreed, dates only to the last few decades. Its very novelty, I reasoned, should facilitate learning when and how it originated. I expected only a few people to claim its origin for their own, but instead, many artisans did so. Both Tejada and Picha, for example, claimed that he or his family invented the art. Why did so many people think embroidery was important enough to claim?

Thousands of times, I asked why women wear *polleras.* One reply was standard: "It's just custom" (*Será pe [pues] costumbre*). Frustrated, I pressed on. What were clothes like in the old days? Who wore skirts like those in this photograph? Did your parents or grandparents work in embroidery? Who are the oldest people living today who know about early embroidery? Who invented embroidery?

My goal was to give credit where credit was due. By finding an inventor, I could rescue him or her from obscurity; an anonymous "craftsman" would become a named "artist."[5] This identification would help me show that embroidery was a vital economic and symbolic activity. Tracing the trajectory of the art would establish how traditions change in Caylloma. Should I discover that embroidery originated outside the province, I could explore indigenous agency, demonstrating how Cayllominos had creatively incorporated "foreign" designs, techniques, and materials in their clothes.

On one hand, I was too successful in locating the inventor. Too many people claimed that identity—for self, family, or community. Complete consensus about "the" inventor could hardly be expected among more than one hundred artisans, much less among thousands of other Caylłominos. On the other hand, I failed to identify a single, or even two or three possible, inventor(s). But another avenue of success was that new questions resulted about invention and the concepts of history embodied in the garments. I was right to ask who invented embroidery, but I was wrong to expect one answer. People spoke about invention in terms of both continuity and change: permanence, antiquity, and heritage, as well as modifications in art, technology, and business. Women wear *bordados* today, people claimed, because their mothers and grandmothers did: *polleras* are what came to us from the past. Nevertheless, when old people looked at the 1931 photographs, they usually acknowledged change. *Polleras,* then, were both the same as and different than before, a relic and a novelty. If the actual garments have changed, why are *polleras* associated with the past?

People expressed the identity of the inventor(s) in terms of family, gender, origins, and place. Most of the supposed inventors are deceased. Custom and tradition are associated with time as embodied in the ancestors, long-dead family members. As relics, *bordados* were heirlooms from personal, family-centered, and community-centered "pasts" more than from "the past." The bitter flavor of nostalgia seasoned Cayllominos' discourses of loss, as they sighed over what they had possessed in their pasts but had no more. Loss of land, power, and autonomy, and rupture of emotional connection to family, community, and home were all expressed through dress.

"The Only Thing We Have from Our Ancestors"

> [Polleras *are] the only thing [we have] from our ancestors; [they are] tradition (* lo único de nuestros antepasados, . . . la tradición*).* — FRANCISCA VALERO
> (Interview, Chivay, March 1992)

In linking *polleras* as a legacy of the "ancestors" (*abuelos* or *antepasados*) with tradition, Francisca Valero expressed a common Caylломino sentiment. Wenceslao Cacya, another Chivay market artisan-vendor, called *polleras* "the clothes that the ancestors left us as a relic (*reliquia*)" (interview, Chivay, March 1992). Valero stated that *polleras* are "the only thing" left. Who are the "ancestors"? Why did they leave clothes?

Susana Bernal explained in more detail why women today wear distinctive clothes. "It is the custom from before, of my mother. There were no pants or skirts, [there was] just what they could sew. It has been that way since the Inkas. I have never seen anything else." *Polleras* characterize both the experience of Susana's lifetime ("never anything else") and greater age, marked in two ways: the immediate past, marked by her mother, and the distant past, by the Inkas. By "just what they could sew," she implied that in her mother's generation, clothes were homemade. People were self-sufficient, not dependent on purchased or imported garments, and they valued local artisanry and skill. Although Susana was the only artisan who mentioned the Inkas specifically in conjunction with *polleras,* in other contexts, people used Inkas synonymously with *abuelos* and *antepasados* to refer to those who lived before personal memory.

For others as well, "mother" connected contemporary use to the immediate past. *Bordados* were a mnemonic device to access childhood memories of the way one's mother dressed or to retrieve stories heard in childhood about earlier events. Rosalvina Cayo, who trims hats in Chivay market, said *bordados* were "the custom of our grandparents" (*costumbre de nuestros abuelos;* interview, Chivay, March 1992). She first stated that embroidery originated when she was a child, then revised her statement, saying it was even earlier. "When my mother got married, she bought a straw hat and embroidered clothes. This was luxurious; all the people looked at her." Rosalvina probably does not remember her mother's wedding in the 1960s.[6] Rather, the mental image that her mother married dressed in the latest style conveyed a sense of pride that her mother could afford "luxury," for Rosalvina's family is far from wealthy.

Parents, grandparents, custom, and place were all tightly interwoven. Felipe Surco, Chivay's principal hatmaker, called wearing *polleras* "the custom of our land of Chivay, of our grandparents" (*costumbre de nuestra tierra de Chivay, de los abuelos;* interview, Chivay, March 1992). His perspective draws on forty years spent creating and trimming Caylloma-style white hats. Embroidery artisan Margarita Sullca maintained that *bordados* are "typical dress (*vestimenta típica*) since my birth, of my people-and/or-village (*pueblo*) . . . [and] the custom of my parents (*costumbre de mis padres*)" (interview, Chivay, March 1992). Now nearly sixty, she has been embroidering for forty years. "The custom of my parents" has literal meaning for her: her father, Tiburcio Sullca, played a pioneering role in embroidery in the 1930s.

"Custom," *costumbre,* at first seemed an empty umbrella term. I was tempted to dismiss it, but it would be a serious error to do so. "*Será pe costumbre*" could be a verbal shrug: "that's the way it is." As people mentioned "custom" again and again, I heard different meanings in the term. Cayllominos used *costumbre* to acknowledge that changes have occurred, to explain them articulately in precise terms, and to point out exactly where they lay. Custom did not mean cultural inertia, an unquestioned continuance from the past, or the absence of change. Because some aspects of *bordados* changed while others did not, Cayllominos could use *bordados* to link past and present.

Rough Stuffs and Fine Fabrics: Changes in Materials and Meanings

"The ancient people put on rough things; now [the material is] fine," said hatmaker Felipe Surco. A significant component of general discourses about *bordados*' past and present features was materials. Only a few fabrics from pre-embroidery days are still used today. Most current materials are not produced locally; many are imported and synthetic. Surco was not alone in contrasting fine and rough stuffs. But despite new materials' alluring flash and dazzle, some artisans dislike them and claim the old fabrics were superior. Older people, less enthusiastic about changes overall, praised specific, long-gone fabrics that younger artisans have never used.

My discussion of fabric, the foundation for embroidery, provides a basis to examine further the overall processes of change in the clothes. These involve increasing commercialization and, paradoxically, "traditionalization," my term for changing attitudes that make new styles of clothes become traditional. Old *polleras* are rare. The following identification of old clothes and fabrics is based primarily on the Shippee-Johnson photographs (1931), as discussed by older people. Among the clearly visible "*gente*" and "*indígenas*," some individuals appear in more than one image. Most Cayllominos had no difficulty determining what fabrics were represented or what kind of people used them.

Among the more than one hundred different materials, *bayeta* and *tela* are particularly significant fabrics. *Bayeta* is a rough wool fabric, and *tela,* the most common Spanish term for "cloth," is everything *bayeta* is not. The differences between them epitomize the changes in Caylloma clothing materials. Sometimes when I asked "what kind of *tela* is this?" I was told "that is not *tela;* it is *bayeta*." *Bayeta,* then, is not one kind of *tela;* the two fabrics are distinct.

In a posed group portrait taken in Lari, thirty-two men stand in straight rows, staring at the camera (Figure 24). Most of them are similarly attired in rustic-looking clothing: pants, vests, and jackets of *bayeta* or another woolen, *jerga*. These fabrics are sometimes patterned, and the garments are often elaborately patched but not otherwise embellished. Such garments were locally made, either at home or by tailors, or traded by artisans from higher altitudes. A few men wear suits of another, smoother, cloth, with neatly tailored jackets. Everyone who saw this photograph attributed class and ethnic differences to the clothes worn, partly conveyed by the fabrics.

Women's clothes also were often made of *bayeta*. In another Shippee-Johnson photograph from Lari, a large group of women is seated around the explorers' airplane (Figure 25). Many people named *bayeta* and *jerga* as the standard fabrics for the women's skirts, jackets, and vests, and even some children's clothes. The photographs also show how sparsely decorated *polleras* were. Skirts had several narrow rows of applied trims (*cintas*) or rickrack (*trencilla*) along the hem; jackets had rickrack borders.

No single term suffices to translate "*bayeta*."[7] A rough imperfect cloth, *bayeta* is typically handwoven in plain weave of handspun sheep wool yarn. In Peru, alpaca fiber may be blended with sheep wool (Markowitz 1992: 91). *Bayeta* has been in continuous use in South America since early colo-

24 Men of Lari

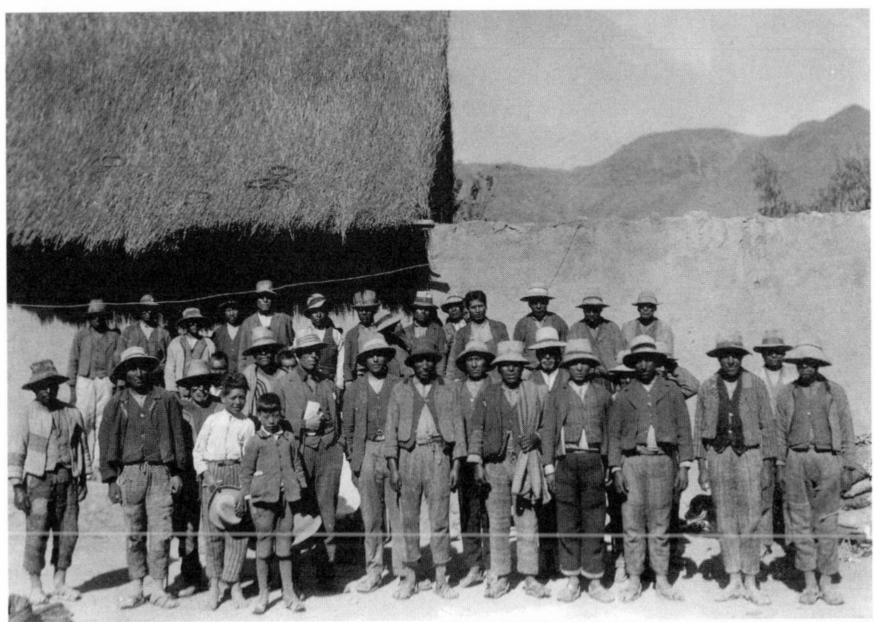

NEG./TRANSPARENCY NO. BB82 (PHOTO BY VICTOR VAN KEUREN), COURTESY THE LIBRARY, AMERICAN MUSEUM OF NATURAL HISTORY.

nial times, when fabric and sheep were imported from Spain. Once sheepherding was established in the Andes, tremendous fabric manufacture ensued made in *obrajes* (weaving workshops that used forced labor), and vast amounts of plain, rough, colonial American stuff replaced imports (Jacobsen 1993:35; Orlove 1977:29–30). Today, every woman who wears *polleras* has at least one made of *bayeta*. The heavy wool is practical for winter. "*Abriga más*," it keeps you warmer, everyone asserted. *Bayeta*'s durability suits it for agricultural and pastoral labors. Because it is cheap, it connotes poverty. It also connotes tradition through age. Older women tend to wear *bayeta polleras* more often than younger women.

"*Jerga*" is woven in small check or stripe patterns, in plain weave or twill. Jerónimo Huayapa, an elderly Chivay vendor, identified *jerga* in several Shippee-Johnson photographs. *Jerga* and other *bayeta*-related fabrics were once common, especially in men's clothes, but now are seldom used.[8] They are almost never seen in women's garments. No Cayllominos I knew wore them. On rare occasions in Chivay I saw older men wearing patterned

25 WOMEN SEATED AROUND AIRPLANE, LARI

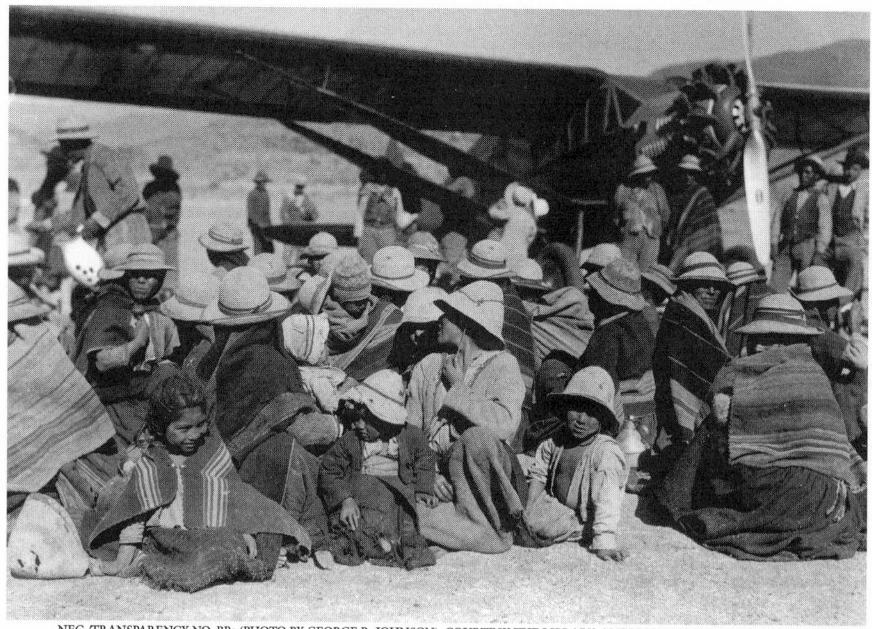

NEG./TRANSPARENCY NO. BB1 (PHOTO BY GEORGE R. JOHNSON), COURTESY THE LIBRARY, AMERICAN MUSEUM OF NATURAL HISTORY.

wool pants; my friends explained that they hailed from higher-altitude communities.

Handwoven woolen cloths are made on two-harness floor looms (de Romaña, Blassi, and Blassi 1987:160, photograph) resembling those introducted by the Spanish in the sixteenth century. Rare in the central Colca Valley, perhaps five such looms exist in Chivay. The cumbersome apparatus, about six feet high and wide, requires a large, permanent location. *Bayeta* is commonly manufactured at home in the higher-altitude pastoral zones around Callalli and Sibayo. Huge quantities are produced throughout the Peruvian highlands, especially in Puno, for national and international sale and exchange. Besides clothing, it is used for pillows and wall hangings (Orlove 1977:97–108). The low tensile strength of handspun yarn used in *bayeta* cannot withstand mechanized looms. Thus, *bayeta* remains within the "homemade" realm, although it may be obtained from commercial sources.

In Caylloma's higher-altitude communities, *bayeta* garments are common again, having been recently revived. For example, men's clothes of white *bayeta* became popular in the late 1980s among activist herders. Lisa Markowitz, an anthropologist, observed one "young man in a full suit of *bayeta* . . . at the inter-departmental herders conference in Callalli. He received many compliments on his attire, which people seemed to appreciate more as a political than fashion statement" (1992:92).

Bayeta, then, has staying power. Still in use after almost five centuries, it is even enjoying a limited renaissance. But why? It is still among the cheapest fabrics, but that is not sufficient reason. The fabric itself is older, associated with the past, with continuity. Scratchy roughness is part of its homespun charm.

Despite the appeal of *bayeta,* most *polleras* are made of "*tela,*" literally "cloth" of any kind. In Caylloma, the term is rarely used generically but almost always means commercial cloth. Today, *percala* (percale, lightweight cotton) and *poliseda* (silky polyester) are two common kinds. Seventy years ago, *tela* meant silk as often as cotton. In her youth, said Eudumila Cáceres, ladies (*señoras, damas*) wore *tela* dresses. The fine cotton or silk outfits of her grandmother and other *señoras* in the early twentieth century were quite distinct from *polleras.* When visiting Caylloma, ladies appeared in high-necked gowns more suitable for the bourgeois lifestyle of urban Arequipa. Chivay's tailors made clothes of other kinds of *tela,* such as *percala.* Old people with decades of clothing and fabric business experience mentioned several kinds that resembled those evident in the old photographs. *Telas* used in Caylloma-style women's clothes were usually cotton, including *tela asargado* and *listado,* striped fabrics, and *tocuyo,* plain or striped. In their shops, Margarita Sullca and an elderly *mestiza,* Leonor Herrera, showed me their remaining bolts of old commercial fabrics, including striped *tocuyo.*

One common *tela* was *percala,* "percale," a smooth cotton fabric, produced industrially and imported from England since the nineteenth century (Flores 1977:59–65). This fabric was formerly a marker of *mestiza* identity, as José María Arguedas noted in *Yawar Fiesta:* stores in Puquio (a fictional town) were run by "*mestizas* who dress in percale and put on straw hats" (1988 [1941]:13).

Fabrics common in the past were assembled into specific meaningful ensembles, constituting appropriate attire for ethnic groups and classes. *Bayeta,* both the fabric and the kind of clothes made of it, marked indigenous identity. *Tela* was always purchased fabric. Different types could be used in indigenous people's clothing, especially blouses and shirts; in *mestizas*' dresses; or in elites' fashionable garments, whether factory made or customized by skilled urban tailors and dressmakers.

My Grandfather Invented Embroidery

Walking down a Cabanaconde street in 1992, I struck up a conversation with Antonio Tejada, a man in his twenties. "If you're looking for embroiderers, come to my father's house," he advised. "Our family has always embroidered." His father would talk about the old days, he assured me, guiding me to the family's home workshop. Antonio's father, Juan Tejada, then in his late fifties, told me that *his* father, Emilio Tejada, invented embroidery. Emilio was a tailor and one of few people with a sewing machine. Juan was proud that his father, the pioneer, taught the art to him. Why did these men claim a place in the history of this art form? Why was embroidery a matter of pride? Why did artisans boast a genealogy that promoted their family's role? What role did gender play? Did mothers and grandmothers invent embroidery too?

In the family workshops that are the backbone of the *bordado* production system, usually two generations work in the same shop. I found no family that traced its shop back more than three generations. Each family member knows only part of his or her own workshop's history. Shops are always splintering and re-forming as children and grandchildren take over the business or, just as often, leave. In many cases, embroiderers claimed the grandparent was the founder.

Details came from interviews with another family, the Sullcas, from which I assembled a detailed workshop history from the 1930s to the 1990s. Family members have engaged in embroidery, tailoring, itinerant peddling, market sales, and keeping shop for seventy years. Tiburcio Sullca was about eighty years old when I spoke with him (interview, April 4, 1992). In Chivay, Margarita Sullca, his daughter, gave me his address in a poor neighborhood of Arequipa, assuring me that her father had been one of the earliest embroiderers; now he was retired. When I found the elderly Sullca at home, he was digging ditches to prepare for the installation of city water pipes. He took a break to speak with me and view the Shippee-Johnson photographs. Although his hearing was poor and his voice sometimes barely rose above a whisper, Tiburcio's sharp eyesight picked out many details and his clear memory evoked the ambiance of art and commerce in Caylloma.

In 1932, Tiburcio Sullca left his home in Sicuani, Cusco, and headed to Chivay. Sullca was already married to Margarita's mother. Initially a traveling vendor, he settled down with a regular post when the new municipal market building opened in Chivay. This founder of the market was also a tailor of local-style clothes and an embroiderer. Sullca dealt in coca, sundries (*chiflería*), and clothes: vests, shirts, and hats for indigenous people and poor *mestizos,* as well as cheap *bayeta* pants. The hats came from Juliaca and Huancané in Puno (near Bolivia). When he traveled there himself, he brought back clothes, hats, shoes, and sandals that he bought "wholesale" in lots of a dozen. To reach the *altiplano* towns, he walked for many hours, or rode a mule if lucky, leaving the Colca Valley through a high pass and heading southeast across the *puna.* At Sumbay, a tiny outpost, he caught the train from Arequipa and rode overnight to Juliaca, where he made his purchases and then retraced his route to Chivay. Sullca often stayed in Chivay and bought from traders like himself or from larger merchants who brought goods for sale or exchange; other times he descended the valley westward as far as Madrigal, a full day's walk. "Selling, selling we went from town to town" (*Vendiendo, vendiendo íbamos de pueblos a pueblos* [*sic*]). Itinerant peddlers were the primary agents bringing goods to villages in the valley and highlands. Some traveled in the large llama caravans Eudumila Cáceres remembered; others walked with mules.

There were also petty vendors who came down from high mountain hamlets and *estancias* (ranches), selling or trading sheep and alpacas—live and as meat, and as fleeces and woven goods—for commercial goods to take back.[9] Dionisia Huanqui, a former herder who traded wool, remembered traveling once or twice a year. In her seventies when I interviewed her, she told how she and her husband descended from their high-altitude *estancia* to the closest village, Madrigal. They walked all the next day, from 4 A.M. to 4 P.M., leading mules forty kilometers to Chivay (interview, Arequipa, April 1992).

Tiburcio Sullca also explained changes in clothes and the invention of embroidery. "I'm a tailor (*costurero*).[10] . . . I knew how to sew for men as well—for men, women, I knew how to do it all. . . . We cut and sewed, right from the cloth. We bought it by the piece in Arequipa and we cut them out," he said, pointing to men's striped vests (*chalecos*) in the Shippee-Johnson photographs. In the 1930s, tailors made *tela* and *bayeta* garments in Chivay on the newly available sewing machines: "We cut them out, *polleras, corpiños,* we sewed everything. We also bought *bayeta;* we embroidered that, but [at first] we just cut *tela* to adorn it and afterward applied those bands to the *pollera,* to the jacket."

"Were there no *bordados* then?" I asked, trying to establish a chronology.

"No, before there was little embroidery, now they are bigger," he maintained. He did not recall the date this "little embroidery" was done except in relationship to his daughter's age (then about fifty).

"She was a girl," he replied, "a baby (*wawa*), when they began to embroider." Thus he indicated that embroidery began in the 1940s.

The bands and trims applied to clothes in the Shippee-Johnson photographs (see Figures 22 and 25) were sometimes narrow handwoven strips. Similar bands, generically called *cinta* (Spanish, "band" or "ribbon") or *watu* (Quechua), are still woven today as hatbands, waistbands for *polleras,* or exercises for beginning weavers. Other *cintas* and rickrack were purchased commercial trims.

Sullca stayed in business for over forty years, keeping his Chivay market post and training Margarita to embroider. In the 1960s, at age thirteen, she told me, she began helping her parents in the market and embroidering on a hand-cranked sewing machine. When her father retired, she stayed with his market post. Margarita married Cecilio Huaraya, from a similar background in Chivay. His parents were vendors of food and drink around the fountain in the plaza. Today, Margarita is rarely absent from her father's former stand; even if only for an hour, she prefers to go every day. She mostly sells embroideries, supplemented by a few "*de vestido*"–style garments. Sometimes she sews in the market, but she also has a store, about five blocks away, where her teenage son, Ramón Huaraya, and a paid employee usually embroider. In the early 1990s, besides working in the business, Ramón was finishing high school. Her daughter, in her twenties, was studying in Lima. Margarita and her husband also own and cultivate fields in Chivay, which largely keeps them at home. Margarita does go to Arequipa once or twice a month for materials and to regional fairs to sell. She and Cecilio occasionally visit their daughter, but usually the daughter sends them materials for *bordados* and other goods to sell in Chivay. Margarita contemplated changing to something less laborious because this line "is a lot of work. We don't earn much. It takes a lot of thought; you need a good head for it." But she was philosophical about continuing: "It's my work (*trabajo*); I just have to keep at it (. . . *tengo que seguir no más*)."

Family connections over time and diversification among clothing-related activities typified Chivay market artisans. Alejandro Cabana is probably the oldest embroiderer still working. Nearly eighty in 1992, he had worked at *bordados* for about forty-five years. With his wife, Florencia Huaracha, he had also maintained a Chivay market stand for more than thirty years. Their daughter, Lucrecia Cabana, began working in the market as a teenager. Even though in poor health, Alejandro still opens the stand and sews there occasionally. Florencia works there more often, but she prefers staying home to sitting in the chilly market. Lucrecia and her husband, Wenceslao Cacya, run a clothing stand near her parents' stand. Stocking only a few *bordados,* they specialize in hats and "*ropa corriente*" (industrially produced clothing) for women who dress *de vestido.* She sometimes helps with her parents' stand.

Opening or closing market stands and moving the business into the home depend on the economy and family circumstances. Bernardo Supo, another Chivay artisan claiming that a relative (his father-in-law) was an originator of embroidery, stressed changes since the early days. Born in the 1920s, Supo entered the embroidery business later than Sullca and Cabana. In the 1930s, after his father died, seven-year-old Bernardo left his Caylloma hometown, Canocota, to live in Arequipa with relatives. Shortly after he settled in Chivay in the 1950s, he met Viviana Casaperalta, who worked in her father's workshop. After they married, Bernardo joined the shop and learned to embroider from her. The shop expanded steadily, and, after her father's death, they became sole proprietors. The huge influx of money in the 1970s from the MACON project benefited embroiderers. The Supos parlayed work, skill, and luck into the largest shop in Caylloma, with ten sewing machines and a staff of twenty-three, including five family members and eighteen paid employees. Twenty years later, it had shrunk considerably. Between their home workshop and market kiosk they have only three employees and do not open the kiosk every day. Supo also diversified beyond *bordados;* he operates the only pool hall in Chivay (interview, Chivay, March 1992).

From these and other, more fragmentary, narratives, a history of *bordados* emerges. Five decades ago, only small amounts of trim, purchased or handwoven, were applied to garments by hand and later, with hand-cranked sewing machines. Several people began to experiment with machine embroidery, facilitated by new treadle machines that left both hands free to control the fabric. Gradually *bordados* supplanted the other trims. At first the artisans embroidered on bands before sewing them onto garments. Now they apply plain bands to the garment during construction, and later embroider through all the layers.

The general trajectory, however, still leaves the question unanswered: Who invented embroidery? One common opinion was that the inventors of embroidery are deceased; another that only a few originators survive. Juan Tejada's father and Viviana Casaperalta's father have long since passed on. In Chivay, Tiburcio Sullca and Alejandro Cabana were among the living pioneers. Of the Cabaneño artisans I interviewed, Melitón Picha claimed to be the first, but he is only about sixty; Alejandro Cáceres, also about sixty, had been embroidering for forty years and had taught many others, including his wife.

The workshop histories seem contradictory, since more than one person claims that he or she, a parent, or a grandparent is the inventor of embroidery. But the contradictions mask pronounced similarities among the claims. The contested histories compete within a common realm of cultural knowledge. The artisans share the belief that embroidery is an important creative domain. As "inventors," artisans simultaneously represent themselves as important, praise their families as cultural innovators, downplay the role of other families, and privilege the creativity of their native land. "Invention," however, did not necessarily mean "making up something totally new." Melitón Picha, who still embroiders, said he learned the designs from a book. Hugo Vilcape, well known for embroidered hats, believed the designs derived from the resplendent costume of bullfighters. Even those who did not claim familial ties to the originator said he was from their hometown, sometimes outside the valley. Jerónimo Huayapa, in his eighties, sells plastic wares and herbal remedies in Chivay market. Originally from Puno, Huayapa believed embroidery originated there: "I think they brought embroidery from Puno. . . . [They did it] by hand, with rickrack, with braid" (interview, Chivay, April 1992). Long-standing inter-village rivalry enters into the origins debate as Chivayeños and Cabaneños compete over their status as home of the best *bordados* today and also of its inventors in the past.

One would have to accept a single narrative, take the artisan's self-evaluation at face value, and privilege the importance of one shop if one were to identify "*the* inventor of embroidery." But that would be a mistake. Few today are of an age to recall clearly the origins of embroidery two generations ago. Moreover, origins are conceptually associated with the time before memory. People do not, cannot, or will not recall a time when women did not wear *bordados.* Rosalvina Cayo's comment, for example, does not encompass a time when *bordados* did not exist, "when I was a child, and before." Embroidery becomes eternal: it seems to have existed forever. Without personal experience, it could never have been any different and so, therefore, how could anyone have invented it? The ancestors must be the inventors—those who went before, those who are known indirectly. Clothes become emblems of desire for permanence, for remaining in one place, and for association with that place—emblems of family and community, of history and home.

Doing Business in Caylloma: *Mistis,* Merchants, and the Context of Clothing Production

Tiburcio Sullca and Jerónimo Huayapa responded to developments in the southern highland region, as did other traders who went there from other parts of Peru. Before *bordados,* an active trade in clothing, textiles, and fiber locked Caylloma into national and international political economy. By the late nineteenth century, the "wool trade" or simply "wool" (*negocio* or *comercio de lana,* sometimes shortened to *lana* or *lanas*) centered on alpaca, primarily extracted by European neocolonial enterprises (Burga and Reátegui 1981; Femenías 2000b; Flores 1977). From the 1890s through the 1950s, *lana* dominated Caylloma's economy. The consolidation and subsequent decline of *lana* coincided with the rise of *bordados.* Gendered and ethnic relations played vital roles in developing the wool trade; their changing constitution contributed to the growth of embroidery as business and as art.

The most prominent family name in the Caylloma wool trade was Salinas, followed by Cáceres and Prado. All three operated large stores on Chivay plaza. For almost half a century, from the 1910s through the 1950s, the Salinas concern was the largest business in Caylloma. As brokers for the large Arequipa commercial firms, especially the Anglo-Peruvian Ricketts and Gibson "houses," the Caylloma merchants obtained wool from the herders through a complex network of small-scale traders (Burga and Reátegui 1981; Flores 1977). In turn, they brought in "national and foreign products," as a sign on Salinas's store proclaimed (see Figure 23).

The differences between the players were drawn in racial terms, especially whites against Indians. Some Caylloma elites proudly claimed indigenous lineage. Others emphasized descent from Spanish conquistadors who settled in Caylloma more than three hundred years before. Those *mestizos* were so well entrenched that they considered themselves natives—Cayllominos but not Indians. The arriviste *mistis* wrested power from both groups. The top traders and agents of wool houses were men, who negotiated primarily with other men to buy wool. Although concentrated in local petty commerce, women were hardly confined to that sphere, and expanding trade created new social and economic opportunities.

Manuel Salinas, in his eighties when I showed him the Shippee-Johnson photographs, explained that his family entered the wool trade in the teens. To work with his uncle Luis Salinas, fifteen-year-old Manuel moved to Chivay from Arequipa in the 1920s. Chivay was his home base for sixty years of commercial activity. He remained there after retiring in the 1980s but increased the time spent in Arequipa. Two interviews, one at his home in Chivay and one at his son's home in Arequipa, illuminated the trade's racial and class dimensions.

> It was unusual for white people to spend time here because in that time [the 1920s] there was the Tahuantinsuyo. . . .[11] [T]he villagers believed that the whites came to take away their lands . . . in those times, but it wasn't like that. Of course there were some, how do you say, exploiters, who liked to seize the best. . . . They threw out the poor Indians. But when we came, it was different, it was just the wool business here. . . . The people here didn't want us, they

> wanted to throw us out. . . . Two or three leaders (*principales*) got their godsons drunk and made them insult us in the plaza, shouting at us: "Get out, foreigners! We're going to throw you out, [back] to your land." I always remember that they did that to us, but later we arrested those men and we said to them, "Why then? If we're not exploiting you here. Look, we're just doing our business." We were giving them some competition. (Interview, Chivay, April 1992)

Salinas's disclaimer, "it was just the wool business," fails to distract us: the trade clearly generated conflicts. Commerce was not a matter of amicable business dealings. During the 1920s, commerce, politics, and ethnicity were tightly bound together. As new traders made their way into Caylloma, many "exploiters . . . liked to seize the best [and] . . . threw out the poor Indians (*pobre indígenas*)." Established merchants, loath to share "their" wool market, set their henchmen against the foreign interlopers (*forasteros*). Within a few years, Manuel related, his uncle was the main player in the wool business, with many "godsons" of his own. Luis became mayor of Chivay, and he jailed those who opposed him.

Manuel was careful to distinguish between his family and the "exploiters." Most others, however, questioned the ethics of all the *misti* families' tactics. Besides consumer goods, including sewing machines and commercial fabrics, the stores sold substantial quantities of alcohol.[12] In July 1931, Luis Salinas hosted the Shippee-Johnson Peruvian Expedition in his "combined hostelry and *bodega* (wine shop) . . . , [serving] bottled beer . . . [brought] from Arequipa on muleback," Robert Shippee reported (1934:111). The emporium not only extended loans and credit, it served as a casino. Jerónimo Huayapa fondly recalled gambling "with the masters (*dueños*) of the house. . . . I liked to play poker, casino, any old game. . . . I knew those *señores*. They were the main men who bought wool. Luis Salinas, José Salinas, and the Cáceres, I conversed with all those *gente* . . ." (interview, Chivay, 1992). Obtaining credit for goods or gambling, of course, indebted the local consumers. The merchants also bought land cheaply and, as government officials, levied fines for minor infractions, requiring land as payment in lieu of cash. These practices crossed into usury, extortion, and violent coercion. Felipe Surco called the Salinas *gamonales* (abusive landowners/bosses) who cheated his father out of the family's land. In many quarters, the Salinas clan was roundly hated.

During the 1920s, communities fought expropriation of their lands with widespread uprisings throughout the southern highlands. Although concentrated in Puno, numerous incidents occurred in the provinces of Cusco and Arequipa. Severe local and state reprisals quashed the outbreaks. Concurrently, shifting local commercial interests occasioned less violent manipulations of Caylloma's political climate.

In 1932, Chivay became the capital of Caylloma Province. This was Luis Salinas's major coup as mayor of Chivay. The former capital, the town of Caylloma, was a mining center. The shift, after more than ten years of campaigning (Manrique 1985:211–212), considerably increased the mayor's political power, which Luis parlayed into increased commercial clout. The new market was his next major project. The modern market building was constructed on an abandoned lot adjacent to the plaza (Jerónimo Huayapa, interview, Chivay, 1992). By the mid-1930s, as the economy began to pull out of the Depression, the new cement structure was in place in the new capital.

Precisely at this time, the young Tiburcio Sullca settled in Chivay. He and his fellow vendors opened the market. "[J]ust us *negociantes* (traders) . . . , we are the founders," he told me proudly. They came from the southern departments of Puno, Apurímac, and Cusco. The new building and new municipal controls radically transformed the marketing system. All petty vendors, many of them women, were evicted from the area around the fountain and forced to rent a space inside the building; uncooperative vendors were fined or denied the chance to do business at all. As the municipality of Chivay and Mayor Salinas tightened control over the space of exchange, they displaced the established trade in wool fiber, cloth, food, and drink but did not initially diminish it. More stores opened in Chivay, often stocked and capitalized by Salinas.

By the late 1930s, Sullca and others from his generation of itinerant traders had solidified into an urbanized stratum of petty merchants, becoming the core of Chivay society. They were neither "*gente blanca,*" since the *misti* wool merchants' ranks were racially and economically closed, nor "*pobre indígenas*" (poor Indians). As middlemen and godsons of the *misti* merchants, they climbed to *mestizo* status, but they remained less white, less prosperous, and far less powerful than the abusive *mistis.*

As the merchant capitalist economy was established in Caylloma Province, power shifted from the town of Caylloma to Chivay. The concomitant shift in relations of consumption and production toward purveying consumer goods, including cloth and clothing, took physical form as the market building. As commercialization concentrated in the new provincial capital, public and private spaces were transformed. Public space, formerly dominated by the plaza, was altered when the market was established. *Ferias* were no longer the primary grounds for commerce and socializing. Exchange space became more private as it moved out of the public eye, and more public as it was drawn into civil society and under city control. Women who played primary roles in local exchange of goods and services were now pulled into the cash economy, paying mandatory fees to the market administration. *Mestizas* also became established in the stores around the market.

Other markers, smaller and less durable than a building, also reveal commercial shifts. Clothes are paramount among them. The wool trade's long chain of middlemen and middlewomen benefited unevenly from the capitalist relations that engaged and exploited them. Almost all alpaca fiber and about half the sheep wool was exported. But as wool went out, other goods came in. Although lack of good fiber arrested artisanal production of woolen goods, *bordados*' development was stimulated by the many new types of *tela,* both national and imported, that became available.[13]

Perhaps most crucial for *bordados,* sewing machines and other tailors' tools reached Caylloma. Around 1910 traders began to bring machines from Arequipa, both imported brands, such as Singer, and national ones, including Carsa. Salinas and other merchants sold them, often on credit. I interviewed Leonor Herrera, an elderly *mestiza* lady and a *comadre* of Manuel Salinas, in her store on a narrow street off Chivay plaza (June 25, 1992). Although she does little business, she resolutely opens shop almost daily. Leonor explained how people used to finance machines with credit. With a down payment (*cuota*) of 150 soles, the buyer signed a contract (*letra de caja*) obligating him/her to increasing payments over three months, 60, 90, and 120 soles. The costly machine became a symbol of prosperity and modernity; paradoxically, as it provided the means for a new livelihood, it simultaneously bound the artisan into a cycle of debt.

New types of artisans, like Tiburcio Sullca, appeared with the new structure of commerce. Men like Emilio Tejada traveled with their sewing machines, tailoring, mending, and embroidering on demand. Domestic production of cloth declined significantly. Even women who made their families' clothes now depended on merchants for cloth and equipment, and increasingly on "*costureros,*" tailors of local-style clothes, like Sullca. By the 1940s, some women and men were skilled producers of the new *bordados.*

As their experiments found favor among local consumers, novelty became customary. Small family workshops gradually became permanent features.

Manuel Salinas carved out his own niche in Chivay's commercial scene. When he opened the store on the plaza, opposite the market, various branches of his family owned almost half the property on the plaza. The commercial and social interests of the largest families joined when Manuel married into the Cáceres family. He never became mayor, but as director of the Department of Public Works and Charity (Beneficencia), he upgraded the bridge over the Colca River, thereby improving transportation.

Around midcentury, Caylloma was even more closely linked to Arequipa by the Madrigal mine and new and improved roads (Chapter 2). The wool trade's golden age was 1935–1950, according to Manrique (1985: 212). In the 1950s, *lana* transformed drastically while the Arequipa textile industry restructured and modernized. Another upgraded road between Arequipa and Callalli bypassed Chivay, improving links between factories and herders. But the merchants adapted, said Manuel Salinas, and wool remained a good business until about 1960.

By then, the *bordado* business had taken off. Ornamented trim was common, but designs were less elaborate than today. Marcial Villavicencio called it "*una cosa sencilla*" (a simple thing; interview, February 25, 1992). Perhaps it resembled embroidery called *de segunda* and *de tercera* today, with widely spaced figures in one or two colors. (I located no clear photographs of *bordados* for this period.) The most lavish embroidery, recalled many artisans, was produced in the seventies, "MACON time," when the irrigation project was headquartered in Caylloma. Intense commercialization accompanied personnel and money flowing into the Colca Valley, including farmers from outlying hamlets and engineers from South Africa. The boom created new possibilities for personal enrichment, especially for the entrepreneurs provisioning the foreigners (Hurley 1978; Swen 1986). While some Cayllominos accommodated the foreigners begrudgingly, others welcomed their money, technology, electricity, and equipment. Abusive MACON staff members ran down livestock in their yellow trucks, ran up tabs in the bars, and left illegitimate children. Twenty years later, Cayllominos still speak of those "*macones*," synonymous with the project itself (Benavides 1983; Swen 1986).

Bordados became a symbol of wealth. As fiestas became larger and more frequent because of the boom, women wore more lavish *polleras.* All over Chivay, embroidery workshops sprang up to meet the demand. The workshop of Bernardo Supo and Viviana Casaperalta employed the largest staff, twenty-three, but it was not unique; several others employed ten or twelve, including the shop of "Chivay Chino," Leandro Suni. Some of the embroiderers directing family workshops today were trained in those old big shops. *Bordados*' popularity reached its zenith before 1980 and has declined since then.

Bordados and *lanas* have intertwined histories. Compared to five centuries of written history and many more centuries of pre-Hispanic history, the half-century dominated by the wool trade seems a very short span. Yet the legacy of that trade extends far beyond wool's direct economic impact. The widespread commercialization and modernization accompanying the marketing of fiber had long-term consequences. *Bordados* were a direct outgrowth of two contradictory trends: the influx of wealth into the province (later exacerbated by MACON) and the shortages of local clothing materials, mainly alpaca, caused by industrial growth outside the province. Their success did not stem from the isolation of the valley or resistance against the incursion of foreign culture and capitalism.

Today, many of the *mistis* who ruled Caylloma at midcentury reside permanently in Arequipa, as commerce in Chivay does not provide a livelihood. Manuel Salinas's store passed to his son, but it is dwindling away. "I opened my store . . . and built the house with my wife. As you can see, it's a whole block. Things haven't gone so badly for me. My son is selling off everything that's left, to go to Arequipa, but we're not going to sell the house." Thus, Manuel concluded the plaintive Chekhovian monologue that was our "interview."

In many such interviews, Cayllominos discussed women's intimate involvement in diverse aspects of the wool trade. This contradicts the impression, given by many studies, that the trade was disproportionately male dominated. Examining the gendered dynamics of *bordados* improves our understanding of regional exchange. It calls into question the claim that "long-distance trade was a male activity, and local marketplace sales of small quantities of foodstuffs was a female activity" (Jacobsen 1993:196 n. 186). But, in addition to local sales, women did participate in many links of the trading chain. They brought wool and animals to market, as Dionisia Huanqui recounted. Women's involvement in commerce was neither small nor limited to foodstuffs; parlaying their roles in production according to increased demand for clothes, women like Leonor Herrera opened stores in Chivay. Men also sold in the market.

The image of extroverted masculinity dominating the southern highlands is not without foundation. Not only did *gamonales* and their *misti* henchmen get Indians drunk and dupe them in casinos and fiestas, they marauded through the highlands on horseback, shooting Indians and burning them out of their homes (Aguirre and Walker, eds. 1990; Poole 1988, 1994). Women were neither paragons of feminine domesticity complementing and stabilizing masculine wildness, nor were they merely consumers in the economy. Women's roles as traders, shopkeepers, seamstresses, and embroiderers were productive as well as reproductive. Less information has come to light explaining how their economic activity articulated with their defense of community interests, but we know that women were combatants in the uprisings of the 1920s (Femenías 1999). All their activities were crucial to constructing the *misti* dynasties that controlled Caylloma and to resisting the new power structure.

From Carpetbagger to Patriarch: Gender, Ethnicity, and the Symbols of Legitimation

> *When my mother got married, she bought a straw hat and embroidered clothes. This was luxurious; all the people looked at her.* — ROSALVINA CAYO
> (Interview, Chivay, March 1992)

> *Q. Did your mother dress you in* polleras?
> *A. My mother? No. She was from Arequipa.*
> — EUDUMILA CÁCERES
> (Interview, Chivay, March 1993)

Bordados as a business developed along with political-economic issues of landownership and capitalist penetration. Cayllominos' decisions about clothing use, having both symbolic and pragmatic dimensions, were bound up with the political economy of cloth trade. The sentiments embodied in clothes, as they coalesced around place and community, were critical dimensions of a patriarchal system that molded ethnic identity as it molded men's and women's bodies. Thus, the gendered dimensions of political and ethnic changes associated with the capitalist penetration of Caylloma depended on a new idiom of idealized patriarchal control—an idiom relying on symbolic legitimation through dress. In Caylloma, women's dress was the primary signifier. Because women could own or control property, and both sons and daughters could inherit it, indigenous female lineage mattered. Yet upper-class women also frequented Caylloma and, with their daughters, perpetuated a different lineage, in which superiority was disconnected from native status. Community identification became linked to motherhood as social and political reproduction were embodied in the indigenous matriarch.

The *misti* "carpetbaggers," as I term the late-nineteenth-century interlopers, arrived without ties to the area. Most of them were men, many were poor, almost all were from other regions or other nations, and some were ex-soldiers fleeing the chaotic aftermath of the War of the Pacific (1879–1883). Whether carving a small niche as a petty trader or growing wealthy as the owner of a commercial house, they needed to belong. Caylloma's *misti* carpetbaggers gained control by manipulating indigenous gender and kinship systems—through marriage and other liaisons, their children's inheritance, and patronage through *compadrazgo* and other forms of kinship. Discourses of race, gender, and ethnicity helped the intruders legitimize political-economic control, in part by communicating value judgments about place of origin and class-related standards of comportment. While some terms are explicitly racial and even racist, others are euphemisms for inferiority and superiority where race remains implicit. In Eudumila Cáceres's lexicon, *gente,* literally "people," are a specific kind of people, non-"Indian" people. Other Cayllominos similarly used *gente* to distinguish by race, origin, or historical-cultural features. As Manuel Salinas pointed out, the merchants and agents of the wool houses were white, at least in their own eyes and those of others in the Colca Valley, although perhaps not in those of urbanites. Also, only a few "white people" (*gente blanca*) or "creole people" (*gente criolla*) lived in Chivay before Manuel and his family arrived from Sabandía, a town next to Arequipa.

> In Chivay before, there were primarily indigenous people here. That is, as they say vulgarly, creole people, the whites—there were few of us, we were all from outside. . . . Of the *gente* from here, there was only . . . Elías Cáceres. (Interview, Chivay, 1992)

Manuel's wife was from the family of Elías Cáceres (Eudumila's second cousin). The *criollos* were presumed to be both white and descendants of Spanish colonizers; however, they were often light-skinned *mestizos* one or more generations from indigenous forebears and rural lifestyles. Oriented toward Europe and North America, creoles marked their race and class by education and fashionable European-style dress, and lived in cities, primarily Lima.

When Cayllominos examined Shippee-Johnson photographs, they used dress to identify "*criollos*" and "*mistis.*" Especially in a Lari group portrait (see Figure 24), one man and one boy stand out because of their dress. The man (eighth from left in the undulating front row) wears a suit (*terno*); beside, and slightly before, him, the boy wears a suit with knee-length britches and boots. Adrián Zavala, a poor, elderly man from Achoma, identified the pair as "Manuel Zapater Neyra and his son Oscar. This man was the sub-prefect of Caylloma." Manuel's cousin, another Zapater, was a wealthy landowner and mayor of Lari, Zavala believed (interview, Chivay, 1992). Others identified the suited man as one of the "*señores decentes*" (decent men or gentlemen);[14] one of the "important people (*gente importante*) or, to put it vulgarly, *mistis*"; a teacher; an *hacendado;* and several types of political official. They often stated that he was not from Lari. Even people who did not identify the two assumed the boy was the man's son because their clothes were similar. Suits and boots, the consensus was, stood for power.

"Decent people" needed "decent clothes." "What did the Salinas men wear?" I asked Jerónimo Huayapa. "Decent men used decent vests of '*casimir*' [fine wool],[15] not *bayeta* clothes," he replied; they wore purchased boots or shoes, not llama-leather sandals or shoes (*polko* or *sek'o*). During the interview, Huayapa, wearing very old clothes, seemed poor even compared to other Cayllominos, yet he associated himself with those decent men. He, too, had worn shoes rather than sandals, he insisted. A well-dressed gentleman in a tie (*caballero bien cambiado, caballero de corbata*), according to Adrián Zavala, sported a Borsalino rather than a "*panziburro*" hat. A very fine Italian hat, as worn by the foreign explorers (see Figure 23, far left), was clearly superior to a handmade felted sheep-wool hat, named for its fuzzy resemblance to a donkey's belly (*panza de burro*).

Judging by the photographs, there were apparently few *criolla* women in Caylloma. Most women in the Shippee-Johnson images wear *polleras* (see Figures 22 and 25). Very few photographs show women wearing other styles, such as one from Lari where two women in 1930s fashions contrast strikingly with the others in *polleras* (Femenías 1997a: 353, 674, fig. 4.5). White women and *polleras* were worlds apart. Manuel Salinas made this clear when he showed me a sixty-year-old photograph of his wife in a simple frock as a schoolgirl in Arequipa. Flora Cutipa, my research associate, asked him if she ever wore *polleras.* "No, she was *criolla,*" he replied, sounding surprised. Eudumila Cáceres was even more emphatic. When she was young, I wanted to know, did her mother get *polleras* for her? "Dress me in *polleras*? My *mother*?!" Eudumila could not disguise the horror in her voice. Her mother was from Arequipa, and Eudumila had also enjoyed the privileges of a private school education there. Even in Chivay they flaunted the latest urban styles. *Criollas* from Arequipa did not wear *polleras.*

The civilized life of urban Arequipa contrasted with the frontier mentality of Chivay. Merchants often married women who, like themselves, were not from the valley. Many *criollo* men, however, led an urban-rural double life of marriage and liaisons, and maintained multiple households. Their wives and legitimate children lived in Arequipa, where the purity of white daughters was chaperoned in exclusive convent schools. Their common-law spouses, mistresses, and servants stayed in Caylloma, where their illegitimate children often went unrecognized. Some pioneering merchants, however, married local women, especially from wealthy *mestizo* families like the Cáceres or, in the smaller villages, from prominent indigenous families.

Focusing on the importance of marriage and *mestizaje* illuminates the connections among political power, political office, and control over land. Caylloma women owned their own property or controlled property by holding usufruct rights to shares of communal land. In practice, both sons and daughters inherited property and rights. Male power depended on customary property rights. Usurpers as well as heirs drew on custom, for both landholding and inheritance depended on legitimacy. Stories of *misti* incorporation into communities and their subsequent development of dynasties followed a single plot, varying only slightly in the individual details. During the post-War-of-the-Pacific upheavals, three brothers, it is told, moved into town. One was the priest, another the merchant, and the third the lawyer or clerk.[16] In most tales, the two non-priest brothers married local women, some with Spanish surnames, others indigenous. The priests also fathered children, whose illegitimacy was usually masked by having the children raised in the mother's natal family, adopted by other families, or raised by one of the priest's brothers; some were left orphans (Quechua *waqcha*). A father who did not recognize his child might well act as his godfather. In the idealized patriarchy that men promoted, all fathers were portrayed as good providers and monogamous; in practice, powerful individuals exposed themselves as flawed patriarchs.

Masculinity structured the politics of belonging, but within strict limits. Politics, as connected to community and state structures of authority, was almost exclusively a male domain.[17] Political leaders practiced extremes of nepotism, as their siblings and offspring rotated through positions, sometimes for decades. Elected and appointed officials came from the same families. Luisa Adriazola vda. de Terán, my landlady in Coporaque, narrated a story of her late husband's lineage in the Terán family that dominated Coporaque.[18] Spanning seven generations, she began with the arrival in Coporaque of three Terán brothers from Bolivia in the 1890s. One brother married a local woman, Carmela Mejía. One of their three children, Juan Zoilo Terán, who became a lawyer or notary, epitomized the Caylloмino rural patriarch. A consummate politician, in a career lasting twenty-five years, he held a dozen different political posts. He fathered twelve children by three different women, only one of them a legal wife, from the *forastero* Bernal family. He also behaved decently, adopting a child who was fathered, Luisa said, by his priest brother. The third sibling, Candelaria, married into the well-to-do indigenous Taco family. All three were raised in Arequipa and returned to Coporaque as adults. Luisa's husband, the son of Candelaria, chose to use the Terán surname because he felt the "native" Taco surname carried a stigma, Luisa explained. Through the 1920s, Juan Zoilo used indigenous and *forastero* family connections to become mayor and then *gobernador* of Coporaque and, finally, sub-prefect of Caylloma. Prolific procreation undergirded patriarchy as dozens of sons and nephews stepped into the shoes of fathers and uncles. Luisa's husband, Edilberto, became mayor of Coporaque. In 2000, their son Hernán was elected a national congressman from a district of urban Arequipa.

Even as *mestizaje* and inheritance played key roles, the symbolism of women's clothes acquired increasing importance. Male authority was limited by female authenticity. Community roots were a crucial factor in legitimizing political domination. Native birth was an important part of this legitimation, which was embodied in the person of the mother, the one who gives birth to a child of the pueblo. Even one born in the community is not as fully "native" as one whose parents and children were born there. Thus, motherhood acquires more importance in each succeeding generation. In a bilateral inheritance structure, where land rights pass through both mother and father to children of both sexes, women's access to property impinges on community membership. The politics of belonging becomes irreducibly female in certain dimensions. Luisa believed her husband was more authentically Terán than Juan Zoilo's children because Edilberto was Terán through his mother. Candelaria's maternal authenticity was unquestionable. Descent traced through a white or non-native mother had less value in terms of community belonging, for she would not inherit. A liaison with an "Indian" man reduced the social whiteness of a female, even if they married, whereas the social stigmas on "purity" did not apply to a man.

Dress was a primary mode of representing the racial and cultural categories channeling political-economic dominance. Patriarchal control was grounded in an ideology of gendered and racial superiority. *Misti* identity, therefore, was phrased as a racial category ("*gente blanca*") or, euphemistically, in terms of comportment ("*gente decente*"). As outsiders, *mistis* needed symbolic legitimation as insiders to claim rights in the communities where they settled. In the Terán clan, a few claimed the status of white *gente;* most of them moved to Arequipa. Luisa showed me an old portrait of the young Candelaria and several cousins; the fair-skinned beauties wear fashionable, high-collared attire. By the second or third generation, female descendants of those who stayed in Caylloma adopted local costume, *polleras.* This helped establish the outsiders' legitimacy. Dress changed them into insiders in the local symbolic lexicon—"the custom of my mother," "our grandparents," "our people." The women who wore *bayeta polleras* were potent, living symbols of localized ethnic authenticity, stimulating *polleras* to become more ornate, even luxurious, extensions of that embodiment. Those women remained in the villages, worked the land, and gave birth to the sons who were businessmen, politicians, and overseers of agricultural and pastoral production. But some wives and daughters were not so transformed. *Criollas* like Eudumila Cáceres were encouraged to remain outsiders and to consider themselves separate and superior. Dressed in fine *tela* gowns, they resided in Arequipa, were properly schooled and finished in elite academies, and infrequently visited Caylloma. The women of local ruling families who wore *polleras,* because they continued to influence inheritance of land, wielded female power. Nevertheless, because *mestizos* actively curtailed indigenous power, there were few male indigenous leaders. Henceforth, *polleras* advertised that local ethnic identity and female gendered power had become subordinate to *misti* patriarchal control, which was represented by *criollas' tela* gowns.

Conclusion: "Tradition of Our Ancestors . . . , Custom of Our Land"

Exploring Caylloma's history has revealed the multiple roles of clothes as economic and symbolic capital. Focusing on gendered and ethnic dimensions of local history has shown how they intertwine with political economy. Gender has permeated the analysis, even when it has not surfaced. Many changes that profoundly affected representative practices depended on the wool trade and commercialization, and date to the 1930s, when the provincial capital was transferred. However, the categories and expression of identity *in* Caylloma are not limited to gendered and ethnic concepts specific to the province or to "ethnic groups" that coexist there. The representation of identity also draws on discourses *about* Caylloma that have been constructed on regional and national levels for many centuries.

Wearing *bordados* is "the custom of our land of Chivay, of the ancestors," stated Felipe Surco. Many artisans and consumers used *costumbre* and *tradición* to explain why women wear *polleras* and attributed the custom to the grandparents and ancestors. Understanding "custom" and "tradition" as historically constructed phenomena depends on learning who the *abuelos* were and how custom and ancestry are associated. These associations extend beyond clothes to broader ideas about the past, ethnicity, and kinship. The traditions of the ancestors are value laden. They encompass nostalgia, artistic achievement, and the promotion of feminine beauty, but not all the associations are positive. Surco, who worked for forty years making and decorating Caylloma women's hats, bitterly recounted how the "*gamonales*" stole his family's lands. Eudumila Cáceres, conversely, recalled that the "*caballeros*" feared an uprising of the "*indígenas.*" Caylloma's traditions entail the relations of domination that white outsiders imposed, indigenous resistance and accommodation, and centuries of bloodshed.

Ethnicity is not a static identification with race and place; it proceeds through dynamic power struggles. The Colca Valley, never an isolated enclave, has become even more enmeshed with international capitalism in recent decades, partly because of MACON. Locally meaningful cultural traditions and ethnic differences were constructed in conjunction with national and international contacts. The ornate *bordados* now considered traditional in Caylloma grew out of innovations arising from inputs of materials, technology, and cash. The continued vitality of ethnic identity and the development of new traditional styles to express that identity embody a profoundly developed sense of history. Cayllominos' history of ethnicity is one of resistance and rejection—not resistance to change as mindless perpetuation, but rejection of domination—and of the assertion of the right to self-determination and self-representation. Our land, our clothes, our people: where we live, how we look, who we are.

Wearing ethnic clothes, the "relics" or heirlooms, is a way to establish continuity with the ancestors. This continuity also implies that asserting ethnic identity is part of the broader set of rights won by those ancestors. The *abuelos* and *antepasados* are not generic ancestors from a neutral past. Rather, Cayllominos' perceptions of what they did and what was done to them, as agents and victims, are perpetuated in Cayllomino identity. They are "*mi abuelo*"—my grandfather—and "*las abuelas*"—the women of my grandmother's generation—not only "*los abuelos*"—the ancestors. Creatively appropriating foreign materials, techniques, and relations, they invented the lavish clothes that embody ethnic pride through the women who wear them today.

Writing about the "invention of invention," Gaurav Desai (1993) points out that there are limits to seeing invention as entirely new. More profitable is seeking to understand reinvention when it is an "episteme of the same, apparently using the same terms as that which is rejected" (Desai 1993:121). Ideas like culture, primitive society, and primitive religion have often had force when they were inventions from the outside, he notes. What happens when "the *objects* of invention begin to take on the role of the *agents* of invention" (ibid.:131, emphasis in original)? Eric Hobsbawm and Terence Ranger, who galvanized the uncovering of inventedness, demonstrate that many practices once thought to be time-honored, or even timeless, have been imposed by outsiders (Hobsbawm 1992 [1983]; Hobsbawm and Ranger, eds. 1992 [1983]). Caylloma *bordados* might seem to be included: apparently ancient, verifiably novel. But we must distinguish among "traditions," examining the reasons for their invention and saliency, and not limit our view to imposition. The people of Caylloma were forced to wear Spanish-style clothes. Unfair credit terms swayed them to buy sewing machines. But their creative efforts, and their views of the past and present, are equally crucial in giving form and meaning to these "traditions of our ancestors."

I spoke with hundreds of Cayllominos about the past embodied in *bordados*. Together we looked at photographs and puzzled out the faces caught in black-and-white. As *criollas, caballeros,* and *originarios* recounted their stories, they filled in the colors of their embroidered history. Cayllominos' memories hold representations of a past that is far from utopian and sometimes painful to recall. Yet many people were willing, even eager, to reminisce at length as pain and pleasure, sorrow and joy burst forth simultaneously; the borders of time blurred in ways that expressed and enhanced the commonalities of sentiment. I did not anticipate that people might burst into tears, as several did, when I showed them a photograph album. Discourses about the past—perhaps once current, perhaps long buried—were revived. For some elderly people, adrift in a swiftly flowing stream of consciousness, the images quickened acute perceptions of a past at times more real than the present.

People were often glad to see these records of their past. While no one recognized him or herself, several people tentatively identified friends or relatives and expressed sadness over those now deceased. As they perused, reminisced, and reflected, negative memories also emerged. Friends and foes momentarily slipped their firm moorings in the past and washed ashore in the present, as the images prompted discourses of longing and reflections on belonging. Anger swelled in their vehement avowals that ethnic, social, and political inequalities had scarred the past. Grandmothers and *gamonales* rubbed shoulders in the crowded space of memory.

For the most part, discourses about the past came easily. The tales people told joined memories of ancestors with contemporary ideas about creativity and competition. Artisans' histories of their grandfathers' inventions were as elaborate as the embroideries themselves, complex, convoluted, and multilayered. Their perceptions of me, and the categories in which they placed me, influenced the stories. Eudumila saw me as a fellow white person, *gente;* others as a foreigner, a teacher—then perhaps I was a *misti* too? These representations of longing and belonging were also conditioned by my position; they related to the politics of my belonging. Despite the influence of my presence and my concern with objects and visual matters, many times I felt myself recede as their stories acquired an independent force. The people I conversed with all have their own vested interests and a sharply honed sense of the politics of their belonging to family, community, and home.

Today, *bordados* are associated with powerful sentiments about the past. They embody memory and continuity from a personal past, through one's mother and grandmother, to the remote past where individual "grandmother" merges with the concept of ancestry itself, "*las abuelas*" or "*los abuelos.*" Documentary evidence of gender relations when the real *abuelos* lived is sparse. Nevertheless, contemporary people's visions of the past include ideas about gender that are significant in conceptions of the past before memory. Caylloma people's memories of the early twentieth century tell us that ethnic identity was linked to native status traced through an indigenous mother's line. Changes in status were closely related to the motif of ethnic conflict in that past. Given that earlier weavers and seamstresses who provided clothes were often women, the emphasis on grandfather as inventor of *bordados* seems to leave grandmothers out of the creative process. Does this signal a shift in women's roles from producers to consumers?

Bordados do more than provoke powerful sentiments about the past. They promote the adornment of women today. The bodies of women wearing *bordados* become microcosms of ethnic space. The very elaborateness of *bordados* sends mixed messages. One might conclude that women's desire for novel attire and the promotion of women's bodies as semaphores of sumptuous display fueled a process of bovaryesque petit bourgeoisization that made women the victims of consumer culture as they indebted themselves for baubles. The paradox is that clothes embody pride in cultural uniqueness, ethnic identity, and skilled artisanry, and all the while still signify political and economic processes that often subordinate those who make and use them. Historical processes conspired to make Cayllominas into objects of desire, accentuated and magnified by adorning their bodies. As luxuriant displays of high status, however, elegant *bordados* indicate rejection of assimilation to elite, "modern," international norms of dress and comportment.

The interview with Eudumila Cáceres was one of my last before returning to the United States in 1993. Eudumila, no longer the pampered young daughter of the wealthiest family in a provincial mountain town, conducts daily surveillance of Chivay plaza. The new stone arch, she complained, obscured her view of the church. Her vision extended farther, though, in time and space—beyond the confines of Chivay, before the arch was built. Llama trains did not chime their gentle "*chirilín*" that day, although sometimes in winter one still sees and hears them. Buses, trucks, and motorcycles roared past, unencumbered by mufflers, while popular music blared out of a store across the way. The pace of life is different in today's Chivay, and so is the ethnic composition of Caylloma's population. As we turned off the tape recorder and shut the photograph album, Eudumila cast a glance around the plaza she knows so well.

"*Ya no hay indios,*" she sighed. "*Puro mistis. Puro pantalón, falda.*" (There are no Indians anymore, only *mistis.* [They wear] only pants [and] skirts.)

Although fewer women in Chivay wear *polleras* than in the smaller villages, I had seen several that day. But to Eudumila, those women were as invisible as the "Indians" in the photographs had been. To her, the more usual modern, purchased dress signified nonsubservient attitudes, a visual statement of refusal to represent themselves as Indians. The "*indígenas*" who rose up against abusive landlords in the 1920s, and who left their images in the photographs of the 1930s, forged a path for the peasants and professionals who now mingle in Chivay's fields, shops, and government offices.

Despite the softness of her tone, the measured timbre of Eudumila's voice still reaches me. Her strident views still distress me whenever my mind hears her say, "there are no people here." The images that she conjured, too, replay in my memory.[19] Addressing history through sets of memories—reminiscences about clothes, claims about the invention of embroidery, interpretations of the structures of ethnic relations—reveals that clothes are more than possessions and more than symbols "of" something else. Memories, photographs, and written documents have given us access to a history of embroidery that is bound up with the politics of belonging that shapes life in Caylloma.

5

Dancing in Disguise: Transvestism and Festivals as Performance

Play with the concept of the unruly woman is partly a chance for temporary release from traditional and stable hierarchy; but it is also *part and parcel of conflict over efforts to change the basic distribution of power within the society.*
— NATALIE ZEMON DAVIS (1978:154–155)

During hundreds of annual fiestas, the Witite dances in disguise. Whirling frenetically around village plazas, every Witite in spectacular *polleras* seems to mirror dozens of women who also wear them. But it is men who don skirts and perform as Witite, the character of a man disguised as a woman, and they do so only during fiestas and folklore events (Figure 26).

The Witite is unique, manifold, and ubiquitous. In Caylloma, he is the only transvestite character in all the dances and dance-dramas, but several men usually perform as Witite in the same event and he is featured in all village festivals. Outside Caylloma, moreover, Witites perform in folk festivals in Arequipa and Lima. The Witite has become the icon of Caylloma, a figure closely and publicly identified with this region. Through ritual transvestism, he embodies ideas about sexuality, race, conquest, and violence that undergird Cayllominos' performance of daily life and depiction of their heritage. With this ambiguous representation, Cayllominos play with the concept of the unruly woman, and thus they struggle over the distribution of power.[1]

In this chapter, I use performance and the performative to explore the interdependence of diverse facets of identity formation and expression. I center on the Witite in order to analyze how gender is performed. Why do men wear *polleras*? is the central question here. By playing this charac-

26 WITITE DANCER

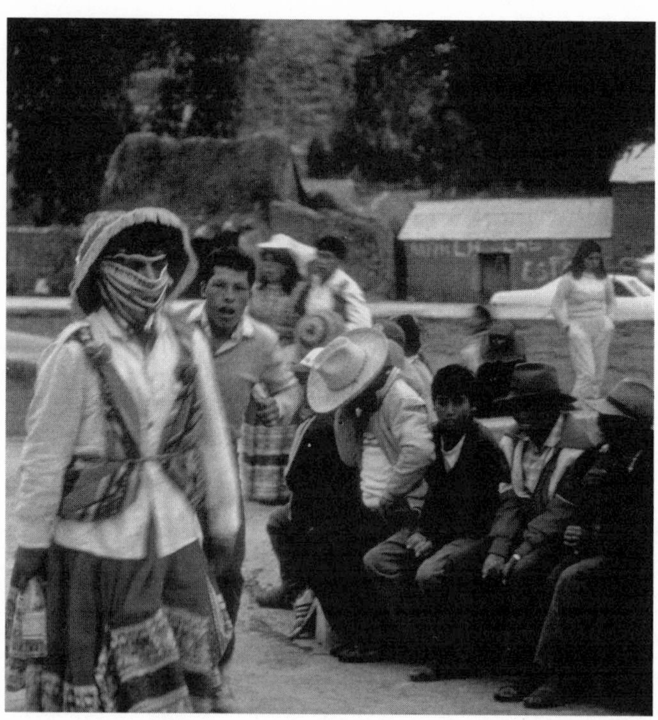

ter, men neither pretend to be women nor aim to persuade anyon[illegible] they are women. Rather, they emphasize that they are *not* women. M[illegible] begin to perform Witite in their teens. By wearing women's skirts, the[illegible] fore, boys learn to be men. Male performance in female clothes, I argue, is a central vehicle through which masculinity is articulated, challenges to masculinity are suppressed, and an ideology of heterosexual male dominance is inculcated in all members of society. Such performance is effective because gender is a primary axis along which power is allocated and contested; examining this specific embodiment of gender, therefore, provides insight into how power operates in society. In addition, because the clothed body is the key symbol of sexuality, spotlighting a male person in female dress forces us to confront how sexuality and gender intersect. The Caylloma experience shows how ritual shapes society through contrast with the quotidian domain. By focusing on performance in festivals, I expand our understanding of social life in general.

My analysis of identity and performance considers the simultaneous need to celebrate festivals and to assert masculine identity. In an area of widespread poverty, in a time of civil war, Cayllominos staged elaborate fiestas with impressive frequency. During them, not only did women wear luxurious versions of their quotidian garments but men appropriated such skirts and danced enthusiastically in them. Where I observed celebrants in a joyous gala, Cayllominos saw fierce warriors. These paradoxes prompted me to inquire how fiestas reshaped the relationship between gender and ethnicity.

My research included performance in fiestas as well as daily life. I have spent countless hours dancing in fiestas, observing dances, and talking with individuals who have danced in, sponsored, prepared, and observed them. At times I have worn *polleras.* I have come to understand the Witite, in particular, and dancing, in general, not only as public performance but as metaphors for the performance of identity. Perhaps as much as people there perform their identities as Cayllominos, I have performed my identity as an ethnographer by dancing in disguise.

Transvestism involves crossing borders established by dress. To understand transvestism I had to cross the borders between lived experience and scholarly analysis, and between academic disciplines. My ethnographically informed ideas about culture, gender, and dress were challenged more than confirmed when I consulted the literature in an impressively diverse array of disciplines. Especially in the last two decades, scholars in anthropology,

ism, queer theory, theater, performance studies, literature, cultural ies, psychology, and sociology have had a lot to say about transvest-. No published studies, however, center on transvestism in Peru, and few even mention it.[2]

In much academic literature and popular thought, transvestism implies homosexuality—but not in Caylloma. When I discussed transvestism with Cayllominos, not one person ever suggested that Witites were homosexual. Indeed, when I asked, everyone flatly denied it. When I spoke with fellow Andeanists, many told me about Witite-like performers in village fiestas where they lived or worked. This anecdotal information helped convince me that transvestism is an important fact of ritual life not only in Caylloma but in much of highland Peru. When I conversed with people unfamiliar with the Andes, most inquired how the Witite was linked to ritualized "third gender" roles or to gay activism. My field research, however, did not point to such links. If transvestism is commonplace in Peru, I wondered, why had I located so few published references? If transvestism and homosexuality are strongly connected in most of the world, why not in Caylloma? If they are not connected, how does Cayllomino transvestism relate to sexuality? And if, after all, they are connected, why do Cayllominos deny it?

All these questions led me to assess the meaning of ritual transvestism in Caylloma, which challenges the presumed transvestism-homosexuality connection that dominates the literature. This reappraisal then made me look long and hard at the stakes involved in performing gender and exploring sexuality. Looking closely at the performances through which Cayllominos asserted their identities led me to ask how and why they did so at a time when severe political repression gripped their country. Questions about assertion led me to consider denial and disavowal; questions about openness and liberty, to secrecy and privacy; and all of these, back to dances and disguises.

Witite sends messages about racial and ethnic as well as gendered dominance. Dancing Witite is emblematic of local discourses that stress racial mixing (*mestizaje*) and violent conflict as inevitable legacies of chronic contacts between outsiders and the natives they have tried, all too often successfully, to subjugate. As local celebrations of tradition invoke this confrontational heritage, they instill dual associations between male dominance over female and outsider over native. By examining the ways that performing the Witite feminizes the native, I uncover how Cayllominos simultaneously perform gender and represent the distribution of power along racial lines as well.

Similarly, my focus on dancing means evaluating how the Witite's performance within festivals articulates with other aspects of identity formation. Gender, race, and ethnicity are intertwined not only with each other but with local and national identities in ways that demand attention. Cayllominos strongly identify with their natal village and a rural way of life. Local pride, which encompasses dances and traditions, has intensified among migrants. Through the privileged ritual domain of the fiesta, Cayllominos celebrate their local heritage even as they perform their identity as Peruvians. They also consistently feature the Witite dance in folklore events outside the province, which represent them in the region and the nation. Based on my own observations and performances, I must assert confidently: these dances are not violent. Their apparently pacific nature was belied, however, by the stories of violence and aggression which people told to explain them. Today the Witite dances are entirely peaceful, everyone concurred, but formerly they were violent "dancing fights." Men killed each other, Cayllominos insisted time and again. These claims led me to inquire how their pride in this tradition relates not only to the glorification of violence and male dominance in the past but to the nationwide climate of violence in the present.

Festivals, Gender, and Performance in Caylloma

At least once a month there is a fiesta in the Colca Valley, and far more in the summer (December–February). Fiestas usually coincide with Catholic holy days and often with agricultural and irrigation rituals of pre-Columbian origin. The contemporary annual cycle makes evident the Spanish colonial legacy. In the sixteenth century, Spanish rulers relocated and reorganized pre-Hispanic communities into grid-form villages (*reducciones*), each having a central plaza with a church on one side, and assigned each community a "patron"—a Catholic saint or aspect of the Virgin Mary—with several sharing important ones; for example, Coporaque and Madrigal have Santiago, the patron saint of Peru and Spain, celebrated on July 25. Today each community celebrates its patron, and numerous other festivals are common to all communities.[3]

During these fiestas, all community members assemble and perform together in the same place, the central plaza, marking it as collective public space. Nevertheless, individual performers vie with each other for prestige in lavish displays of dance and music. The elaborate garb worn at fiestas is a luxurious version of the locally distinct daily wear. The similarity of clothed appearance fosters a sensation of shared identity even as differences in the quality of dress and the quality of performance stress competition.

Fiestas require tremendous investments of time, energy, and resources. Far more collective than individual effort is required to make the project materialize. Numerous social roles and group behaviors, which underlie or support public presentation through dance, have a collective character and so are public, but in a different way than performing in the plaza. Because fiestas are so frequent and the ritualized performances are constantly repeated, festival concerns are quotidian as well as ritual. Cayllominos are concerned with fiesta preparations all year long.

While I lived in Caylloma, fiestas were inescapable—loud, boisterous, raucous events. My friends insisted that I attend and urged me to wear *polleras* to do so. Fiestas were still celebrated with relish and gusto in all the villages, despite widespread poverty. The urban experiences of migrants have rejuvenated, rather than undermined, fiesta celebrations. Not only the Cayllominos who live in Arequipa and Lima, but even those in Bolivia, Chile, and the United States, flock back to their native soil, especially in February to dance at Carnival.

Respect, dignity, and pride are expressed and earned in fiestas; these positive features contrast sharply with the racism and discrimination that indigenous people face in urban centers. These cultural productions are manifestations of the political struggle and cultural activism of Andean communities, I maintain, building on the work of Mendoza (2000), Poole (1990), Rasnake (1988), and Turino (1993). By attending to the actual identity of *cargo* holders in Coporaque and the large number of *cargos,* I arrived at a view of the *cargo* system rather different than those presented in much literature on Andean fiestas. While I agree that fiestas simultaneously encourage community solidarity and foster inequality, I pay special attention to the relationship between gender and power. Gender shapes every aspect of the multiple roles that people play in fiestas, including, but not limited to, *cargos* (offices or burdens). Women hold a few high *cargos;* they hold many lesser *cargos;* and they carry out many supporting actions. In Caylloma, the flexible manner of gendering *cargo* roles challenges the gendered division of labor. Women hold *cargos* on their own. Men hold a *cargo* in which they represent themselves as women. Marriage, although a factor in filling other *cargos,* is not the principal requirement. Even when a woman is co-*mayordomo* with her husband, she may refer to herself as *mayordomo.*[4]

Fiestas are sponsored by individuals whose ability to undertake sponsorship is based in class, race, and gender status. Thus, fiestas both shape and conform to the hierarchical ladder of *cargos* that fiesta participants assume as they take their turns in succeeding years. Because *mayordomos* (sponsors) are the highest *cargos,* they have been treated as the stars of the enterprise (Rasnake 1988; Sallnow 1987). This focus, however, has created a distorted image of fiesta presentation—one which slights women's contributions—and thus impedes our understanding of power in society. Even in a small-town fiesta, several thousand people may participate; only a handful are sponsors and several dozen other people occupy other *cargos.* The *mayordomos'* responsibilities and expenses, while considerable, vary depending on the fiesta. Many other *cargos,* although less prestigious and less demanding than *mayordomo,* are necessary for fiestas to proceed.

Gender, migration, and political-economic reality converge in Caylloma festival *cargo* practices in other ways that contradict existing fiesta literature. In Caylloma, the ideal is that each community member should fill the *cargos* in a specific sequence; in practice, the sequence is not always followed. Many legal residents of the Colca Valley, who own land there, do not actually live in their native villages but spend most of the year outside the valley. Because there are few male *comuneros* (community members) who are permanent, year-round residents, communities often not only allow but encourage migrants and temporary residents—many of whom are women—to take on *cargos.* Therefore, while *cargos* are still closely related to the politico-religious positions of authority that men assume, *cargo* obligations do not necessarily dovetail with the "real" political obligations of civil authority.

In Caylloma, *mayordomo* is the highest *cargo.* One path of upward mobility requires individual *comuneros* to hold less burdensome *cargos* set aside for younger, often single, people. The Witite is among the early *cargos,* which a boy often assumes first in his teens. He may move next to the larger *cargos,* especially after marriage, or continue to dance Witite. Another path is to share a *cargo.* For Carnival, the primary cargo is called *cabecilla* rather than *mayordomo;* it is shared among several people, not necessarily related and possibly unmarried.

The gendered aspects of festival practices—both performance and support activities—are important primarily for two reasons. First, they intersect in complex and sometimes contradictory ways with concepts of gender appropriateness—ideas that are temporarily restructured during festivals. Second, the gender dynamics of festivals are embedded in the distribution of power in other domains of social life. Women engage in a wide range of social relations; no single role dominates over all others. Gender structures fiestas overall, not only through marriage, but because of the depth and breadth of female networks.

Delia Bernal Terán is one young migrant woman I met. In 1992 at age eighteen she returned from Lima to be a *cabecilla* of Carnival in Coporaque, one of three young people who served as co-sponsors. Delia is the youngest sister of my *comadres* Nilda and Candelaria Bernal, who live in Coporaque. Delia had worked in Lima as a maid for six years, in a home where Nilda formerly worked. Like her older sister, Delia decided to visit Coporaque during Carnival. When I finished fieldwork four months later, she was still there, living with her parents. She believed her employers in Lima had kept her position open for her, and she thought she might return. Perhaps, however, she too would stay at home, meet a young man, and marry. Fulfilling a prestigious ritual position strengthened her ties to her hometown. Her obligations to her sister and parents brought her home to visit; the possibility of settling down kept her there after the fiesta.

Carnival: *Pujllay* and the Work of Play

Carnival (Spanish Carnaval or, more commonly, Carnavales), the largest fiesta celebrated simultaneously in the entire Colca Valley, takes place in February during the summer.[5] According to the Catholic calendar, Carnival ends before Lent begins on Ash Wednesday. In the Colca Valley, however, some communities begin celebrating on the Monday or Tuesday before Ash Wednesday, and others, several days after Lent has begun. The flexible scheduling correlates with completion of several related activities, enabling villagers to participate in Carnival in more than one community over the course of one full week.[6]

The continuance of Carnival in Caylloma today and the Witite's inclusion in it both point up the gendered and ethnic contradictions it embodies. Carnival means boisterous, even lewd, behavior—a last hurrah of indulgence before the Lenten restraints. The atmosphere of wild abandon, however, is also serious stuff. Far from being merely a "free-for-all," Carnival provides a social space for alterations of hierarchy, usually called inversions (Babcock, ed. 1978; Bakhtin 1984). "Play" is more than, and other than, reversal or temporary release, as Natalie Davis (1978) has pointed out. Carnival can be either a mask for or an alternative to political disobedience for both men and women. Even in its apparent formlessness, Carnival can provide a formal means of protest and thus change the distribution of power (Davis 1978:154).

"*Pujllay,*" the Quechua word for "play," is widely used as a synonym for Carnival throughout the Andes (Rasnake 1988:182, 242; Ulfe 2001). Pujllay is play, but creating this structured play requires hard work. Behind the public spectacle lies an equally impressive display of sociality and hospitality. Sponsors and other major participants begin to make arrangements for food, clothing, musicians, dancers, and decoration at least one year in advance, preferably two or three years. During the current year's fiesta, sponsors for the following year are publicly named. Even more than his or her personal material resources, each individual's decision to commit to this costly obligation is influenced by social resources. Strong gender and kin networks are imperative, for they provide the support that will enable a sponsor to fulfill his or her obligation.

Anyone in a community may participate in a fiesta, people from other communities regularly attend, and an atmosphere of openness and liberty holds sway. Nevertheless, participation is structured. The contemporary political-economic reality of significant outmigration affects participation overall and sponsorship in particular. Carnival crystallizes the push-and-pull that urban opportunities and rural roots exert, especially on young adults. Festivals often have two main sponsors, one from each of the two sectors (Quechua *saya,* Spanish *parcialidad*) into which communities are divided. Because many community members are kin of more than one sponsor, however, festivals create contradictory obligations to support several kin groups. Carnival, no matter how communitywide, also represents each of the two sectors. And, although it creates and expresses kinship bonds, it can also highlight family conflicts.

Carnival is a very big deal. This became clear to me in 1992 when I spent three days celebrating Carnival in Coporaque. About a week before the festival, relatives begin to arrive from as near as the next village, as far as the United States. No matter how many vehicles the bus companies add, nothing seems to relieve the standing-room-only character of rural travel in the Andes. Relatives shout boisterous, jubilant greetings to passengers as they alight in their hometown; other travelers, eager to be on their way to more distant villages, loudly harangue the bus drivers. Chivay doubles in size from 5,000 to 10,000; many celebrants there also attend Carnival in a smaller town. Coporaque's official population is about 1,100. Normally, some 300 people are in the village, but about 1,500 are present during Carnival.

During the pre-Carnival week, people are busy completing many annual activities. *T'inkachiy,* a ceremony to insure animal fertility, is performed in outlying pastures (Bernal 1983:119; Gelles 2000:101–103; Paerregaard 1989; Valderrama and Escalante 1988:167; also Sallnow 1987:133–140). Two days, of Comadres and Compadres, are set aside for reaffirming those kinship ties. People work together to prepare all the food; women brew *chicha;* and artisans labor long into the night to finish sewing elaborate outfits. Here too, gendered structures of interaction play significant roles. Even though men and women share many tasks, most people consider preparing special food and obtaining fancy clothes to be women's work. Grandmothers and *madrinas* rely especially on younger women to help them, but young men may be obligated as well.

No matter what street I walked down, people pulled me into their homes to eat and drink *chicha* (corn beer) with their families. Most celebrants I met were young people, especially young women and teenage girls, who had come to "dance"—literally, in the plaza, and more broadly, to participate in various ways. Some youths frequently returned to their parents' homes, especially if they lived in nearby Arequipa; many others had not been home for years. Few if any had become rich, but against all odds, many had amassed enough cash, or arranged for enough credit, to make the fiesta happen—and to make it huge.

Desire drives the Andean Carnival, which embodies fundamental contradictions of generational conflict because it is the principal time of courtship. Sexual and material desires coexist uneasily as physical drives wrestle pragmatic concerns. In the Southern Hemisphere, Carnival occurs in midsummer, so it is a celebration of fertility realized rather than one of latent fertility at winter's end, as in the Northern Hemisphere (see Sallnow 1987:131). Sexuality permeates this festival of fertility, as cultural performances both celebrate and enable reproduction of humans, animals, and plants (Allen 1988; Harris 2000). Fertility eclipses reproduction: sexuality moves from potential to real; desire is fulfilled. For young people expressing their emergent sexuality, "to dance" is largely a synonym for "to court" or "to flirt." For those aiming to prove their preparation to enter adult society, "to dance" means "to hold a *cargo*" or "to be in charge" (*estar encargado/a*).

During Carnival, females enjoy liberties far greater than those they have the rest of the year if they live in the village in their parents' home or under their watchful eyes. Dancing in the plaza, young unmarried people attract suitors but may also displease their parents should they catch an unsuitable mate. Married people likewise risk inciting their spouse's jealousy.

Throughout my fieldwork, stories like Nilda Bernal's were very common. Nilda formerly worked in Lima as a maid but has lived in Coporaque again since the mid-1980s, when she returned home for Carnival. When she returned home to dance, the money she earned as a maid in Lima helped support Carnival. After dancing with a local man during Carnival, she began dating him. The match was ended because their parents withheld their approval. Nilda demonstrated her loyalty to family, in part, through marrying a different man, whom her parents considered an acceptable spouse, the following year. With Juan, she later cosponsored a major fiesta. Thus she earned family and community approval as she moved through appropriate adult actions and *cargos.*

The work of play in Carnival goes deeper than the men's and women's specific tasks. Performance of local cultural traditions strengthens family prestige and pride in heritage. Most young people leave Caylloma because there is no work there or because their parents believe there are better opportunities in the city to study, earn, or both. Even those who return infrequently rarely sever all ties. The senior generations' wealth lies largely in land and animals, which young adults expect to inherit. By playing large roles in fiestas, young migrants support parental values even as they threaten parental control by choosing their own mate. To claim a future place in their home community, because they cannot buy land, they can and do buy culture—by paying for fiestas. Children go through the ritual of Carnival, dressing up and dancing and feasting, even after they become adults, as a way to claim their own place in their community.

Dances and Disguises

The Witite dances first and foremost at Carnival. This fiesta is always celebrated with many dances, among which the Witite is primary. While most villagers perform the dance, only a few men portray the character. As Witite's costume and manner of self-presentation shape his role and performance, they help to shape Carnival itself. To understand how Witites perform, I also had to analyze how women, as well as men who are not Witites, perform. By considering these together, I came to understand the role of Witite within the carnival realm, as it is emblematic of the carnivalesque and the festive. Conversely, anything festive, ritual, or inverted might be equated with Witite. Dress uniquely shapes the relationship between gender and the festive.

My analysis drew not only on personal participation but on acceptance of Cayllominos' characterizations of my performance as Witite-like. The house where I lived in Coporaque was well positioned for my participant observation. Set high on a corner of the Plaza de Armas, it offered an ideal vantage point for watching festivities, which helped me decide if and when I should join them. I could also take a back exit to another street, thus avoiding the most boisterous festivities in the plaza. Fiestas meant splitting my time between the plaza, watching, conversing, and dancing; other people's homes, partaking of elaborate meals; and my room, writing and reflecting (but very rarely sleeping). When I first dressed in *polleras* for a fiesta, I borrowed garments from my *comadres,* and my neighbor Agripina helped me dress. Tweaking the too-short *polleras* into position, she decided to pin up the top one. Not only would it stay in place while I danced, but, she wisecracked, it would make me look like a Witite.

During every fiesta for a day or two, as it started off slowly, I would hear the musicians warm up and watch them march around town playing distinctive Carnival tunes and other traditional local anthems, accompanied by a few diligent dancers from the sponsors' families. I went visiting and found friends at home, preparing vast quantities of food and *chicha,* and sewing final stitches on costumes. On the second or third day, most people finished those tasks and went to the plaza. When a fiesta is in full swing, forget sleep. Every time I attended one, after several days of hearing the music round the clock, I would lose my ability to tell if it was actually still playing. The beat echoed so loudly in my head that it seemed I was carrying the band with me.

When a fiesta gets under way in earnest, the dancers assemble to begin the dance. In 1992, the Witite dance in Coporaque began with male dancers (some in Witite garb) and female dancers (almost all in *polleras*) organized in separate lines on opposite sides of the plaza. From the yard of my house, I watched the band assemble near the center of the plaza, close to the church. The dancers entered the plaza through stone archways, which crown the streets stretching away from the plaza's corners. The dancers at the head of each line met at the center of the upper side of the plaza. Each line then passed the other, moving in opposite directions and curving inward until the male and female lines formed two concentric circles around the plaza's central fountain. At that point, the lines dissolved and men and women paired off to dance as couples.

Upon entering the plaza, the men's line, with about twenty dancers, quickly reached its position around the fountain. The men had to circle the fountain several times, however, before the women's line, with about fifty dancers, reached that position. When the lines broke up into couples, many women danced with each other rather than with men. Some Witites, as they often do, danced alone. Women rarely do so; they usually dance in couples or trios with men, women, and/or Witites (Figure 27). All throughout Tuesday, more dancers joined the group; by Wednesday night, several hundred people danced together for hours.

The Witite dance itself is simple but powerful. There is no complicated choreography or intricate footwork. So few and simple are the steps

27 DANCERS WHIRL ABOUT.

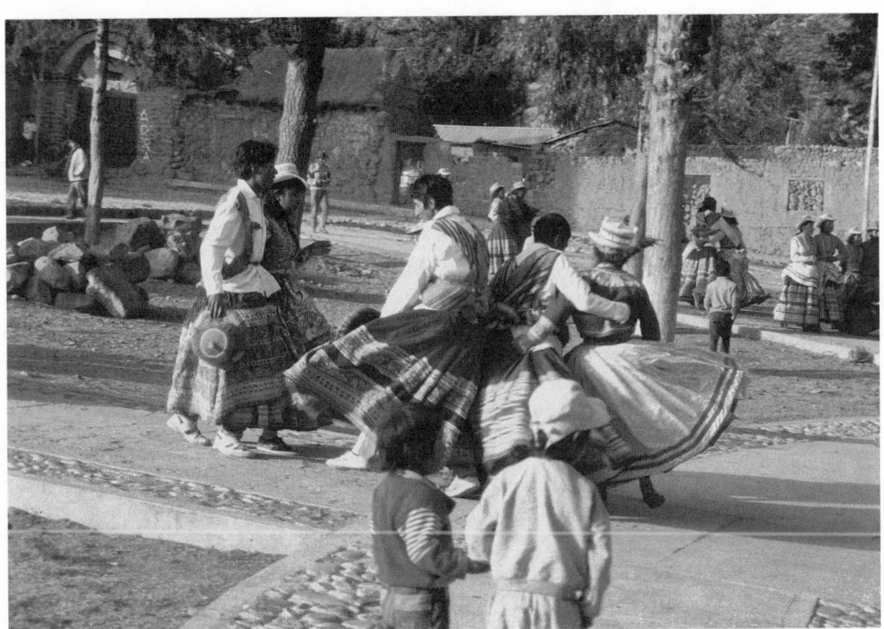

that even tiny tots (and *gringa* anthropologists) have no problem learning and participating. The music and the dance compel attention, as the *bombo* (drum) keeps a deep, even beat. Much of the power derives from sheer numbers of participants. In vast collective motion, hundreds of dancing bodies move in sync. Everyone does the same thing, makes the same motions: all progress forward and in a circle, usually counterclockwise, stop on a dime, and whirl about together. There are only two different steps: short running steps forward, and steps in place in a circle. Done to a four-count beat, the patterns vary only slightly: eight steps (or combinations of eight) forward, four steps whirling about, repeat twice, eight steps forward, whirl. (You can get really dizzy.) Side by side, with an arm around the partner's waist, as couples pull each other around into the whirl, their upper bodies bob and twist wildly, with the free arm waving and often brandishing a bottle of beer or cane alcohol.

The circular motion around the plaza seems to sweep away difference. From far away, all *comuneros* are drawn to their hometown, to its very center, where they dance the same steps, wear the same clothes, and eat the same food. Anyone can join in. The performance emphasizes inclusion, collective behavior, and solidarity.[7] But the circle continuously breaks apart and re-forms, and from time to time a new line breaks off and snakes down the street. Dancers move off to different spaces, usually the homes of friends and relatives. Thus the performance also stresses exclusion: in relations between performer and audience as well as among audience members, and in distinctions between individual performance styles. Most of all, the Witite himself stands out.

The Witite dance alters, rather than merely fills, public and social space. The plazas of Caylloma's villages are nearly empty except during fiestas.[8] Through the practice of dance, public space becomes gendered and sexualized as the dancers occupy the plaza. More women than men always dance. Women's figures and images fill the plaza. As they whirl about, their ornate, flying skirts accentuate their ethnic identity and project their sexuality as the bodies form collective movement in dance. Among similar figures who wear similar Caylloma clothes, the sameness of all is accentuated as the individuality of each is diminished. This vast sea of whirling *polleras* creates a strong visual impression of female space. A closer look shows, however, that it is far from exclusively female. Some men dance. Most men wear standard male attire (pants and shirt), thereby affirming their male identity. The Witite presents himself in female garments, which makes him appear not to be male, thereby apparently affirming the importance of female identity. Nevertheless, he challenges that importance by appropriating things that belong to women. He asserts male dominance as he claims the right to take women's things.

The costume transforms the actor who plays Witite, masking his face and sheathing him in skirts. Cayllominos use the term *disfraz,* "disguise," but they know the dancer's identity. The figure can be considered disguised only up to a point because public performance, in fact, puts the individual in the limelight, bringing him recognition and even fame. Disguise, therefore, is a fiction in which all participate. Audience members are also performing roles: spectators who suspend disbelief. Individual dancers distinguish themselves as Witites through the quality of their performance. High energy, reckless abandon, and total absorption in the dance are prized above all. A few excellent dancers continue as Witites long after they fulfill their initial *cargo,* achieving such an elevated status that *mayordomos* hire them to dance at fiestas, paying them with money, food, and alcohol. Being a Witite does not make most dancers stars, however, but enables them to serve their community and distinguish themselves. In recent years, the Witite has assumed an integral role in folklore. The Colca Valley's four high schools send dance teams to local, regional, and national competitions, another vehicle through which many teenage boys perform Witite. Thus, individual distinction goes hand in hand with family and community service and prestige.

Dress is crucial to the way the Witite establishes his character. Cayllominos usually call his dress *disfraz,* "disguise" or "costume"; *baila disfrazado,* "he dances in disguise"; *lleva disfraz,* "he wears a disguise." When a man dons the regalia, he consciously initiates playing the role of Witite. The garments comprise a unified costume with narrowly prescribed elements. Although each dancer is unique, the individual costumes vary little, primarily in colors and fabrics. Uniqueness stems from the dancer's manner of self-presentation; each projects a highly individualized style of wearing the costume and dancing. Although Witites communicate norms of male dominance by appropriating women's clothes, because their costume is not identical to female ceremonial dress, the specifically male and gender-ambiguous elements of the ensemble are also significant.

The female garments that Witites wear are: *pollera,* carrying cloth (*lliklla*), and hat strap (*anqoña*). I believe that *polleras* are the most important garment associated with women. In fiestas as in daily use, women wear two or more layered *polleras;* they pull up the lower half of the uppermost *pollera* and tuck it into the waistband. Witites also wear several layers, but they secure the edge of the top layer with large decorative pins—the style Agripina recommended for me.

Llikllas, rectangular woven carrying cloths, are women's possessions in which females carry babies or burdens on their backs. Men sometimes borrow them to carry supplies and tools. Boys, but not men, may carry babies in them. All use only one *lliklla,* folded diagonally and tied over one shoulder and under the other, or around both shoulders. Witites, however, wear two *llikllas* at once, each folded and wrapped around the torso and one shoulder vertically. Over both cloths, they wrap a braided sling around the waist, thereby creating pouches. A special hat (*montera*), exclusive to Witites, is made of fabric over a hard, straw armature. Long, thick silky fringe hanging from the brim obscures the Witite's eyes and upper face. Sewn to the *montera*'s underside are several bands, *anqoñas,* finely handwoven and with beaded edges. Because *anqoñas* are commonly used by women and rarely by men, they emphasize the impression of femaleness. In normal daily wear, each woman's hat has only one *anqoña.* Each Witite, however, wears three or four bands at once, criss-crossed, obscuring his face (see Figure 26), and enhancing the aura of disguise.

Two objects are specifically male: tunic and sling. The tunic (*polaca*), which may be white or a khaki-colored army uniform, is worn untucked over the skirt, partly covered by the *llikllas* and belted with the sling. Witites never wear the woman's embroidered blouse and vest; women never wear the *polaca.* The sling (Quechua *warak'a,* Spanish *honda*) is hand-braided by males, used by males, and is conceptually male, being associated with storms, lightning, fertility, and sexual potency.[9] Both a tool and a weapon, it is associated with beneficent protection and with violence. Men and boys sling rocks to shoo dogs, herd animals, and kill birds (which eat grain crops). In today's dance, men occasionally brandish an empty sling. When they, rarely, sling at each other, their ammunition is usually locally grown fruit, especially unripe quince and prickly pear cactus (*tuna*) roots, and dahlia tubers. The use of natural objects strengthens the sling's associations with fertility and Pujllay's celebration of summer. But in the past, Cayllominos claim, Witites hurled rocks at each other.

> The . . . Witite inspires respect because he is haughty and imposing. The clothes he uses seem to change the dancer's personality: he seems taller and has a mysterious air. . . . In the dance . . . he

> stays outside the line. . . . When he turns around in the crowd or begins to dance in place, he seems to look at the rest defiantly, as if to say, "Here I am, and what do you say [to that]?" Really, this is the true Witite dancer. (Bernal 1983:193)

Cayllominos' emphasis on the dancing fights in Carnival led Alfredo Bernal to see the figure as primarily warriorlike or militaristic. Bernal, the only other anthropologist who has written extensively about Witite, downplays the *polleras* and does not portray the dancer as primarily representing a female. Stressing that the hat is helmetlike, the tunic military-style, and the sling a weapon with ammunition, he concludes that the Witite is a "war dance"—one he believes has pre-Hispanic roots (1983: 193–194).

Bernal identifies "the true Witite dancer" as an isolated performer with a haughty, defiant air (1983:193). He bases his characterization partly on observations of performances, but also on his own knowledge and, especially, his expectations of what the character should convey. This aspect of the performative is key. Bernal downplays the female garments, I believe, because he thinks they make the character seem feminine, unmanly. I argue, on the contrary, that the character seems masculine not only in spite of but also because of the skirts. This dependence develops from his appropriation of the objects but also from his manner of self-representation while wearing them. Bernal's interpretation, like mine, is based in the performative—the character's style of dancing, mannerisms, and possibly parodic stance are keys to understanding ritual transvestism.

Through an aggressive exhibition, the Witite shows that he is a man who flaunts masculine bravado, despite the fact that he wears a woman's skirt. He is important precisely because he represents a self who is neither solely male nor female. Even though the Witite's aggressive stance seems to counter the female costume he wears, male and female characteristics are not mutually exclusive. Cayllominos tend to place positive value on female comportment that is subdued, dignified, and composed. I frequently heard both men and women express negative opinions about women who were too bold, danced with many men, and/or spoke too loud or too often. Nonetheless, aggressive behavior is not the exclusive province of men. Because aggression is also a key element of female behavior, it is usually circumscribed. During Carnival, however, Cayllominos not only accept that women act differently but expect them to do so. As aggression is then released into the domain of culture, it is revealed as a human characteristic—

neither male nor female, but wholly cultural and intimately Caylloмino. Although female behavior is sufficiently liberated to take on aspects of the aggression customarily associated with men, this freedom does not replace the strictures on women's normal behavior. Wild behavior is appropriate in the dance and in the plaza, but less acceptable in other public spaces or at other times.

Natalie Zemon Davis (1978:154) has written eloquently about play, power, and "the concept of the unruly woman." Her views are apropos of Witite's performance in the contexts of ethnic, gendered, and cultural aggression. Pujllay purports to be play, and thus displaced from the serious realm of normal life. But the work of play is part of the ongoing construction of daily life, which is why such play is more than mere temporary release from social norms. If unruliness merely destabilizes male domination, then it could ultimately serve to consolidate it. Wildness does characterize women, so aggressive performance may extend beyond Pujllay and, thus, fundamentally threaten the social order. How can play overturn patriarchy? The unruly woman presents an image of a real alternative to male dominance (see also Barnes 2000; Franco 2000). Witite is not merely an aggressive male in female dress, a wolf in grandma's clothes. He also stands for the unruly women who really are women, and he does so by dancing alongside them. These very contradictions are vital to Witite's continued viability in contemporary Caylloma. They are often expressed in discourses about his origin.

Performance, Violence, and History

Witite stories abound throughout the Colca Valley. The tales feature Witite as the symbol of subterfuge, usually connected with conquest, sexual relations, marriage, escape, abduction, or rape—or manifold combinations.[10] When Cayllominos explained to me why Witite is present in Carnival today, they emphasized two distinct things: the origins of the character and the ways the dance has changed. They made it clear that his roots are in the past, a time when gender, race, patriarchal domination, subversion, and violence intersected differently than in the present. The stories share this core: a man disguised himself as a woman in order to trick another person. Cayllominos usually placed the Witite in the distant past, an ancient era before the memory of living people. They identified this past as the time when the Inkas subjugated the Collaguas and Cabanas who ruled the Colca

Valley, or they sometimes conflated the pre-Hispanic and colonial periods. Local folklore holds that Mayta Capac was the Inka who conquered the valley; this emperor's likeness adorns monuments in Coporaque and Chivay. According to Bernabé Cobo (1979 [1653]:119), a Spanish chronicler, when the Inka married Mama Tancaray Yacchi, a daughter of the Collaguas *cacique* (local nobleman), this matrimonial alliance integrated the Collaguas into the empire.[11]

Long ago a man dressed as a woman in order to abduct a woman from her home, recounted Dionisio Rosas, my neighbor in Coporaque.[12] The man and woman both lived in the Colca Valley, but he was of local origin (*originario*) or an Indian (*indio*) and her parents were white or Spanish (*españoles*). Her father refused to let the *indio* even visit the girl, much less marry her. Since she lived in her parents' home, how could the young man be with his beloved? Around the town, women came and went freely, constantly visiting each other's homes. Therefore, the man disguised himself as a woman and went to visit her. Once inside the house, he managed to abduct her. These events took place in the time of Mayta Capac, said Dionisio. Not only that, he elaborated, but the Inka himself had played the same trick. He too had disguised himself as a woman to make off with the *cacique*'s daughter.

Dionisio's first story of trickery and abduction occurred between an Indian and a Spanish family; the second variant, between the Inka and a local leader. By adding the second example, he emphasized that the instance was not unique and that the events occurred in the distant past. His unorthodox chronology adds an intriguing twist. The Inkas preceded the Spanish in the valley by at least a century: in the time of Mayta Capac, ca. A.D. 1420, no Spaniard had yet arrived in Peru. In his view of history, Witite's ancient origin is thereby verified.

Mestizaje figures centrally in both stories. In the conceptual and chronological mixing of Inka and Spanish, ideas about power embedded in the Witite are likewise related to marriage arrangements. Dionisio's account presents two contexts in which stealth and trickery were acceptable in gaining a female mate. *Rapto,* the term he used for "abduction," also can imply "rape" (usually called *violación*); either way, it connotes male violence against women and the unwilling participation of the woman. Another approach to the arrangement, however, also merits investigation: a tradition of "marriage by capture."[13]

Alfredo Bernal mentions that local tradition attributes the Witite's origin to an episode of abduction: "[T]he daughter of some landlord families . . . is courted by an indigenous man; in order to obtain her, the youth disguises himself as a woman and abducts her" (1983:184). He insists, however, that no such abduction ever happened. In colonial times, he continues, there were no large estates (*haciendas*) in the Colca Valley, so there were no such landlords (*terratenientes*). Therefore, neither courtship nor abduction of this type was possible. But the size of the landholdings is not really the issue. Other Cayllominos did mention the importance of power and class, conceiving of a past in which landowners clearly dominated the landless. Bernal, himself a Colca Valley native, apparently wishes to avoid the implication that men abducted women, and maintains, instead, that marriages were arranged between families in a "gentlemanly" manner.

The "suitor," as Dionisio described him, bypassed the traditional marriage negotiation between parents. The young Indian tricked the parents as much as he did the girl. Racial and ethnic difference figures prominently in his narrative as the main reason that the white, Spanish parents objected to the match. The man gained access to the woman's home by disguising himself and taking advantage of acceptable patterns of gendered social interaction. He manipulated gender to cross racial lines, tricked everyone, and made off with the woman he desired.

When I began to analyze the relationships among trickery, conquest, and marriage, I had trouble coming to terms with the suggestion of rape. These stories bothered me because they do not merely leave the suitor's intentions ambiguous, but in fact reduce them to a secondary matter. Did the "robber bridegroom" intend to marry the woman or just to make off with her for a temporary sexual encounter? These stories matter for understanding gendered relations of power in Caylloma, and so it matters if people claim that the woman agreed or not. On one hand, the man removed the woman from the protective custody of the parents' home. As this interprets sexuality as a domain that depends on protection for its restraint, female sexuality can be a significant motivator: if desire were mutual, the woman might have tried to escape and her parents to prevent her. On the other hand, the man appropriated female behavior and dress to trick the parents, which implies that he manipulated norms of social behavior. Ultimately, in interpreting this tale in relation to Witite's contemporary meanings, I had to juggle two readings: it is both a tale of abduction, in which a male imposes his sexual desire against the wills of the female and of the elders, with violence at least an implicit factor, and a metaphor for sexual awakening, in which abduction and escape represent the unleashing of desire.[14]

Male violence against men, however, as well as against women, is a factor here. Stories of the Witite character's origin explore patriarchal structures of domination, implying that male violence against women was a way to impose that domination. While the origins may be lost, in discussing early versions of the Witite dance, explicit claims of violence between men are a recurring theme.

Oral history accounts from former Witites shed light on this violence. Alfredo Bernal (1983) collected them from two elderly Coporaqueños who had danced Witite some forty years before. Luis Condo and Alejandro Taco Apaza said the dance was then quite violent. They characterized it as a "dancing fight" in which men vied "to see who was the best" as they "fought between equals." Both men agreed: slinging was the way to win.

"The Witite dance was . . . terrible," Luis Condo declared bluntly. At age sixty-seven, Condo, a man from Coporaque, explained how Witites danced in his youth (in Bernal 1983:188).

> [We] Witites . . . danced disguised. . . . [We] slung at each other, aiming for the nape of the neck—one, two, even three times! Whoever had the best aim was the best team. No doubt, it was a dancing fight. That was the object of the dance because Pujllay always caused some injuries. Sometimes I cannot explain why we did it. Why did we sling at each other? It was just to see who was the best. We always sought to distinguish ourselves; being all from the same *pueblo* (people/village) and Christians, we seemed enemies.

Rivalry between opposing teams was a central element of the dancing fight.[15] Each of the performing teams represented one sector (*saya*) of the community. Guided by captains, team members fought by slinging fruit or rocks at each other. The dancing fight had a formulaic pattern, including greetings and measured distances. Combatants were to be equally matched; thus victory between teams and individual members could be accurately assessed.

> [T]hey went out to dance in the streets and plazas. . . . [T]hey fought between equals; he who slung the best always won, but only we men danced. The act of slinging at each other was the cen-

tral part of the dance. Dancing in couples is recent. . . . (Alejandro Taco, in Bernal 1983:189–190)

Violence was an integral part of the performance. "Pujllay always caused some injuries . . . ," Condo recalled; "we seemed enemies" (Bernal 1983:188). The combatants intended to inflict damage: "we slung at each other, aiming for the nape of the neck" (Bernal 1983:188), where a solid blow can kill or paralyze the victim. Although the fights were staged and the teams evenly matched, the outcome was not predetermined: they played to win. The conflict in these fights extends into, rather than breaks from, daily life and thus its significance moves beyond ritual. Such fights *are* violent, they are not representations *of* violence; the acts of violence they contain are real, as Orlove (1994:147) has pointed out about similar fights staged throughout the Andes.

Both male and female Cayllominos frequently mentioned the Witite tradition to me as a custom about which I should know more. When I inquired about its history, several people said that in the old days, the slinging sometimes got out of control. More stones than hard fruit found their way into the slings. Dancers sometimes blinded, or even killed, their opponents. State authorities used those deaths as a reason to intervene. They reviewed dancers' ammunition before each dance began (Bernal 1983:201) and ejected individuals who carried rocks. When their policing did not diminish the injuries, they forbade the slinging altogether, probably in the 1950s or 1960s.[16] My research in Coporaque municipal archives indicates that state authorities attempted to ban fiestas as early as the 1930s.

In the past, the Witite dance during Carnival was the domain of men and the fights were between men. Caylloma's women did not perform in it with men but had their own dance. The single women danced together in a performance that was associated with service to the Catholic Church, which encouraged the women to dance as well as to care for agricultural fields that pertained to the local church. The women in charge obtained their own musicians and sang their own songs (Bernal 1983:196–197). Women's songs in Quechua formerly were regular features of Carnival and several other fiestas but are no longer sung, according to a catechist from Coporaque (Seferino Huaraya, personal communication, 1992).

Today, outbursts of violence punctuate Carnival. Fights break out between individuals, frequently buttressed by excessive alcohol consumption. The dances themselves are not fights, however; they are not primarily about violence. Outlawing the fighting apparently sparked two related developments: a less violent type of social encounter evolved, which is the contemporary Witite dance; in it men and women danced together, and the separate men's and women's dances were discontinued. Only within the last few decades did the dancing fight give way to social dances. Most recently, the folklorized versions were introduced, completely nonviolent and ostensibly apolitical productions.

Disguise, Demeanor, and Domination: The Subversion and Inversion of Hierarchy

If play with the concept of the unruly woman is a chance for release from hierarchy, Witite makes us ask: How effective is temporary release? Does subverting authority in fact challenge that authority? If so, to what extent, and under what circumstances? Dress always shapes gender because donning appropriate gendered dress both confirms and challenges cultural conceptions of appropriate gendered behavior. The transvestite plays crucial roles in society precisely because he or she can create and inhabit new gendered and cultural domains. By pushing the boundaries of gender appropriateness, cross-dressers call into question the very meaning of male and female (Garber 1992). In crossing out of normative heterosexual bodily representation, transvestism is transgression. Wearing the dress of the "opposite sex" does not necessarily speak of sexual behaviors; nevertheless, it has serious implications for gender identity and identification.

The Witite's temporally and ritually confined transvestism compels us to attend to the boundaries and hierarchies that dress implies. The Witite is primarily a role within the culturally defined structures of a *cargo*—one that not only is a first rung on the socio-political ladder but depends on public expression for its effectiveness. Transvestism occurs within these bounds. Witites differ from "berdaches" or "third gender" persons because they do not wear female dress daily, carry out other female tasks, or assume a feminized lifestyle for long periods of time.[17] Except in a festival or dance, it would never be appropriate for a man to dress publicly as a Witite. He would not do so, for example, in a political meeting—a formal event where women customarily wear elaborate *polleras* (Chapter 6). According to all Cayllominos with whom I spoke, Witites are not homosexual. Gay activism in Peru is centered in, and almost completely confined to, Lima.[18] In rural communities, neither have I met any out homosexuals, male or female, nor have community residents told me about any. This transvestism, therefore, seems disconnected with nonheterosexual identity. In fact, one common explanation stresses that the Witite dress, far from implying homosexuality, helps young men court girls by reducing parental objection (Gerardo Alfaro, personal communication 2000). In addition, Witite's diffusion into folklore alters his significance as ethnic icon.

Since everyone "knows" the Witite is male beneath his skirts, why does he continue to wear them? What new gendered domains does this transvestite create? Witites use a "feminine mask": their disguise creates a "carnivalesque body" (Russo 1986:225; see also Bakhtin 1984) that, as it is distorted or subverted by dress, also distorts or subverts the social hierarchy that created it. Wearing women's skirts gives a Witite an experience that he shares with women but not with men who do not wear *polleras.* The boundedness of Witites' *pollera* use as a disguise or costume, however, mitigates against potential long-term effects, and does not necessarily make males empathize with female conditions. As males appropriate female identity, they validate male dominance and patriarchal structures of authority, which are key features of Andean social hierarchy. At the same time, this appropriation creates spaces for resistance—both female resistance to the sexual controls of patriarchy, and ethnic resistance to the political controls of white society.

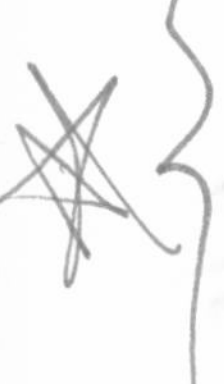

Taking on the Witite *cargo* is a rite of passage through which young men advance toward male adulthood. In these liminal spaces—ritual, festival, and transvestism—Witite plays with sexual desire. His actions must remain "play," however, because as a male in *polleras,* he embodies the inability to reproduce. He is not female in that his figure is ultimately sterile and he could not fulfill another adult male's heterosexual desire. Thus, the carnivalesque body of Witite simultaneously embodies heterosexual attraction and its denial. These contradictory characteristics are not only expressed publicly *in* Carnival, they *stand for* Carnival.

Witite means the subversion of identity: a man assumes the dress of the (supposedly) most subordinate member of society, the indigenous woman. A key element of the story is that women moved freely because others did not notice them. Thus, transvestism accentuates female subordination because it emphasizes women's invisibility. Another key element of the story is that racial difference shaped all the characters' actions. Witite did not fool the parents of just any girl; he was an Indian youth who used subterfuge to fulfill his desires at the expense of a Spanish family. Rather than vanquish domination, he evaded it. Thus, transvestism also accentuates indigenous subordination because the story does not paint the Indian man as a combatant against the Spanish or whites. Even as the story seems to glorify Indian ingenuity in achieving a goal by escaping, it reinforces negative associations of indigenous identity with dishonesty, the conquered with the female, the colonized with the cunning.

In contrast, the elderly men's narratives stressed the dancing fights. As each highly visible fighter opposed another like himself, revenge settled individual scores. The men fought within the bounds of the *saya* teams and, ultimately, social structure did not change: there were still *sayas,* still *cargos,* still *comisarios.* This constancy may support the idea that rituals are merely a "safety valve." If ritual release from authoritative structure is temporary, does ritual always heal the whole social fabric? Far from it. What follows need not be a return to the status quo. Such interpretations of social "rupture" in public events block full understanding of its significance because they depoliticize even the most overtly political events, disregard real historical incidents, and downplay local actors' agency (see Bakhtin 1984; Scott 1990; Turner 1974). The evidence I have presented here, beginning with Alejandro Taco's statement that "there was no justice, justice was done personally" (Bernal 1983:189), suggests a different argument. Refusing to allow state authoritative structures to constrain them, Cayllominos dispensed justice according to their own needs and values. They reconstituted social order in their own terms and accentuated their own control over social forces. In doing so, they asserted that the state system was itself unjust. Through public, local resistance to state domination during Carnival, the men of Caylloma not only showed their awareness of injustice, but performed their resolve to shape their own political fortunes.

Did Cayllomino men "really" kill their opponents or their oppressors? Cayllominos insisted that dancing fights caused deaths, and that these deaths were the reason the fights were outlawed. Thus, they conveyed their understanding that the state wanted to control not only social disorder within the fiesta but the communities' right to stage the fiesta at all. The state considered local cultural traditions important enough to ban. For purposes of this analysis, the fact that Cayllominos assert that they killed others matters more than if they did so. The dances they perform today, and their insistence that the dances have had political meanings, express their awareness that resistance itself is a local cultural tradition.

What role does gender play in Cayllominos' claims about justice? Witites and women intertwine in multifaceted "maskings of maskings," much as Natalie Davis has shown for early modern Europe, when some "unruly women" who took to the streets in protest were women and others, cross-dressed men. Their actions destabilized normal gender relations, even though the limited exercise of liberty occurred within a ritualized time and space. It is precisely the instability of an inverted gender hierarchy that creates spaces for "conflict over efforts to change the basic distribution of power within the society" (Davis 1978:155).

In Caylloma, the mixed messages of cross-dressing apparently indicate that it works only in one direction: performing in *polleras,* the Witite appropriates female garb. There is no corresponding female character who similarly appropriates male costume. It is acceptable for a man dressed like a woman to dance with wild abandon. Is it equally acceptable for a woman to dance that way? I don't think so. Inversion does not just occur within Carnival, it is the essence of all carnivals because it embodies the fantastic. Carnival's very ambiance is defined by displaced gender norms; this displacement does enhance women's position and even changes the power structure, but the structure is not thereby eliminated. Men do not become women by wearing their clothes and they do not ultimately cede male power. Women dance in Carnival wearing their own clothes. Females who emphasize their appearance as female draw more attention to their performance and to their bodies. As these wild unruly women display unprotected female virtue, they also imply unrestrained sexual activity.

The dominant woman "embodies the most despised aspects of 'strong' femininity, and her subordinate position in society is in part underlined in this enactment of power reversal" (Russo 1986:216). What is "sanctioned play for men . . . is always risking self-contempt for women. . . . [I]n the everyday . . . world, women and their bodies . . . are always already transgressive—dangerous, and in danger" (ibid.). By removing the woman from the parents' home, Witite initiated her sexual awakening. Yet the woman already had the potential to express sexual identity. Her parents had to prevent her from expressing it in order to maintain social order. The story affirms that the natal home is the proper place in which to guard female purity—the very purity she is always in danger of losing.

Conclusion

At the first fiesta I ever attended, in Maca in 1986, I saw Witites dance. Although their appearance struck me as odd, I accepted them as one coequal element of the complex performance. At every fiesta I have attended since then—probably one hundred in all—I have seen Witites dance. I learned to ask in advance how many Witites there would be, where they were from, and so forth. While I lived in Peru, their participation came to seem as natural to me as to Cayllominos. Once I returned to the United States, however, my distant vantage point denaturalized Witite and jump-started my analysis of dress and gender in Caylloma. As I wrote, I had to rely on one parenthetical phrase, "*polleras* are worn only by women (except when men wear them in fiestas)." My analysis of that exception does not conform neatly to any one interpretation that any one Cayllomino offered me.

Why do men wear *polleras*? Why do men dance in *polleras*? Focusing on "dancing" helps answer these questions because of its multiple meanings for Caylloma festival participants, for it is in festivals, and only in festivals, that both men and women wear *polleras.* Dancing alone, the Witite gains prestige, playing the culturally sanctioned role of one masked figure among many even as he distinguishes himself as a specialized unique performer. Dancing in couples, young people court and flirt, separating themselves from the group and forming pairs that may become permanent. Dancing in a circle, everyone can participate because everyone knows the steps. Dancing in their hometown, migrants who have left Caylloma's villages rejoin their communities. Dancing in *polleras,* the anthropologist joins the circle, only to be called Witite.

Attending to the other side of "dancing," the backstage of the festival, shows that the people who make the dancers' clothes, cook their food, and serve their *chicha* enable the performance to happen. By correlating performance with social costs, I have shown that large expenditures of money and social resources are valuable investments in social and cultural capital. Paying hundreds, even thousands, of dollars for clothes, food, alcohol, and music is by no means squandering scarce resources, although sponsors sometimes must incur debt to do so. Rather, in difficult economic and political times, "dancing" is one of the multiple strategies of daily survival and future advancement which people must pursue.

Living in Peru as an anthropologist and joining fiestas as a dancer, I found myself compelled to explain the currency of the local cultural performances that continued apace in a nation plagued by violence. Probing the Caylloma case of apparent gender-bending in fiestas forced me both to consult a substantial body of scholarly literature and to depart from it. Being a feminist anthropologist and employing feminist theory was useful but inadequate. Focusing on transvestism required me to tap diverse approaches to diverse sexualities—it required me to become an unruly scholar.

Beginning with a specific performance limited to the festival context, I learned about identity formation in many different domains. In embodying ideas about race and ethnicity, Witite complicates our understanding of gender. Ethnicity structures Cayllominos' strong identification with their rural homes and their use of traditional dances to express local pride. But Cayllominos are also Peruvians. Because all Peruvian rural communities stage fiestas, continuing this traditional ritual also encourages community members to celebrate their national identity. Therefore, the Witite dance has been extended into folklore events and represents Cayllominos regionally and nationally. Even as Cayllominos urged me to dance in disguise, and my participant observation convinced me that the dances are not violent, their claims that veiled aggression is represented pushed me to uncover the "dancing fights." Why did they insist that the dancing men formerly killed each other? Slipping behind the peaceful mask, I confronted the connections between the celebration of tradition and the acclamation of violence generally and male dominance specifically. The local exegeses which emphasize *mestizaje* and its relationship to violence identify Witite's origins in conflicts between natives and outsiders—that is, in Caylloma's lengthy history of invasion and conquest. Claiming that Witite embodies a proud warrior, some Cayllominos, especially men, even identify him with the Inka himself. While this insistence represents a defense against their relative lack of power in Peruvian society, Cayllominos also place the tendency to violence in the past. No one claimed that Witites are warriors today. Rather, people clearly conveyed that they value not only peace but justice. Nevertheless, the Witite is no anachronism. He conjures images of trickery, fighting, conquest, and abduction.

Dancing Witite, I found, invokes two kinds of dominance: male over female and outsider over native. Performing Witite not only feminizes the man, it feminizes the native, thereby associating masculinity with non-native whites (usually glossed as Spaniards). In performing gender, therefore, Cayllominos also represent power as racial and ethnic inequality. The literature on transvestism and on Peruvian ritual initially failed to help me understand what I saw and heard because no substantial study of transvestism in Peru had been published. Juxtaposing "explanations" of transvestism that assumed that it signified homosexuality with recent anthropological contributions that rejected such shaky assumptions, I reconsidered why this association had been so commonplace and had gone so long unquestioned.

The racializing of gender in Peru, whereby "women are more Indian," has been documented (de la Cadena 1995). The Witite case, however, encourages us to inquire into the gendering of race, whereby all Indians are glossed as more female. Octavio Paz famously wrote that masculinity became a fundamental, irremediable problem at the point of conquest, as Spanish men raped native women, so that all Americans became "*hijos de la chingada*," "children of the fucked or the screwed over" (Paz 1989 [1950]; see also Bartra 1987 and Franco 1989:xix, 131).

Highland Peruvian transvestism, an active component of ritual life, is not necessarily connected to homosexuality, third gender(s), transgender(s), or gay activism. In discussions of transvestism, all Cayllominos denied such connections, and at first I took the denials at face value. Ultimately, however, I had to acknowledge that my questions brought risks—those associated with exploring sexuality—and that ethnographic endeavor must leave some secrets. Cayllominos insisted on staging cross-dressed performances even in the darkest days of compromised democratic rule, so dancing in drag might indicate that freedom of expression transcended political repression. But their alternative explanations for drag, I came to believe, also indicated an underlying reluctance to discuss homosexuality—a different, but equally necessary, disguise. Even if an individual performing Witite was "really" gay, I was probably not going to know it. Nobody was likely to come out to this foreign anthropologist because it was just not safe. Much has been written of the "safety valve" that temporary ritual release opens, but there is no safety in being or appearing gay in Peru. But if feminized representation takes on an acceptable cultural neutrality—if it is anesthetized as folklore—then all sexual hierarchy is destabilized and transvestism can mask sexual identity for all.

When I visited Coporaque in 2000, Delia Bernal was living once more in Lima and had not married. She spends several months each year in Coporaque. Young migrants like her still return home—to finance fiestas, to work the fields, to care for their parents—in short, to dance. For both men and women, fiestas embody gender contradictions that simultaneously support and challenge traditional culture. Young people often invest in fiestas—in the entire fiesta system, not just in one fiesta—because other paths to survival and advancement are blocked. Women play primary roles in buttressing the often-shaky social institutions that have eroded along with the rural subsistence base. They even sponsor fiestas, far from only "helping" *mayordomo* husbands. At the same time they apparently acquiesce to parental authority by participating in traditional fiestas, they also subvert that authority by asserting their independence.

When they support fiestas and perform dances, all young people, but especially young women, learn about patriarchal domination over their social and sexual relationships—and about its limits. The Witite stimulates this education. As he covers his "true" identity, this trickster uncovers ways to challenge patriarchy. Feminine in appearance but manly in demeanor, he challenges parental authority even as he supports the patriarchal structure, for he emphasizes that, in choosing a mate, male privilege matters more than female desire. Nevertheless, by using female garb, Witite promotes recognition of women's value. Performing in lavish *polleras* to display wealth and attract men, women are subjects with their own desires as well as desired objects. Through dancing, girls replicate the symbolic action of escaping from the parents' home with the duplicitous Witite. By disguising their desires in skirts, boys learn to subvert authority as well as to invert gender.

The ambiguous Witite, resplendent in *polleras,* is anonymous in his disguise but famed as a cultural icon. The conqueror of women, he represents himself as a conquered woman. These contradictory roles exemplify a cultural tradition that apparently validates subterfuge and manipulation more than confrontation and challenge. A trickster, Witite's mutability is his constancy. He keeps alive collective memory of Caylloma's past, when political rivalries were so severely repressed throughout the year that they were overtly and violently expressed through performance of a specific cultural form on a specific day. Although the violence diminished when armed confrontations were banned, rather than fade away from one fiesta, Witite sprang up hydra-like in many. Pried apart from that political violence, the character has been transformed from combatant to dancer, and the dance itself, from fight to folklore.

6

Marching and Meaning: Ethnic Symbols and Gendered Demonstrations

Impersonating Authority

Spectators assemble in Chivay's central plaza. In rows of chairs outside the Municipal Hall, local authorities sit chatting with representatives of NGOs while residents mill around. Children chase dogs and climb trees. Adults soon fix their attention on the scene before them.

A table and chair are arranged in the street. The Judge takes a seat. A woman in Caylloma-style *polleras* approaches timidly and stands before the table. She has a baby tied in a carrying cloth (*lliklla*) on her back, and her young daughter hides in the *polleras*' folds.

"Your Honor," the woman addresses the Judge in a soft, respectful tone. "I've come to make a complaint against my husband. I pressed charges against him, but the police won't do anything. He beats me, he won't support our children, and he goes with other women." Elaborating these grievances, her composure disintegrates; her voice rises until she is shouting. She calms her agitated baby by bouncing it on her back (Figure 28). "You can do something. Issue a court order in my favor. Make him support us. Please, Your Honor, help me with my case!"

Why does this woman plead with the Judge before the assembled community? Is justice dispensed in public in Chivay? A closer look reveals that the "Judge" is a woman: she wears a man's dark business suit and tie, her hair is bound up in a cap, and her face is disguised by a painted fake mustache. The "Baby" is a plastic doll. In this skit, women play all the parts. The Coporaque Mothers' Club is performing on the International Day of Nonviolence against Women. Accepting the satire's premises, the audience engages with its humor and its graver message.

The pompous Judge, rather than take the Wife's charges seriously, rebukes her for neglecting her Husband. He is a busy, underpaid public servant, he whines, and she is wasting his time. After arguing halfheartedly, the Wife agrees to pay for the court order.

28 THE WIFE IN *POLLERAS* ADDRESSES THE JUDGE.

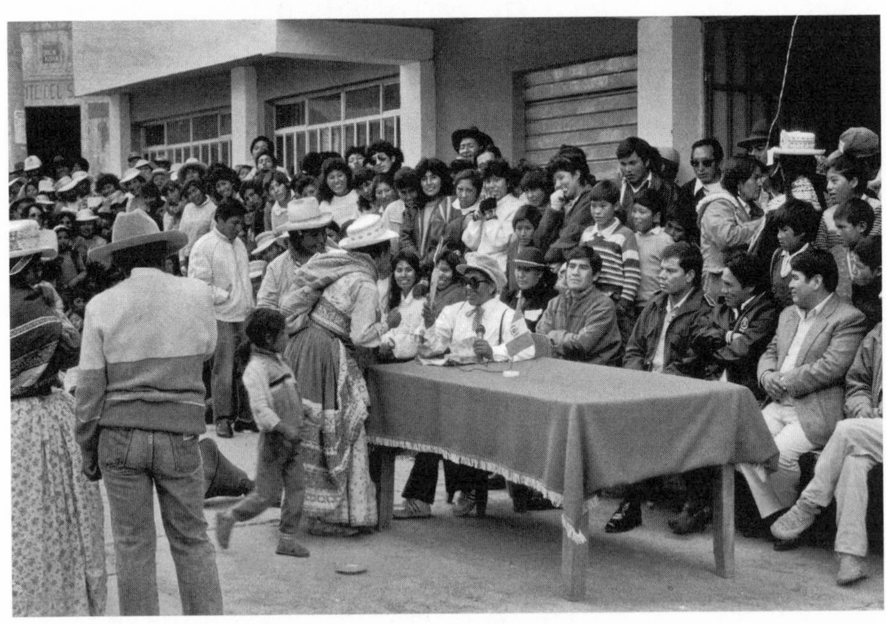

"Here!" She slaps a few bills on the table. "Consider yourself bribed!"

Next the Wife and the Husband appear before the Judge, who mildly admonishes him. He is not supporting his children, the Husband admits, and he is involved with another woman. Enter the Other Woman, also in *polleras,* hugely pregnant. Expecting him to support the new family-to-be, she angrily disputes the Wife's claim to the Husband. Then the Judge switches sides and orders the Husband to support his original family. This only fuels the Other Woman's rage.

"Homewrecker!" shouts the Wife. When the skirmish turns physical, the Husband unwisely attempts to "resolve" the dispute. Separating the women, he hits each in turn until one falls to the ground; the plastic Baby goes flying. The Wife helps the Other Woman to her feet. Uniting in defense, they push away the abusive Husband and berate the ineffective Judge. Finally, the Other Woman sobs out her confession: the father of her unborn child is the Judge, not the Husband! He initially dismissed the Wife, hoping to foist the Other Woman and her child onto the Husband and thus evade his own paternal responsibility. His deception exposed, the performance ends.

The skit was a roaring success. The audience enjoyed the drama tremendously, egging on the characters, who in turn camped it up. Both men and women laughed, although sometimes uneasily, at the exploits. In only ten minutes the performance effectively addressed several serious family and judicial problems. Every element rang true for the audience members with whom I spoke later. This satire about domestic abuse and inadequate child support, enacted in a public forum in the early 1990s, would not have been staged only a few years before.

This was only one of many changes in the presentation of gendered political issues. Skits, marches, and assemblies were sponsored by the Federación de Mujeres Campesinas de Provincia Caylloma (Federation of Peasant Women of Caylloma Province; hereinafter, FEMUCAPC or the Federation). The Coporaque Mothers' Club participated in the Federation's province-wide meeting in Chivay. These large-scale events are nonviolent collective representations staged for political ends. Recognizing that existing structures of authority privilege men's participation, and that the political process benefits men, Cayllominas have initiated new strategies challenging those privileges.

The skit used dress to communicate ideas about gendered politics. In three important ways, this public performance showed how Cayllominas have created new political spaces, and how *polleras* have been deployed in them. First, it portrayed corruption as linked with male bias in the judicial system. Because many Peruvians lack faith in the system, the audience could predict that the male Judge would accept a bribe and side with the Husband. Women, particularly, hesitate to seek redress, especially for gender-related grievances. The Wife won only because she bribed the Judge and the Other Woman shamed him.

Second, it depicted triumph through solidarity. The women shared two bonds: ethnicity and motherhood. Both wore *polleras;* one had a baby, the other was pregnant. Setting aside competition over a man, both women acted to defend family interests, not to advance individual goals. Together they exposed the Judge's corruption and distortion of the system and fought the Husband's domestic abuse. Beginning as rivals, they triumphed as allies.

Third, it drew attention to the intimate bonds among authority, masculinity, and ethnicity. Women in *polleras* bested a man in a suit, using garments which usually occupy opposite ends of an ethnic, gendered, symbolic, political spectrum. The woman acting the Judge "cross-dressed" as a man. If the Judge were a woman, this skit would not even make sense, much less be funny. In Peru, national political positions have long been inseparable from male identity. Very few women run for office; even fewer are elected. The skit's black humor increased with the audience's recognition that playing the role of a judge is the closest a peasant woman would ever come to being one.[1]

Dress was also the primary gendered and ethnic symbol in other public political events. The increasing appearance of political actors in *polleras* in public offers a lens for examining recent national political transformations, as Marcia Stephenson (1999) has noted for Bolivia. Like many Peruvian women, Cayllominas have used numerous "formal" and "informal" channels to claim a share in national institutions and increase their use of the legal system. Some have continued to act in "traditional" women's political style, networking and supporting husbands who hold political office. Others have demanded female access to male positions of authority, simultaneously participating in exclusively female structures of authority as alternatives to the entrenched male-biased institutions.[2] Public performances provide an ideal arena for analyzing how the personal overlaps with the political, often considered a crucial feature of "women's politics." Exploring how women represent "women's issues" in public space and discourse, I find that the appropriation of the physical space of plazas and public buildings is central to the ways they accentuate personal-to-political connections. More generally, *pollera* politics addresses legal and civil rights women have as Peruvian citizens, human rights, and women's rights. Performing their concerns in public space draws attention to women's bodies as contested sites of reproduction and domestic security.

My perceptions of gendered politics in Caylloma public life were fired by attending village council meetings in Coporaque and meetings and marches in Chivay, especially of the two main provincewide women's organizations: Mothers' Clubs and the Peasant Women's Federation. They were also kindled by conversations with many male and female political representatives, among them mayors, a district attorney, a former judge, and members of the Federation and a valleywide farmers' association (APACOLCA, Asociación de Pequeños Agricultores del Colca). Staff members of Peruvian NGOs, especially CAPRODA, which sponsored the Federation, also explained their programs and goals. In addition, in text and images in printed materials, including Federation documents, CAPRODA pamphlets, and Arequipa newspaper articles, I found ample, and sometimes troubling, representations of the ways that gender informs politics in Caylloma.

Theoretical considerations of the body politic undergird my analysis of the ways *polleras* represent the power of ethnicity and motherhood. Focusing on the involvement of the Women's Federation president helped me grasp the broader implications of Caylloma women's organizations. One meeting and one march, in particular, revealed how ensembles of garments behave as political emblems when authenticated in the public domain. Ideas about gender promoted in texts and graphic media, however, rarely square with actual uses of dress. Such contradictions demonstrate how the politics of dress in Caylloma clash with national ideologies of clothing, race, and ethnicity.

Public Culture and Domains of Representation

Dress and the Gender of the Body Politic: Authenticity, Authority, and Autonomy

The actions of authorities and parties, the most frequent subjects of political analyses, have limited value for understanding political practice. It is more fruitful to explore how the domains of gendered and ethnic authenticity and autonomy intersect with political authority. Clothes shape the body politic. Dress links authenticity to authority, for women use *polleras* to indicate that they are entitled to represent their communities. Furthermore, dress links both concepts to autonomy when women claim rights to address critical issues in exclusively female organizations and events.

Gender is one area where Cayllominos' distinct ideas about what makes someone an authentic political actor, representative, or leader do not always correspond with regional or national discourses. The factors that empower local actors also generate conflict with state organizations and NGOs. Communities participating in extralocal organizations constantly struggle for autonomy. At the same time, community autonomy often conflicts with gender autonomy, which in turn is supported by feminist ideologies and practices which some NGOs promote.[3]

Dress can play unique political roles because it is a kind of public space, linking gender and the body politic through visual representations of identity. Self-representation through dress goes beyond personal choice. While public space is most obviously comprised by places where people have the right to appear, assemble, and speak, it is also constituted by intersecting personal spaces. Dress is the first level that mediates between personal and political domains—the human body and the body politic. As the immediate space that surrounds the body, dress extends the individual body to join with the collective physical presence of multiple bodies.

I frequently noticed that most women wore traditional clothes at formal political events in Caylloma, but men rarely did. This is especially apparent because, except at specifically women's events, men usually outnumber women by a huge ratio. Men are also more likely to speak and call attention to themselves. Markedly distinct male and female strategies for authenticating status are part of the gendered division of symbolic labor: appearance is a kind of "work," which men and women do quite differently. Through dress, this symbolic labor occurs in two domains of political representation. First, dress represents the individual—the gendered body and the person. Second, the person represents the group or community. These connect as the body personal—in which dress is synecdoche for identity—is joined to the body politic—in which person is synecdoche for community.

In political theory, "corporeal representation," or the "image of the body politic," means that "one body or agent is taken to stand for a group of diverse bodies" (Gatens 1996:21). Because there is no general body, a privileged part of the body takes on the role of a metonymical representation of a complex body, for example, "head of state." Moira Gatens traces the analogy between parts of the body and the state, as well as the concept of the whole body as representative, to Hobbes. By extension, she reminds us, "Western" political thought has considered "natural authority" to be male and, thus, the authorized political representative to be the male "head of household" (ibid.). Yet because many different bodies are present within the corporate body, a coherent body image cannot effectively be formed to represent the corporate whole (ibid.:25).

Thus, I question maleness as an inherent quality of the body of representation and address the implications of positing that femaleness is central.[4] In Caylloma, the female body has become representative of the political body, but in certain circumstances and privileging specific parts of femaleness. A woman in *polleras* is stating visually, "I am in touch with my roots and close to my home; I am your kin—sister, daughter, and mother." Each woman makes and projects decisions about her political identity as a member of various communities: family, ethnic group, village, region, and nation. Her female identity intersects unevenly with those dimensions of group membership. From the Cayllomino perspective, self-representation in *polleras* corresponds to ethnic divisions of communities more than to race. Because each community (or area of several communities) uses a unique clothing style, *polleras* legitimize the representative who wears its clothes. Cayllominos read the local distinctions so closely that dress cannot stand for a generic or composite Indian identity. Thus, when a woman appears in public in the local *pollera* style, she visually states her membership in one specific community.[5] This condensed symbolic association is another instance of synecdoche through dress. Political representation in a democracy means that a representative stands for his or her community: the person embodies authority. So, who is entitled to represent? Who qualifies as leader, not just member? If the female body is treated as partial, and women's political being as autonomous, to what extent can the woman in *polleras* represent the entire community or political body?

Motherhood is primary among the meanings attached to the bodies of women but not of men. This attachment endows women with unique force in broader political arenas. Conversely, because women concern themselves with the domestic domain and reproductive issues, their concerns are often labeled "natural." Such a false "naturalness" depoliticizes the domestic sphere. As motherhood factors into "women's issues," it structures how "personal" topics become politicized as well as feminized.[6] In Caylloma, as in most peasant communities, almost all adult women are mothers. Nevertheless, adulthood is not the same as motherhood; each entails distinct duties and responsibilities. For political purposes, however, motherhood as a quality *within* femaleness has become primary, to the extent that it *equals* femaleness. In Caylloma, women's political participation is channeled almost exclusively through Mothers' Clubs. Motherhood and family have become political themes connected to the private and public meanings of the body.

Public Image, Public Office: Representation as Visual and Political Discourse

One March afternoon I visited Zenobia Taco Inca at home. The president of the Women's Federation for much of the 1990s, Taco self-identifies as a native of Coporaque, where both sides of her family trace their origins to pre-Columbian times. Outside her house at the edge of town, I looked down on the mottled brown fields where stunted, withering crops testified to the drought's devastation.

Today I hoped to discuss Zenobia's involvement with the local Mothers' Club and the Federation but doubted that she would be home. Some days, Federation work took her to other Caylloma communities. Most days, however, formal political activities were less demanding, and she was usually busy working in her family's agricultural fields with her husband; three children, ages four to twelve; and aged father. Zenobia was home, however; she had the flu. Coming out into the patio, she greeted me and invited me inside. Feeling chilled and not expecting to go out, Zenobia wore *bayeta polleras* over jogging pants. Motioning me to take a chair, she resumed her seat on a sheepskin on the dirt floor in front of the open door and picked up her mending. With no electricity, she needed the sunlight to sew.

I often visit Zenobia when I am in Coporaque. She brims with ideas about how to change the status quo. Today the flu had zapped her usual resolve and she was more contemplative. We chatted as she bent over her four-year-old's overalls.

"I'm patching my little son's pants," she told me. "These children grow so fast, and we can't buy new ones every day. You can patch clothes, but you can't patch bellies," she sighed.

The harvest had already begun, after many months of no rain and severely rationed irrigation water, so the yield would not improve no matter how much it might rain from now on. Her children would go hungry, she was sure, without the food aid obtained through the Mothers' Club. The federal government's Glass of Milk (Vaso de Leche) program guaranteed them breakfast. Through the Women's Federation, they could obtain seed to plant next spring, because there would not be enough seed from this year's harvest. All three programs were organized for and by the women of Caylloma. Compared to the problems Cayllominos faced, however, they amounted to a pittance.

In long double days, women in the valley labor from dawn till dusk in their fields and then manage their households. Cooking and taking food to the fields, encouraging the children to study or do chores, preparing bundles and sacks of harvested grain to take to market—women have such full schedules that they seldom have time to sit and talk about what concerns them. Scarcer still is time to organize to address these concerns.

Taco had learned that, despite its importance, political activism imposed yet another task on already overburdened women. The Federation she worked so hard to organize demands more time and effort than she has. Planning the agenda for an upcoming Federation meeting, she worried about generating more support from other members. Her political work benefited all Cayllominos, but it took time away from her fields and family and brought complaints from her husband and gossip from her neighbors that she neglected her children. Zenobia was so discouraged she contemplated resigning as president. After conversing for almost an hour about her dreams and worries, I left, wondering more about her health than Federation politics.

But several weeks later her usual high energy had returned. Attending a provincewide meeting of the Federation, I stood in the back of Chivay's Municipal Auditorium, looking over a shimmering sea of hats on the heads of a hundred seated women. The delegates, all women, came from communities all over the province. Once my eyes became accustomed to the dim light, I recognized the speaker in front.

"Unity!" cried Zenobia. Her bright red *polleras* swayed as she paced across the stage. Speaking boldly through a microphone in Spanish and Quechua, she encouraged the *compañeras* to stay united. The food and seeds they would receive would help them through the winter. More important, through filling leadership positions and participating, women would advance their goals. Without unity, the women elected to those posts could not go on alone. Working together, they would make the Federation succeed.

If impassioned oratory was a hallmark of Zenobia Taco's political style, so too was her uniform of luxurious *polleras.* In wearing them proudly in the meeting, Taco was not alone. Most wore *polleras;* a few wore pants and sweaters. I attended several meetings of the Organizing Commission and the Federation. Far more women used *polleras* there than in daily life. At the meeting just described, for example, a few women were resplendent in top-grade finery; others were less elegantly attired. *Polleras* appeared in a dazzling array of styles. Some showed beneath the table where officers sat on the auditorium stage. The hat was the most succinct signifier. Almost every woman wore her local style of hat. Exceptions were NGO staff members, representatives of Arequipa women's groups, and me.

Zenobia had presence. All her garments were correctly chosen, coordinated, and perfectly positioned; her carriage was elegant. A Cabaneña representative, in contrast, wore the correct *polleras* and jacket, but her blouse was not the appropriate embroidered one, and because her *corpiño* (vest) did not fit snugly, the blouse puffed out below, as it never does on women who wear *polleras* daily. In this hyperpublic display, habituation influenced self-representation and revealed how accustomed a woman was to wearing *polleras.* Style in composing, inhabiting, and performing an ensemble showed not only personal but communal identity. For three years Zenobia Taco was president of the Organizing Commission. When the Federation was finally constituted, she became its president, too (Figure 29). Taco is a Coporaqueña, in part because her parents were born there and her children as well. Motherhood, kinship, and community membership combined in constituting her right to represent Caylloma. The *polleras* typical of her community were sufficient to signal that right, but her manner of wearing them, signaling habitual use, strengthened her claim to authenticity.

Polleras and Performances in Women's Organizations and Events

During the early 1990s, Peruvians nationwide contended with social problems ranging from the endemic crisis to a cholera epidemic. The ideology that women are more attached to family and children caused many of the problems to be labeled "women's problems." State institutions operated social programs on dwindling resources, church and NGO-sponsored asso-

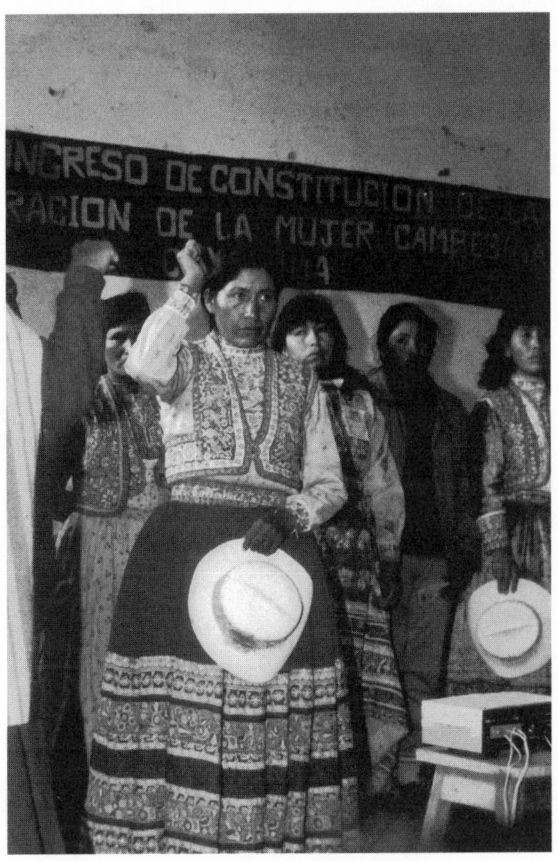

29 Zenobia Taco is sworn in as president of the Women's Federation.

ciations extended their poverty-relief programs, and political parties incorporated women's issues into their platforms.[7]

Politicizing issues considered especially relevant for women has created the new women's politics. By establishing separate organizations, women have seized opportunities to hold positions of authority in democratic structures. Participating in "*concientización*" (consciousness raising) and "*capacitación*" (training) programs, interacting with NGO sponsors, appearing together in public, speaking in public (sometimes using formal oratory in Spanish), and making decisions democratically are aspects of this process. Gender has become an effective basis for social mobilization and resistance, both by increasing participation and by giving structure to "a set of issues around which men as well as women can press for change"

(Eckstein 1989:27). Nevertheless, when these issues are separated as the bases of political mobilization, although "women often mobilize for men's and household concerns, men infrequently mobilize for issues defined as women's concerns. If anyone struggles for 'women's issues,' it is generally only women" (ibid.).

In Caylloma, the gender-based autonomy of participating and occupying positions of authority in women's organizations is inextricably linked with ethnic authenticity. At the same time Caylloma women enter the "formal" political domain, they accentuate their apparent attachment to old values and lifeways. Acting upon common interests also accentuates conflicts, as new political processes simultaneously create openings and problems.

Issues of gender subordination within patriarchal families color every aspect of Cayllominas' political involvement. A few women participate actively in community- and state-linked structures, for example, as members (*vocales*) of a district council (*consejo*). Formal female representation, however, usually means participation in a women's organization: a Mothers' Club or the Peasant Women's Federation.[8] In fact, only members of the Clubs can join the Federation, which is the primary means to expand political participation beyond the community level.

Mothers' Clubs

The Club de Madres is the cornerstone of a series of *asistencialista,* "voluntary," organizations for women first established by the state, the Catholic Church, and NGOs in the late 1960s in urban neighborhoods, especially in Lima, and also in peasant communities (Barrig 1994; Blondet 1990: 34–44, 1991:96). The Church is still the primary sponsor. Clubs expanded greatly in the 1980s to provide education and work for "unemployed" urban women as well as food aid.[9] Education includes literacy, religion, and nutrition. Employment "training" is usually limited to sewing and knitting, or sweeping and planting flowers in the parish. Volunteers from the parish and students from the public university give talks about various civic and moral topics, but the women's interest is rarely piqued. Despite its importance as a building block of women's organizing, the Club's extreme paternalism stifles independent political action. The emphasis on food aid distribution especially enforces relations of dependency.

Because Clubs in rural communities usually replicate the structure and programs of the urban ones, they often fail to meet rural needs.[10] Participation can link rural women with national and international institutions, and with urban members of similar organizations. However, it can also distract women from involvement in other areas of social and political life and is sometimes discouraged by husbands.

In Coporaque's Club, women organized around common goals, planned programs, managed group finances and projects, and worked together democratically. In 1991–1992, Maximiliana Terán was president and Felícitas Bernal, vice-president. Both women were in their late forties, mothers of large families and grandmothers of a baby or two, and respected within the community. Club activities included establishing a seed bank, planting house gardens, building a headquarters, and establishing a lunchroom (*comedor*) in the new structure. Although members were glad they would get seed, they were less enthusiastic about growing lettuce, which they rarely eat. The lunchroom also had limitations; since most local women prepare lunch at home, the diners would probably be the teachers and the nurse. On the other hand, at biweekly meetings, women were able to discuss problems of mutual concern. Of more than one hundred members that year, said Maximiliana, about twenty were quite active in the Club and beyond.

The Peasant Women's Federation

> *[Our goals are] to achieve our rights as the women, mothers, and peasants we are, at the local, provincial, regional, and national level.* — FEDERACIÓN DE MUJERES CAMPESINAS STATUTES (1991)

The Federation emerged in Caylloma and Cotahuasi in the 1990s, after its initial organization in urban Arequipa in 1989, supported by CAPRODA. With its stated objective of achieving women's rights, the Federation is the only large-scale organization for women that is active in Caylloma.[11] It also links the province with the region via branches of the national organization elsewhere in the department of Arequipa and throughout southern Peru, and via national meetings that officers and delegates attend.[12] Federation goals include consciousness raising, acquainting women with their legal rights, and improving women's economic status.[13] It has presented public fora calling attention to these topics and has staged large-scale public displays, including the skit described above, and marches against violence.

In a few short years, the Caylloma Federation made remarkable strides, successfully establishing itself as the legitimate representative of women's interests, creating new links that join Caylloma's women to the state, and helping counteract harmful state policies. The Federation aims to strengthen the position of all women, stressing their similarities and uniting them to work toward common goals. Although some goals were achieved by increasing local representation and awareness of common interests, conflicts within the group were impediments to such achievement. These often originated in intercommunity, class, and ethnic conflicts preexisting in Peruvian society. The Federation ideal is democracy, but members and leaders often have their own ideas about democratic practice.[14] Furthermore, while empowering women to speak and act, Federation participation has not necessarily engendered more traditional political consciousness or practice, namely voting. "I don't get involved in politics" (*No me meto en la política*) is still an oft-heard refrain.

During 1990–1993, the FEMUCAPC was transformed from an Organizing Commission to a full-fledged association registered with the Peruvian state. Crucial to this development were three provincewide meetings in Chivay: two annual Commission meetings and the Constitutional Congress. In April 1991, the Commission held planning sessions, discussions, and elections. At the November 1991 Congress, the members wrote a platform and elected new officers of the board of directors (*junta directiva*). I attended both 1991 meetings, including closed-door sessions, as an invited observer. Watching how work-a-day democratic tasks were accomplished, I saw ideology clash with practice because of differences in intraregional relations and ethnic identity.[15]

The Federation's administrative units correspond to national political divisions. Several Federation delegates are chosen in each Caylloma town or village (District or Recognized Peasant Community), and sometimes one or more of its *anexos* (outlying hamlets); they attend provincial Federation meetings. The main delegate is always the president of the community's Club and the other delegates are usually its officers. Board officers are elected by the whole membership at an annual meeting. Each community has one board member. In addition, a member (sub-secretary) is elected from each of the province's three large sectors: Upper, Middle, and Lower Zones. Despite similar basic needs in all Caylloma communities, different areas have different political, economic, and ecological characteristics, and so have different internal compositions and external relations. These complex relationships are also played out in the Federation.

In participating, women draw on their status as citizens, mothers, and peasants. The Federation's name and structure, and the Clubs' membership requirements, support these criteria, which, even as they overlap, also contradict each other. As citizens, women are encouraged to think of themselves as representatives of legally constituted communities, involved in national processes.[16] As mothers, women apparently are qualified by virtue of their bodies and family duties. Because Federation delegates must be Club members, motherhood becomes elevated to the most important factor in women's participation. Motherhood overrides not only citizenship, but all other criteria linked to female identity and marital status.[17] "Peasant" status, which is also required, remains an ambiguous identity not defined in the statutes.

Two important aspects of identity—ethnicity and race—are ignored in Federation policies. The Federation has no membership criteria involving ethnicity, only class: "peasant." But ethnic politics is a significant factor in power relations in the Federation, as revealed at community and regional levels. Both "*mestiza*" and "Indian" women inhabit almost every community. Differences between them factor into alliances that join *mestizas* in all communities, at the expense of Indians. *Mestizas* usually have more education and experience in public speaking, better command of Spanish, and more familiarity with state and NGO bureaucracies. The structure of political participation favors those who speak persuasively and have more social resources (if not more money).

The board declared its differences with both sponsors and members in the April 1991 meeting. It resigned en masse. Zenobia Taco, as president, led the resignation. This radical move expressed her belief that the membership did not sufficiently support her and the board. The unity she called for in her speech on the morning of the first day proved elusive; that same afternoon, the board resigned. The subsequent raging debate continued for two more days. The controversies underlying the resignation were structured along ethnic and regional lines. Women from the Lower Zone perceived the Middle Zone, where Chivay is located, as dominating the Federation. This led them to challenge the Board, in part prompting the resignations.[18] The membership finally persuaded half the board members to complete their terms. Several *mestizas* were included among those filling the vacant positions.

During the discussion and election, officers' and members' discourses revealed how ethnic differences corresponded to local and sectorial differences. As the representatives of each of the three sectors opposed those of the other two, all used the same criteria to criticize the others: class, ethnicity, and motherhood. For example, one officer claimed that the women seeking board positions were not members in good standing of their communities. These return migrants, she said, did not own land or farm their own fields; instead, they were paraprofessionals employed as *promotoras* (organizers/teachers) for several organizations and NGOs. Thus, as *mestizas,* they were neither peasants nor "authentic" Cayllominas. Others disparaged them as mothers, saying their children did not live with them.

In these challenges to authenticity, cultural knowledge through dress was a contested domain. "Knowing how to wear" was used to evaluate ethnic authenticity as a basis for authority. On the first day of the meeting, I noticed two women in pants and sweaters. They took every opportunity to address the membership, speaking loudly and forcefully in Spanish, and pausing frequently to ask the delegates if they understood. They never spoke in Quechua. The next day, however, when the post-resignation elections were held, both appeared in full embroidered regalia. Because they seldom wear *polleras,* their authenticity as insiders was cast into doubt in symbolic terms. After the Congress, Taco harshly criticized one of them, Melania Jiménez, for faulty *pollera*-wearing. "*¡Ella no sabe llevar!*" (She does not know how to wear [them]), she dismissed her rival's performance. While Taco's judgments were founded in class and racial aspects of ethnicity, underlying them was the ongoing regional rivalry. Jiménez is from Cabanaconde; the former vice-president of the Commission, she was elected Lower Zone sub-secretary. Claims of the superiority of any given part of the valley consistently include ethnic markers, including *polleras.*[19]

Contention notwithstanding, Federation members, officers, and advisors spoke optimistically and enthusiastically about unity among women as peasants and mothers. *Polleras* functioned as a primary symbol of women's legitimacy to represent a community. By wearing elaborate *polleras,* candidates for office demonstrated their qualifications as representatives. But the conflicts that erupted impeded the voiced desire for unity. Ongoing discord between upper and lower valley was replicated in the Federation. Conflict was appropriately symbolized visually by *polleras* on two levels: dressing "*de vestido*" versus "*de polleras,*" and wearing the *pollera* styles of different communities and sectors. The Federation largely smoothed friction by relentlessly emphasizing unified action to achieve specific goals, including the performance of public, collective representations.

Marching against Violence

Every afternoon the wind stirs up dust, rattles the metal roofs, and sways the branches of the slender pines. Today Chivay's plaza is filled with hundreds of women in *polleras* holding placards, assembling in clusters of twenty or thirty. Outside the church a dozen women struggle against the wind. No sooner do they unfurl a long blue banner than it starts to curl out of their hands. A tall woman grasps its center, and another woman pulls one edge tight. Others line up alongside them, and all begin to walk in a procession. Together they straighten the twisting banner so everyone can read it: "Constitutional Congress of the Federation of Peasant Women of Caylloma" (Figure 30). Behind them, groups of women fall into place. Their cardboard placards proclaim the names of Caylloma's villages. Butcher-paper signs express the march's message: "No to violence. Yes to life." This blustery day is November 25, the International Day of Nonviolence against Women. The women of Caylloma have joined together to march in opposition to violence.

Each village's delegation took its turn around the plaza, finally passing the Municipal Hall, where the province's authorities sat on a reviewing

30 A MARCH AGAINST VIOLENCE

CONGRESO DE CONSTITUCION DE LA
FEDERACION DE LA MUJER CAMPESINA

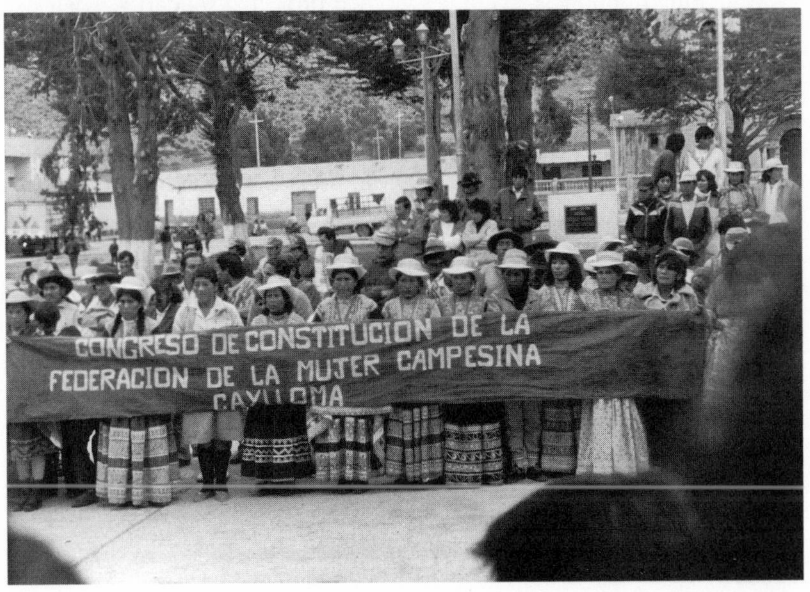

stand. Next to them sat Peruvian soldiers stationed in Caylloma under the state of emergency. Holding the banner were officers of the newly confirmed Caylloma Federation and related groups, including the Cusco Federation. As they paused before the assembled authorities, their presence visually condensed the group's diversity and unity. Ankle-length Caylloma-style *polleras* marked Chivay, Callalli, and Cabanaconde; Chuquibamba, in neighboring Castilla Province, was signaled by knee-length *polleras.* As the women circled, a brass band creaked out a rusty melody and a throng of spectators cheered. Fists raised, some marchers shouted "¡Viva!" But many marched in silent camaraderie amidst the clamor of the band and the rustle of paper as the wind whipped their signs. From start to finish, the march was entirely peaceful.

The women were united in two purposes. The first was to speak out and act out against violence. The Day of Nonviolence, a United Nations initiative celebrated in fifty countries, was observed in Chivay for only the second time in 1991. The organization of the march by community reflected the organization of the Federation. Coordinated in advance with provincial authorities, the march received their full cooperation. The second purpose was to convene the two-day Constitutional Congress for the Federation. Also endorsed by the province, the Congress's meetings and a dance had taken place in the Municipal Hall. The march was its final event.

Marching in public, Caylloma's women projected solidarity. Their use of similar dress enhanced the spirit of collectivity. The women marchers took a courageous stand, challenging the patriarchal domination manifesting as domestic violence within the generalized violence ravaging Peru. This march occurred only four months before Fujimori's *autogolpe,* and within a zone under military occupation. Still, a programmed march like this one differs from a spontaneous demonstration. The gendered autonomy that the FEMUCAPC explicitly mandates is conditioned by interaction with other political structures. Caylloma authorities, including Chivay's mayor, approved the march and then watched it. Official approval constrained the scope of the issues it challenged. There were no signs criticizing the government. Although autonomy empowers women in the Federation, adherence to narrowly defined "women's issues" also defuses its wider impact and dulls its political edge.

Inscribing Ethnicity: A Pamphlet Series

Polleras appear in a series of illustrated, photocopied pamphlets. Inscribing gender and ethnicity in text and graphics, dress is the key to communicating the legitimacy and authenticity of the political actors depicted. The Legal Woman Series (Serie Mujer-Legal) pamphlets, which publicize the joint Federation-CAPRODA legal aid program, are distributed throughout Arequipa's highlands, primarily at Mothers' Club meetings. Their themes include women's rights, human rights, and Peruvian citizenship. Specific issues address freedom from domestic abuse, access to the legal system, and paternal responsibility. In this low-tech, accessible format, women are clearly shown in *polleras:* these contemporary Peruvian citizens are not modernized *mestizas* or generic peasants dressed "*de vestido,*" but ethnic "Indians" dressed "*de polleras.*" Representing the clothed body as a primary site where authority and authenticity intersect, the images evince the instrumental, political uses of clothing, and imply that the value of women's bodies is distinct from that of men's, even when both are ethnic bodies. The following three images vividly represent politics in *polleras.*

"*Basta ya de violencia.*" (Enough violence already.) One drawing shows women marching, much as I witnessed, with a banner reading "No more abuse!" and placards denouncing domestic violence (Figure 31; Serie Mujer-Legal No. 8). The women in braids wear "ethnic" dress with the various jackets, blouses, and hats that mark Caylloma, Castilla, and Puno.

In the second and third images, women exercise their equal rights to political participation (Figure 32; Serie Mujer-Legal No. 1). The two drawings show the voting process and its possible result. The caption explains that women have the same rights as men to vote, elect, and be elected. In the voting scene, as one woman deposits her ballot, other smiling women, men, and children wait in line. The women, who wear hats with ribbon bands and streamers, are from Chuquibamba. In the other scene, a woman holds elected office. "Alcalde" (Mayor) reads the sign. Her hat and jacket indicate that she is from Caylloma; a woman in *polleras* has assumed the post of mayor.[20]

Both pamphlets emphasize women using legal channels as a way to effect change, and promote female solidarity by showing women together. The election pamphlet especially encourages attention to female authority. To persuade readers that political authority can be embodied in women and not just in men, it shows the mayor in Caylloma *polleras.* This message

BASTA YA DE VIOLENCIA, LAS MUJERES QUEREMOS EL AMOR Y LA PAZ
Por esto, compañeras, muchas mujeres en todo el mundo y también en nuestra Region Arequipa, celebramos el dia 25 de Noviembre como
EL DIA DE LA NO-VIOLENCIA CONTRA LA MUJER
AMOR SI GOLPES NO
SI ALGUIEN TE GOLPEA ¡DENUNCIALO!
BASTA DE VIOLENCIA
¡NO MAS MALTRATO!
25 de Noviembre :
DIA DE LA NO VIOLENCIA CONTRA LA MUJER

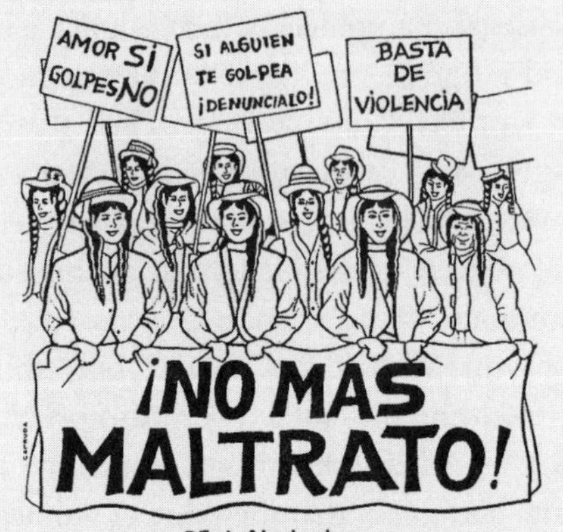

31 Women in *polleras* participate in a political demonstration.

8º
Las mujeres tenemos derecho a votar, elegir y ser elegidas para cargos públicos y ejercer funciones, a nivel de la Comunidad, el Distrito, la Provincia, la Región y la Nación, igualmente que los hombres.
ALCALDE

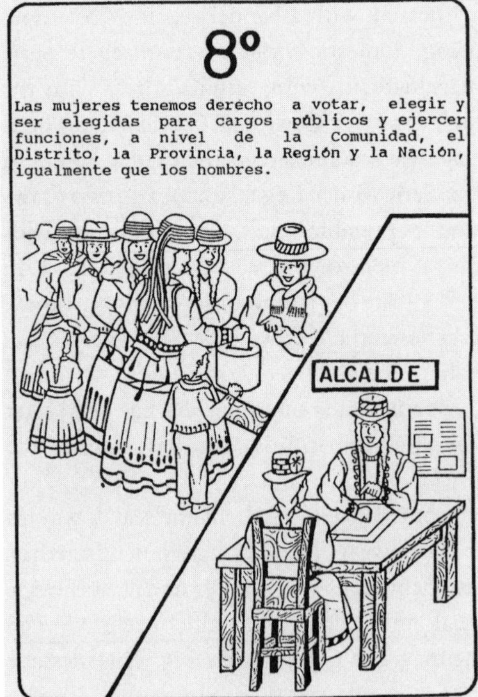

32 Men and women voters; a woman mayor

contrasts with the skit, in which authority was represented by a man impersonated by a woman dressed in male clothes: the Judge.[21] In the last pamphlet, authority was represented by a woman *as a woman,* dressed in female ethnic regalia: the Mayor. Because political representation was identified with maleness, in the skit women had to convey political authority by impersonating males, thus accentuating the fact that, as females, they were denied authority. The pamphlet offers a different message: a woman can have power and authority.

Mayors are elected officials. To get elected, a woman draws on the support of her community. Judges, however, are appointed, not elected, and thus do not require the same degree of community support. The pamphlet depicts the woman as a mayor, not a judge. This is an important distinction because the position of state authority she holds is not a state-appointed position. Her community-based power, signified by her *polleras,* is invested in her person as the elected representative. The realm of the possible remains imaginary because of the type of authority represented, and also because the pamphlets are propaganda. The alternative vision of political authority they promote remains at odds with political reality.

Impersonation, Appropriation, and the Politics of Authenticity

The slipperiness of authenticity is vividly displayed in political performances as women's dress reveals the boundaries of ethnicity. The new women's politics has changed concepts of authenticity and authority. The politics of belonging dictates that each woman affiliate primarily with her community, but that she do so by representing herself as female within the male sphere of political action. She makes this "unnatural" change palatable to her constituents by accentuating her "natural" appearance as mother and as "native" community member.

In Peru, mobility across ethnic boundaries is severely limited. Elite dress is largely "modern," "Western" dress. The business suit is the uniform of political actors, both men and women, at the national level. Upper-class, urban, professional women wear a suit with a skirt; *polleras* are associated with rural indigenous identity. In political events, Cayllominas showed their awareness of class differences within that domain, as *mestizas* wore elaborate, first-quality *polleras,* not everyday ones. Nevertheless, not one Cayllomina represented herself as an elite, suit-wearing professional.

Polleras are ethnic signifiers of political representation because each community has its recognizably unique style. Ethnic identity in this respect is predominantly local identity. But ethnic identity is also racialized in Peru. Dress indicates "Indian" identity as contrasted to white and *mestizo* identity. "Indian" dress, therefore, stands for community, and "white" dress, for nation. In this contrastive pair, Indian is the opposite of Peruvian, not part of it. Dress reinforces the idea that indigenous and national identity are opposed because white dress is largely homogeneous nationally (and transnationally, as white elites from different countries dress similarly).

As the primary emblem of female solidarity, political use of *polleras* apparently transcends ethnicity, yet ambiguity reappears between solidarity and appropriation. In a symbolic inversion, women revindicate an emblem of oppression by transforming it into an emblem of pride. "Indians" take pride in their unique, luxurious dress. *Pollera* politics is also a symbolic subversion: "*mestizas*" also seem proud to wear "Indian" dress. While this appropriation seems anomalous, since indigenous identity is routinely degraded, the localization of ethnicity leaves them few alternatives for representing authenticity.

Impersonation could explain the expanding use of *polleras*. Impersonation is drag: a kind of border-crossing in which representation depends on appropriation, requiring the viewer to recognize contradiction. Perhaps the use of dress in political meetings is similar to that in the skit. That is, *mestizas* who wear *polleras* at Federation meetings are apparently pretending to be somebody (or some bodies) they are not: Indians. These Cayllominas cross a racial line: they appear "Indian" in order to appear female. Why would gender identification take precedence over racial identification? Is it more important to be female than to be non-Indian? With the nationalization of *mestiza* identity and dress, the only way they can visually signal their community affiliation is by appropriating the highly localized *polleras*, which are glossed as indigenous. In fact, *mestiza* women are not impersonating Indians. Rather, they are showing that they are indigenous, that is native, in the sense of being born and raised in the community. Local origin thus becomes deracialized and made palatable as ethnicity.

In the skit, humor hinged on audience recognition that impersonation had gendered dimensions. Women pretended to be people they were not in real life: political authorities. They performed this pretense by cross-dressing, donning male dress suitable to male roles. The female actors manipulated gender through such appropriation to accentuate the equivalence between maleness and authority, and to signal female displacement from spaces of authority, thus calling attention to the limits of their appropriation. As women wear clothes that are not "really" theirs, they also represent themselves as more authentic. We are presented with a paradox: *polleras* seem to have become both more and less authentic emblems of identity.

Although I privilege the "native" gloss of "indigenous" in these instances of public representation, I must point out the limits to the power embedded in the symbol of *polleras.* The fact that Indian dress is the dominant symbol in these political situations might seem to imply that Indians have the dominant position in Caylloma politics. This is not the case. Rather, most political representation is channeled through *mestizos,* whose privileges include education, Spanish-language use, and connections to broader political structures. Focusing our gaze on dress, however, we discern the limits of *mestizaje.* Caylloma *mestizas* do not overreach their symbolic grasp by representing themselves as upper-class urban elites. Although holding back may result from internalized proscriptions, it is more significant that white dress is not the dominant symbol in Caylloma women's politics. White clothes cannot provide community identification, which is necessary for Federation participation. In public fora, *mestizas* need *polleras* to represent themselves as authentic community representatives. They must cede part of their class and race advantage to stress solidarity.

Not all uses of *polleras* constitute impersonation. Still, *pollera* use is not entirely open to all. Indigenous women must use *polleras,* otherwise, what would *mestizas* have to appropriate? If *polleras* were not primarily emblems of ethnic authenticity, appropriation would be meaningless. We need to consider not only what *polleras are* but what they *do. Mestizas* demonstrate their sense of entitlement through dress. Most *mestizas* are natives of communities, who were in fact born there, and differences between *mestizas* and indigenous women are largely questions of categorization, sometimes involving parentage as well as class. On a daily basis, *mestizas* deliberately choose not to wear *polleras;* this is part of what makes them *mestizas.* The same woman may change ethnic affiliation during her life, or be categorized differently by different people. While ethnicity is audience- and context-dependent, nevertheless, *mestiza* use of *polleras* cannot be dismissed as exclusively instrumental. Changing identities is not as simple as changing garments, as effective use of clothing depends on the body knowledge and habituation that come from repeated wearing, from practice.

Even when confined to ceremonial occasions, the way women use *polleras* invokes habitus. This constitutes the set of sensations through which people come to feel "at home" in their *polleras.* Lifelong habituation engenders culturally appropriate posture, stature, and gesture, all of which naturalize the appearance of a woman in *polleras.* A woman who only wears *polleras* occasionally does not share in that habitus. Zenobia challenged a competitor's authenticity for what I call "flawed habituation," defective cultural knowledge: "*no sabe llevar,*" which means both "she doesn't know how to wear," and "she's not accustomed to dressing" in *polleras. Mestiza* women are less capable of wearing *polleras* properly, and women who lack this capability are *mestizas.* Habituation, however, shapes vision as well as the body. All local women see *polleras* constantly. Even women who do not wear *polleras* daily, and so wear them uncomfortably, understand the necessity of *polleras* for representing themselves in politically legitimizing terms. *Polleras* have become the uniform of the female political actor.

Conclusion

Within public culture and performance in Caylloma, ethnic symbols are crucial to political action. One primary aspect of political representation is the physical presence of women and men in public spaces, especially the plaza. Meetings and marches both reflect women's concerns and influence them to think and act collectively. These performances help create new spaces where women engage in new political actions. The Federation, more broadly, offers alternative political culture, encouraging women to participate in the forefront of political action, whereas other political organizations relegate them to the background. It also redefines relationships between women and the communities they represent. As elaborately clothed women come together in meetings and marches, they create one social body, both by acting as a group and by displaying their ethnic regalia. They demonstrate that a female body can signify the body politic.

The establishment of separate women's political organizations in Caylloma has intersected in complex ways with traditional family structures and institutionalized male dominance. The fact that women's politics is linked to motherhood and focused on children and family simultaneously politicizes and re-domesticates women. At the same time, motherhood and native origin have been elevated as symbols of indigenous identity and assigned prominent roles in ethnic identification. With the increased emphasis on maternity and native authenticity, women become the embodiments of community identity, and femaleness comes to occupy a large share of ethnicity. The link between community and identity is likewise symbolized by women's bodies and the garments surrounding and shaping them: *polleras.*

The gendered and ethnic dimensions of Caylloma politics are geared first to community needs. As representatives of communities, women must be attuned to their constituents' demands, for their power is rooted in their community. Whether Indians or *mestizas,* women must endorse traditional roles, representing themselves as wives and mothers as well as community members. Local support is a necessary but not sufficient condition for the success of a female political actor, however, because she must travel in multiple political circles, negotiating local political structures through articulation with national and international ones. Federation delegates represent their province in national meetings.

Dress departs from its traditional meanings and uses to acquire new meanings in new public arenas. Those new meanings, nevertheless, originate in the traditional. Many Cayllominas still wear *polleras* in their daily lives, habituating their bodies into wearing them over the life course. In the ongoing contesting dialectics among local, racial, and class aspects of ethnicity, and between gender and ethnicity, identities encompass internal contradictions. Increasingly, as *polleras* have come to represent these multiple identities, they have become political uniforms that are appropriate even outside Caylloma. As symbols of ethnic strength, however, they do not challenge the class and race barriers that still prevent rural women from appropriating white, elite attire.

Autonomy for women is a double-edged political sword. Emphasizing autonomy may reify separation and further marginalize women's politics (Molyneux 2001:160). The Women's Federation as a social space, and likewise the plaza filled with women as a physical space, may ultimately be reduced to "a space full of women but empty of politics" (Kirkwood 1988: 24). In today's Peru, however, it is a hard, cold fact that political action is often dangerous and stigmatized as subversive. For both reasons, women often claim "I don't get involved in politics." While female authority will clearly gain equal footing with male authority only when women occupy state-sanctioned offices, issues of co-optation and collaboration with authoritarian regimes contaminate that objective. Yet as long as female autonomy is only exercised within women's organizations like the Federation and remains oriented to family and community, its wider impact is limited. Mayors wear suits, not *polleras.* The mayor of Caylloma in *polleras* is still a fantasy.[22]

7

Making Difference: Gender and Production in a Workshop System

Learning to Sew in a Workshop

Susana Bernal opened her Chivay market kiosk in the early morning, after she sent her children off to school. Benefiting from proximity to the bus stop, vendors accommodate travelers' last-minute demands. By nine o'clock, after the Arequipa-bound buses departed, the frenzy yielded to the calmer atmosphere of regular customers' routine transactions. Then Susana and her fellow artisans settled behind their machines and began to embroider (Figure 33). I also began fieldwork sessions then, sometimes conducting formal surveys, other times casually inquiring about sewing techniques or social events. Visiting Susana at her kiosk was a central feature of that work.

One day in April Susana found time to train me. Learning to embroider on the machine, one of my primary fieldwork goals, was tantalizingly elusive as weeks passed and other tasks absorbed us both. After months of schedule-juggling, the agreed-upon week arrived, and I eagerly awaited Susana's return from tending her fields in Coporaque. At long last I would pass from observer to participant. Today I would learn to sew *polleras.*

My anticipation was tinged with apprehension, however. Susana dismissed my suggestion that she teach me in the afternoon in her home workshop. Women with children end their market shift around noon and go home to cook before school lets out at 1 P.M.

"At home those children don't let me do anything," she claimed. Morning in the kiosk would be better. I couldn't hide my dismay.

"Everyone will see me there! They'll laugh at my mistakes."

"Why would they laugh at you? You'll do fine."

So, that morning I found myself sitting in her kiosk.[1] Its public location had commercial advantages. On the outer ring of the fenced-in yard, hers is the last kiosk in the row, on the same corner as a bus stop. Through the chain links, waiting travelers discuss their imminent journey or the price

33 Gerardo Vilcasán at work in his Chivay market kiosk

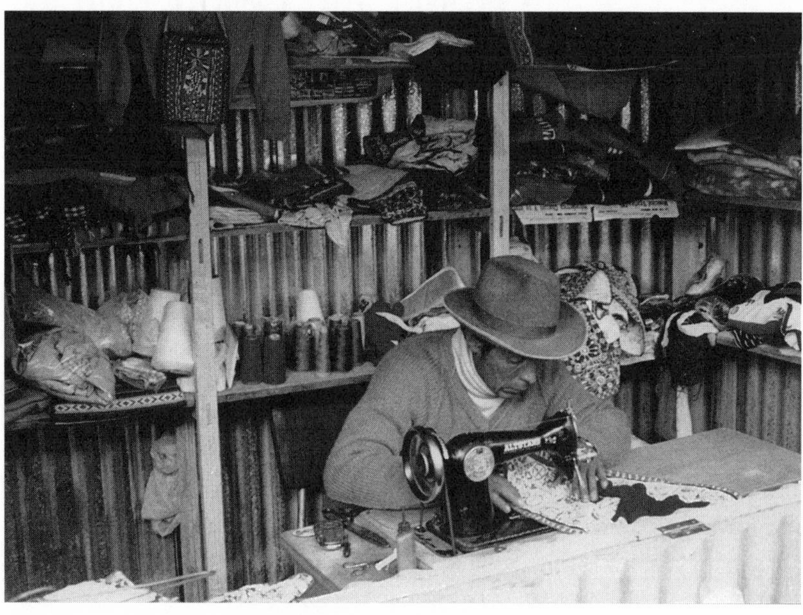

of merchandise. As a traveler and customer, I had often done so. Now, as a worker, I gained a new perspective. People wandering through the market paused to observe my efforts. Although a chest-high counter separated us, rarely have I felt more exposed.

For three mornings, Susana and I worked on two *polleras* for which she had orders. After Susana demonstrated each task, I followed her example. She trained me like any other apprentice, beginning with simple but necessary tasks. A tolerant teacher, Susana gently corrected my mistakes and, as she observed that I grasped the basic techniques, gave pointers to make sewing easier. In eleven years as an embroiderer, she had taught dozens of apprentices to sew, many with no experience.

First we cut polyester fabric into strips for trim. Next she had me sew long straight seams on a *bayeta pollera,* then apply the slippery bands to the rough *bayeta.* Although I had learned to sew at age twelve and had never stopped since, I knew nothing about treadle machines. I began enthusiastically, but failed to achieve the even tempo produced by regular foot pressure; the machine jammed and the thread glumped up under the fabric. As we examined the crooked rows of trim riddled with broken stitches, we joked.

"What's the señora like who commissioned the *pollera*?" I asked.

"Oh, just a señora. She brought me the *bayeta* herself."

"Well, she had better be a blind lady, because no one else would wear this *pollera* with such crooked trim!" I resigned myself to picking out the faulty stitches. Reapplying the trim, I gripped the fabric tighter so it would not slip. Fieldwork requires a sense of humor, but even more a willingness to make a fool of oneself through new experiences. My wounded pride, nonetheless, played a role in my endeavors to succeed. It is one thing to do poorly at something absolutely new, which for a city girl in a country town is almost everything. It is quite another to do poorly at something you think you mastered long ago. Demoralized and frustrated, I advanced slowly. But by the end of the morning, I grew accustomed to the machine's quirks. Developing my own pedaling technique, I attained the elusive rhythm and fell into the comforting monotony of sewing.

Once Susana thought I would do no irreparable damage, she returned to her daily business. During the midmorning lull, vendors do their own errands and neighbors watch their kiosks. Today Susana needed blue fabric for trim. Damiana, her neighbor and cousin, had nothing suitable to lend or trade. With her four-year-old son, Susana went to buy fabric. When they returned, the boy was feverish. She asked me to staff the kiosk while she took him home and put him to bed. Because he was too young for kindergarten, Susana often brought him to work. He played with other vendors' children or napped inside the kiosk. I was concerned about his health and my likely shortcomings as a substitute vendor. She would never leave him home alone. She reassured me that she would stay only until he fell asleep; her sister-in-law, visiting from Coporaque, would stay with him. In addition to being an embroiderer, Susana's husband, Leonardo Mejía, was a substitute schoolteacher, which required temporary residence in a distant community near the town of Caylloma. He was lucky to be hired two years in a row; the downside was being away from home several months at a time. In his absence, Susana relied on Leonardo's siblings and her own.

I worked for Susana in her kiosk for only a few days. From sewing straight seams on one *pollera,* I advanced only to sewing hem binding on another. Through working, I learned technical steps in clothing production and where that production fits in a social economy. By sitting in Susana's kiosk, following directions, observing and imitating her actions, and watching her juggle work and family, I learned how the steps in making *bordados* intersect with the construction of identity as a woman and an embroiderer—with making difference in gendered and professional terms.

The *bayeta pollera* that I helped Susana sew was a typical commission or order (*pedido*). A woman brought her own fabric to the artisan and asked her to embroider and assemble a suitable *pollera,* thus setting in motion a chain of events and relationships. Susana passed the fabric to me, the *operario,* who began the construction process. She, the experienced embroiderer, drew the designs and completed the embroidery. Susana also depended on others to help her fill the customer's order: the *operario* sewed and staffed the kiosk in her absence, neighbors and fellow vendors supplied her with materials, and relatives assisted her with family responsibilities. To accomplish her productive work of embroidery, she had to coordinate the reproductive work of child care and meal preparation, and her other productive work of farming. In an area where family-operated workshops predominate, not only do customers prefer to buy from relatives and friends, but artisans rely on kinship exchange patterns in dealing with each other. Both customers and producers are usually farmers, who use part of their income from selling agricultural produce to buy clothes. While enmeshed in global capitalism, Caylloma's political economy also relies on traditional kinship and gender relations. By interacting with her network, Susana managed to get her embroidery work done, take care of her family, improve her embroidery skills, expand sales to different markets, and even teach an anthropologist to sew.

The interdependent practices of production, reproduction, and exchange, I argue, uniquely intersect in the *bordado* business. This chapter stresses production, centering on relations of production and reproduction within the family workshop (*taller*). Chapter 8 stresses exchange. My analysis shows how relations of production and exchange in the *bordado* business take particular forms for women as they overlap with reproductive activities. My central question, How do people make *polleras*? has these corollaries: Is anything different about how men and women make them? How do different workers perform productive tasks? How do these tasks correlate with skill, prestige, and remuneration?

I have found that petty commodity production (PCP) and feminist theories best illuminate such cultural concepts of "work." Because production is shaped by the spaces in which it occurs, including homes and Chivay market, I have analyzed workshops as productive sites. Workshop organization has multiple permutations, as the chronicle of Susana's and Leonardo's workshop reveals. In focusing on staffing, I have elaborated technical elements of *bordado* production, the acquisition and transmission of skill, and the gender-attribution of tasks and of attitudes toward teaching and learning—all of which shape the gender of labor.

Production, Exchange, and Knowledge: Analyzing Gender in Workshops

Countless times, people told me one notable "fact" about Colca embroidery: the men do it. I heard this claim from embroiderers in the valley, especially men, and from many nonembroiderers, including urban Arequipeños who knew the valley only as tourists. Women, however, rarely report any such thing in the exclusive, confident terms that men favor. They did not claim that women *or* men are the embroiderers. Several times men pronounced themselves *the* embroiderers even as a woman nearby was cutting out or sewing a garment. From answers to survey questions about the tasks that individuals perform, I concluded that half the embroiderers are women. Why would men claim something that was obviously untrue? Why did women agree?

In Caylloma family workshops, as women and men, as workers and kin, embroiderers produce a good whose cultural value derives from the production process. Because garments are handmade, no two are exactly alike. They are produced according to cultural knowledge, which is shared among all users and producers, but also according to gendered knowledge, which has exclusive aspects. In an ideal gendered division of labor, men and women have specific roles in the clothing production process. Through their multiple, constantly changing meanings, however, the underlying concepts of gender, family, and household both sustain and challenge those roles. Ideologies and definitions of "work" incorporate reproductive responsibilities that often fall to women, influence participation in the labor force, and shape the way the workshop system is structured.

A husband-wife team is the core of the embroidery-production unit. Cayllominos consider each shop to have a "head" or "owner" (*dueño*), so in my surveys I asked everyone to identify the *dueño.* Usually, the husband identified himself as such. Only a few workshops are headed by women, according to the responses of both men and women. This suggests a system of patriarchal households, each of which maintained a separate shop under the father's direction. The model did not match the practice. Even in workshops which ostensibly had a male *dueño,* women often had more responsibility and more work. Discrepancies in self-identification as "worker" and "owner" stemmed from contradictory ideologies of work, authority, gender, and marriage.

One important factor in my analysis is space, because work often has been characterized as production according to the place where activities are done as well as their intent. As spaces, the household and the workshop overlap, yet are often treated as distinct. As concepts, the household and the family are distinct, yet are often considered synonymous. Caylloma embroidery encompasses characteristics of household, workplace, and family.

In the Caylloma *bordado* production system, work and workplace intersect in ways inseparable from gendered practices and ideologies. Women engage in a capitalist economy, but in ways that do not rigidly separate home from workplace. Work by women who are not adequately categorized as housewives or wage laborers is a gray area in economic theory, but this type of small-scale enterprise plays a large and vital part in the Peruvian national economy (Babb 1998 [1989]).

Two aspects of Colca Valley workshop production are obvious: a good is produced and it is not exchanged only within the family. Because the system is based on unwaged family labor, rather than wage labor, it is tempting to classify embroidery primarily as reproduction rather than production. It might be considered domestic production, but this too emphasizes its subsistence-oriented facets, which are few. Analyses of small-scale enterprise as petty commodity production (PCP) are useful in helping us understand the productive dimensions of embroidery.[2] To understand how domestic production overlaps with petty commodity production, in attending to work space, I stress the public dimensions of the workshop system. Because much of the production, not only the exchange, of objects takes place in the public spaces of the market and stores, rather than in the confines of the home, I do not consider it primarily domestic production. To distinguish between domestic production and family production, I stress the necessity of separating the concept of family from that of household. Precisely in that separation lies a reconceptualization of the domestic. In addition, because relations of production and exchange are issues of social relations and hierarchy, they inform us about broader relationships among gender, power, and authority.

Petty commodity production and domestic production are both characterized by unwaged labor and rely heavily on family labor and organization. However, PCP cannot be considered merely domestic production writ large. Difference in scale generates different modes of exchange and qualitative changes in relations of production within productive units—units which may, but do not necessarily, coincide with the family or the household.

The term "household" has caused numerous problems because it contains so many inherent ethnocentric and androcentric biases that its analytic usefulness is severely limited, if not actually disabled.[3] "Family" and "domestic group," although closely related, are not synonymous, and a theoretical split of "domestic-political/jural" (or "public-private") into separate domains cannot always be justified. Utilizing critiques of the household concept which focus on its gendered dimensions, I aim to shed new light on Andean productive systems (Femenías 1990).

Examining Cayllomino artisans' activities facilitates understanding how petty commodity production structures workshop systems. Gender plays a decisive part in Cayllomino culture and economy, as it usually does where women play important roles in economically valued activities (which are often textile related; e.g., see Schneider and Weiner 1989; Stephen 1991). Women's active roles in social reproduction are, in turn, crucial in developing and maintaining gendered domains, whether individual, family, or institutional. In artisan communities, reproduction overlaps with learning, which takes place both within families and through apprenticeships served outside the family. Defining reproduction broadly enough to include some aspects of production and exchange challenges the validity of orthodox views, which locate value primarily in production. In Caylloma shops, reproduction, production, and exchange coexist and overlap in part because they utilize kinship networks, in which reciprocal exchanges generate productive tasks.

Embroidery is a business, but not one that results in capital accumulation. Rarely do shops earn enough to reinvest in the business itself, although some artisans and merchants intend to enlarge or expand it. Slim earnings mean that massive expansion, which fundamentally transforms relations of production into a factory system where owner opposes worker, is unlikely to occur.[4] It also means that some workers become alienated, which may sow the seeds of class consciousness.

Workshop, Home, and Kiosk: Productive Practices in Multifunction Spaces

A physical site where clothes are produced, the workshop is also a business, the purposes of which are to make garments, exchange them (usually outside the family), generate income, and occupy one or more persons. All workshops use family labor. Although all have some common characteristics, there is no single typical workshop (see also Femenías 1991a). My discussion of shop space encompasses physical features and organization of the space; operations or tasks performed in it; reasons for using one kind of space rather than, or combined with, another; reasons for changing to, or adding, a different kind of space; and social and gendered relations associated with those spaces. I am particularly concerned with ways that the physical arrangement of productive space relates to gendered and social arrangements of living space and how all of these influence people's decisions about involvement in embroidery production. Restructuring the private and public aspects of work alters a person's identity as a worker and as a man or a woman, even when she leaves the home to work only a few hours daily.

My classification is a flexible template based on standard organizational patterns. Fundamentally, a workshop can be any place where garments are made that contains a sewing machine and a person who knows how to operate it. Becoming familiar with the variety of productive arrangements convinced me that embroidery workshops are distinguished in three basic ways: technology, labor, and production, which generated the guidelines for my survey.[5] First, isolating sewing machine technology, I surveyed only shops that had one or more machines used for embroidery. Second, I specified personnel and labor. A workshop has personnel with the skills necessary to make embroidered garments from start to finish. Family labor is primary, usually unwaged, and sometimes supplemented with paid labor. Third, I isolated shops as places where production dominates over exchange. Numerous stores and stands sell garments made by artisans and/or materials used in garments but do not make those garments themselves; others primarily sell industrial, factory-produced clothes. I surveyed a few for comparison.

Homes and kiosks are distinct but related workshop spaces. All workshops in private homes share some basic similarities in the way they organize space, but there are significant differences between communities. It is in Chivay that about 80 percent of the valley's *bordado* production occurs. My surveys provided approximate percentages and revealed how much the categories overlap: More than 50 percent of Chivay's production is done in the market building, another 35 percent in separate workshops, and the rest in homes. In this urbanized town, there are many commercial venues, and economic differences influence the physical arrangement of domestic space, as people with surplus space either establish a workshop or rent space to others.

In terms of a domestic domain, home implies living space, affective bonds between residents, and primary function as reproductive domain. Nevertheless, home is the first place most embroiderers establish a productive space. Relatively low start-up costs encourage people to enter the business once they have mastered basic skills. Embroidering at home is also attractive because it can be alternated with other tasks, including child care and its close corollary, teaching. In most homes, living and sleeping areas are combined in the same room, where other activities also occur. The workshop is usually part of the living/bedroom(s) or the kitchen, and sometimes both. Establishing a home-shop involves rearranging physical space, which also alters practices and relations of production, thereby creating new social spaces. Home-shops must accommodate the machine, supplies, and stock. The machine is best located near a good light source, usually a window or an open door; it is rarely set up outside. A storage area for regularly used supplies, tools, and materials, and recently finished garments is usually in the room with the machine, and less frequently used materials and the stock of finished garments are kept in a separate room. A typical home lacks sufficient free space to dedicate an entire room to the workshop. To expand a shop, the family may spread the production and storage space among the existing rooms or add a room within the house compound if there is enough land. Space influences scheduling and economy of scale because working year-round is likely to improve earnings. Increasing production requires artisans to devote more space to sewing, have more machines and personnel, enlarge their stock, and, in turn, devote more space to storage. During the off-season, they try to amass a stock, which is usually modest because the vagaries of fashion and the economic crisis mitigate sales success.

Many embroiderers want to have a space dedicated to embroidery which is also an accessible exchange location. The desire to add more personnel, to separate domestic and/or agricultural responsibilities from embroidery, and/or to enlarge storage space also leads artisans to establish a workshop which is not a residence: a kiosk or stand in the market.

Chivay market is a nucleus of production as well as commerce (Figure 34). Open seven days a week, it is the only sizeable market in any community in Caylloma Province and the surrounding rural area outside Arequipa. Not only are more *bordados* available, but the production and exchange of clothing of all kinds is most densely concentrated there. More *bordados* are made in Chivay market than anywhere else in Caylloma (and the world). About 80 percent of embroidery producers in Chivay have a market kiosk or stand. Artisans with stands often accomplish much of their production and sales elsewhere. Kiosks are used primarily for exchange and secondarily for production. Many people have both a home workshop and a kiosk. Food is the most commonly traded item, followed by clothes. Of 150 market stands, about one-third deal in clothes of all types. Of those 50, 18 deal mostly in embroidered clothes—about 12 percent of all market stands. At most of these stands, artisans both make and sell *bordados,* but even vendors who do not primarily sell clothes display the colorful garments.

Inside the building, the stands are open. One main section is shared about equally by clothing vendors, who occupy about 90 percent of the stands that ring the walls, and produce vendors, who occupy two central, double islands. In each clothing stand, goods are stacked on a wooden shelving unit and a counter of planks and crates, with the most enticing, attractive items hung up. Interspersed are a few stands selling plastic dishes, herbs and dyes, cassettes, and sundries. In another section, meat vendors and a restaurant area occupy the entire space. The roofless yard outside is three times larger than the building. The wood-frame kiosks have metal roofs and walls; they are arranged in rows into two large blocks, of forty kiosks each, surrounded by a fence with four gates. A central open area is filled with large tables, each with several stands.

Working with Susana impressed on me how much more public a kiosk is than a home-shop. To embroider there, each artisan places a stool or chair and a machine and performs her craft before anyone strolling through the building or yard. Although kiosks and stands never function as residences, they have attributes of private spaces: each is individually rented, unauthorized persons cannot enter without permission, and, upon leaving, the occupant locks it (or secures a stand with a cloth cover). Each vendor operates her own kiosk, but all share market membership. The market is a pub-

34 CHIVAY MARKET AND CHURCH

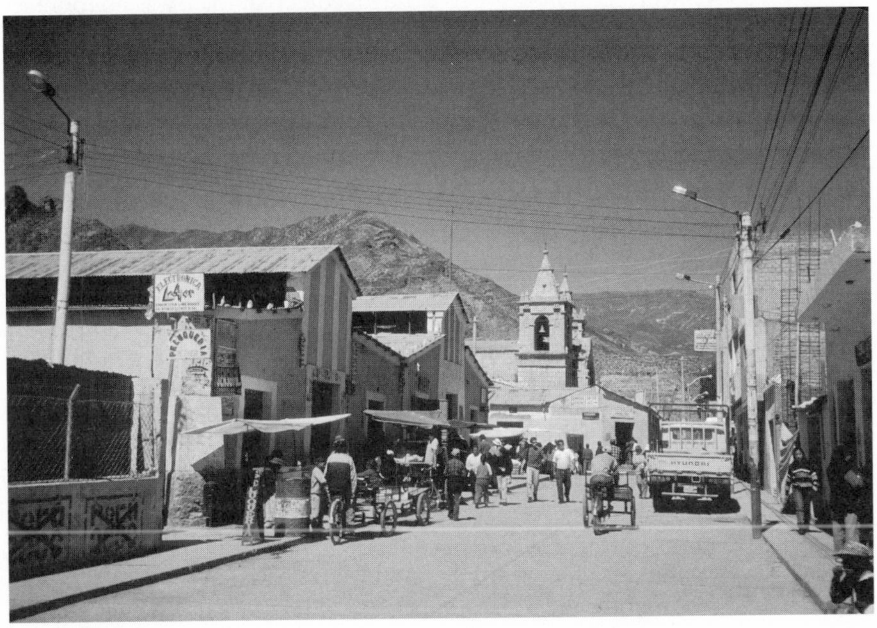

lic space, operated by the municipality of Chivay and open to all comers. Each vendor's responsibility for her own business includes paying membership dues. Privacy and community combine because each vendor/artisan can simultaneously carry out some domestic duties, especially child care, and benefit from fellow vendors' services and support. Small favors and transactions constantly occur during a market day. A sense of community among marketers moderates the individuality and competition.

Susana's and Leonardo's Workshop: Chronicle of a Business

Susana Bernal and Leonardo Mejía have operated an embroidery workshop for fifteen years (as of 2000). We met in 1985. Over the next eight years, they moved their shop and residence five times in two communities, Susana opened a Chivay market kiosk twice, and Leonardo lived and worked as a teacher in two other villages.

Both were born and raised in Coporaque and lived there most of their lives, although Leonardo lived in Arequipa for several years. In their last Coporaque residence, a house on the plaza, they used the large front room as a store, but later made it a workshop, storage room, and living room. To one side of the tiny patio behind it, which had a sink, was their combined bedroom-kitchen, crowded with three beds. Although the plaza location was convenient, the houses are so close together that there was no room to expand. Expecting to maintain their primary household there, they bought a lot three blocks away and planned to build an adobe house.

They moved to Chivay in 1988 to improve their business and their children's opportunities. By opening a market kiosk and living near the market and transportation, they could sew and sell more, including in other towns. Chivay has a high school, which Coporaque does not, so the two girls and two boys would get a better education. Since moving, however, they continue to rent the Coporaque house because they must maintain a residence there. Leonardo twice served as assistant mayor and they have fields which take them back at least weekly, with longer stays necessary for fiestas, sowing, and harvesting.

In Chivay, the first residence/workshop they rented was conveniently located two blocks from the market, but it had more drawbacks than they could overcome. Set at the back of the compound, it had only two tiny rooms, and the furniture, machines, and six family members barely fit inside. After four years, a tavern moved into the street-front room, generating constant noise and traffic. Anticipating that the landlady would rent their rooms for beer storage, they moved.

The next residence, rented in 1992, was a house on a small park six blocks from the Plaza de Armas. It also had only two rooms but was much larger than the previous house, providing sufficient space for the store and workshop. Besides a small kitchen, it had a large room where a curtain divided the living/bedroom area from the store, a common arrangement among small store proprietors. The workshop occupied part of both rooms, with one machine in the kitchen, and two others in the bedroom and the store. They opened the store a few hours daily, usually during lunchtime and after school; the girls attended customers. The earnings were meager, so as they sold the food and sundries, they bought embroidery supplies. The store area functioned as storage for the business, from cases of soda to embroidered garments, and as work space for cutting garments and sewing.

Their next move should prove permanent: they bought a house in 1993. With their slim savings and a microfinance program loan, they purchased a two-room street-front house on Chivay's main avenue. At the edge of town, ten blocks from the plaza, it is farther from downtown than the previous house, but the main street location is advantageous. Their first project was to add another structure with two rooms in the patio. Within three months, the adobe walls were up and the metal roof nailed in place. Susana's father came from Coporaque to help them stucco the walls and finish the rooms. The four children would sleep in the larger room, and the other would be the kitchen. The two existing front rooms would become the parents' bedroom and the workshop.

Susana simultaneously operated her market kiosk, which she opened in 1991. She kept a machine there to embroider while she sold. One night an after-hours robber took most of her stock; she closed temporarily and moved the machine home. Besides appreciating the advantages of the market location, Susana enjoyed running the kiosk independently of Leonardo and working with other vendors instead of staying home. She considers the kiosk hers, but the home-shop is shared with Leonardo. At home, before the new rooms were built, production was complicated by space constraints. One machine was in the bedroom, so after the children went to sleep, she and Leonardo had to sew in the kitchen. A year after the robbery, with her stock replenished, she reopened the kiosk. Once her girls were teenagers, they could take care of the younger boys overnight, after their aunt helped them cook. In addition to producing in both shops, Susana began to travel and sell in other towns.

Wives and Workers: The Gender of Labor

Staffing and Production

Gender and kinship relations thoroughly structure the production process. To establish a workshop is simple, but to guide it to success is difficult indeed. One person with one machine can earn a little money selling the garments he/she makes to family and friends. Earning a modest living as an artisan depends on deployment of social and material resources, perseverance, and discipline, as well as talent and skill. Making *bordados* is shaped by gender in part because it requires qualitatively different kinds of cognitive knowledge. First, knowledge of the female body is required to cut and tailor garments to the appropriate size and style. Second, knowledge of sewing is needed to use the machine to create appropriate garment and embroidery designs.

In staffing workshops, readily available skilled labor is paramount for completing garments in a timely manner. In this kin-based system, about half of workshops use only the labor of both spouses, and another 20 percent regularly tap the labor of their offspring. Additional labor is usually provided by other relatives. Occasionally *operarios* are hired. Staffing needs are shaped by the tasks required to make an embroidered garment, which owners assign according to the worker's current knowledge and ability to learn new skills. Eight basic tasks in the production-and-exchange process are: buy, sell, measure, cut, assemble, embroider-draw, embroider–fill in, and teach. Other kinds of labor support the workshop, providing the embroiderers with time to sew and teach.

Gender correlates with the value assigned to various tasks. Drawing, the single most gender-segregated task, is overwhelmingly a male activity. Measuring, cutting, and teaching tend to be female tasks, but the gender gap is far smaller than for drawing. In evaluating gender-specific tasks, men tend to value "male" tasks most highly, but women share their opinion surprisingly often. Women also emphasize the importance of other skills, like cutting and fitting, which men may downplay or ignore. Gendered values extend to teaching and learning, which often proceed through apprenticeship. The gender of labor links performance to production, as artisans and persons are produced through learning and accomplishing their work.

"Work" itself was also gendered. "I don't work," answered many women in the surveys when I asked, "Who works in the shop?" Often they were sewing even as they spoke! Men rarely demurred. Defining "work," "worker," and "owner," although a vexing problem, opened the door to my understanding gender in shops. Among the fifty workshops surveyed, the largest has six workers, and is the only one with so many; most have two or three; and five have only one worker. About two-thirds are nuclear family based. Typically, a married couple works with one other relative, usually an adult child. Siblings and cousins are frequent contributors in one-third; another 20 percent use other relatives, especially in-laws. Three generations work together in the same shop only in 12 percent of cases. The use of hired workers is uneven. Only one workshop I surveyed, Ocsa, uses only *operarios* and no family members; 10 percent use them regularly, and several hire them occasionally.

At first glance, men overwhelmingly dominate shop ownership. In 90 percent, a man is an owner. There is a sole male owner (*dueño*) in about 30 percent; shared ownership between spouses in more than 60 percent; and a sole female owner, always married, in less than 10 percent. For workers, the overall male:female ratio is roughly equal, but unevenly distributed. Three-quarters of workshops have equal numbers of male and female workers, but the rest show a pronounced gender imbalance, usually having more men. Ten unmarried men work alone or with their brothers. The Condori workshop is the extreme: five men and one woman (the owner's daughter).

In establishing who was the *dueño,* the wife often stated that her husband was, and then explained that she did all the work because he never sewed anything. In the most disturbing case, only three minutes into the survey, a female artisan-vendor named her husband as *dueño,* then burst into tears and told me that he, an alcoholic, had abandoned the family so she ran the business alone. Among married couples, both husband and wife sometimes claimed to be the owner. Three married women specifically identified themselves as heads: Damiana Sarayasi of Chivay market, Rosalía Valera of Coporaque, and Clorinda Maqui of Cabanaconde. Their husbands, who did not, are not from Caylloma and claim limited knowledge of sewing.

A typical disagreement about who worked in the shop occurred between Susana Bernal's brother and sister-in-law. Saturnino Bernal and Leandrina Ramos run a two-person shop in Chivay—according to him. Leandrina maintained, however, that they employed a third person, Saturnino's sixteen-year-old nephew. Ernesto, the son of Saturnino's oldest sister, Felícitas, had recently learned to embroider in his parents' shop in Coporaque, where he lives with them. Sometimes, however, he assisted his uncle and aunt in Chivay, where he attends high school. Staffers generally did not mention this kind of casual labor. Susana has another brother, Hilario, who sometimes lent a hand, especially while Leonardo was away teaching. I found Hilario in her shop several times, diligently cutting garments and drawing designs, but Susana never said he worked there and did not include him in her survey answers.

Generational relationships also influence how relatives are defined as workers. The oldest generation, who began the embroidery tradition about sixty years ago, is rarely active now. Only seven people I surveyed are over sixty years old. Two-thirds of embroiderers are between twenty and forty. Typically, adult children of embroiderers stay in the business, taking over when the parent retires. The Tejada shop of Cabanaconde is one of the few three-generation shops. Juan Tejada, several adult sons, and some grandsons work together. His youngest children learn alongside grandchildren the same age. His wife, Eufemia Bernal, sells *bordados* but does not sew. Again, these arrangements are not exclusive, and another son sometimes contributes labor to his father's shop, but "work" is what he does in his own shop.

At the other extreme is the single-worker shop. In the surveys, only men said that they "work alone." This meant they could complete most or all of the tasks by themselves. Occasionally, they do so. More often, "alone" means one artisan draws and designs the garment and a relative does the remaining tasks. This characterization relates to the male propensity to value drawing. It sometimes means that the artisan prefers to remain undisturbed in the workshop. The "Chivay Chino," with two shops in Arequipa, works at home; his wife staffs the shop near San Camilo, the central market. "He doesn't come out of his house," she told me. Emphatically a solo actor, he dislikes being distracted while sewing.

Non-kin labor is rarely used. The term "*operario,*" glossed as "operator," "worker," or "apprentice," is applied exclusively to nonrelatives, contracted orally for specific periods (Figure 35). Most commonly, they work for board, especially as novices, and later earn money for piecework. Rodolfo Cayo, one of four siblings with market kiosks, learned embroidery as an *operario* in Cabanaconde. While an apprentice (*aprendiz*), he was not paid with money, only with room and board. His job was to sew straight seams and apply trim, but after hours on his own, he copied garments and so learned to draw. The lack of pay often propels apprentices to strike out on their own as soon as they grasp basic skills. To avoid losing skilled workers,

35 JUAN DE DIOS CHOQUEHUANCA APPLIES YARN TO A *POLLERA*.

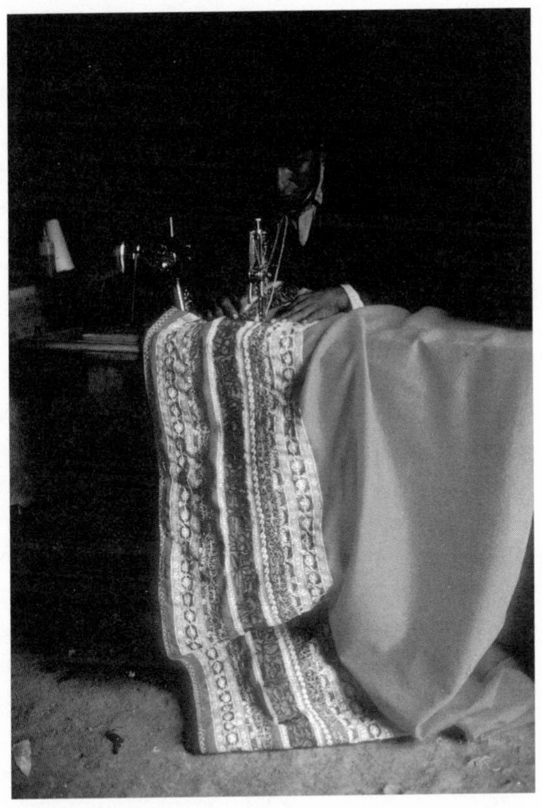

owners postpone teaching specialized skills, especially drawing, until an *operario* has been in the shop for a while. One-quarter of embroiderers surveyed learned as *operarios* in other people's shops before establishing their own shop.[6] In a few cases, an *operario* married someone in the shop: another *operario,* the owner's child, or the owner.

In the workshop development cycle, young embroiderers, as they become adults, may continue to work in their parents' shop or go to work in someone else's shop. Because most shops are operated by couples, and because married women sometimes run their own workshops but single women never do, marriage is more important for a woman than a man in creating an independent workshop. Contradictory forces tug at married women embroiderers because they are also farmers and mothers. Once their children have their own families and businesses, artisans may retire and/or emigrate to the city to live with children there. Frequently, however, grandparents who no longer "work" in the shop just alter their responsibilities, giving their children time to sew and sell by assuming non-embroidery duties, including child care and house building. The socialization aspect of child care is an important component of the embroidery business. Caregivers often supervise learning, helping children and grandchildren acquire skills such as measuring cloth. Access to social and kinship networks enables all embroiderers, but especially women, to accomplish all their productive and reproductive tasks.

"I Learned All by Myself": Apprenticeship and Social Reproduction

Embroidery is learned but not taught. When I asked how people learned, they commonly replied, "I learned all by myself" (. . . *solito/a no más*). Not only did no one teach her, claimed one woman, but her parents did not want her to learn. Because she had always wanted to sew, the child used her father's machines when he was out. (She conceded his legitimate concern about damage to equipment.) Discussions of "traditional crafts" often make the "handing down" of skills from generation to generation (usually, "father to son") central to the very definition of "tradition." Pride in mastering a family craft, exclusivity and even secrecy in joining a guild, and prolonged apprenticeship periods are often mentioned as important influences on skill transmission.[7] The role of gender in characterizing craft-related skills and the overall socialization process, while also major factors in skill transmission and value, has received less attention. Cayllominos' "*solito*" claims indicate determination and pride in achievement even in the face of opposition, but their attitudes toward learning also reveal how they value teaching and knowledge. How is knowledge passed on when one (or both) participant(s) does not believe that "teaching" is the activity that is occurring?

It is relatively easy to achieve technical competence at fundamental tasks. Novices learn each task in sequence based on the artisan's assessment of its difficulty and her need to get it done. For example, Susana had me sew straight seams. Although this enabled me to practice, she needed to have them sewn; it was a real *pollera* to be sold, not a sample. After basic sewing, the next steps are a proving ground, as the apprentice learns to decorate garments, develops a feel for the craft, masters a variety of techniques, and becomes a versatile member of the staff. With experience, artisans perfect the nuances, attaining skill and perhaps art.

Apprenticeship follows two general trajectories. Over three-quarters of artisans surveyed learned from relatives, and the rest as *operarios* in other shops. Typically, the embroiderer grows up in an embroidering family. In the workshop day in–day out, observing her parents or siblings embroider, and trying to make herself useful, a child begins unaware to acquire skills. In the workshops I visited, most parents were tolerant of children's intrusions into their work, despite occasional exasperation. They were more comfortable than I with letting children handle dangerous objects like scissors! Gradually I also let children help me work. When I collected fabric and trim samples, the youngest Condori daughter, age six, was a somber, dedicated assistant. She helped me choose fabrics and, holding huge tailor shears carefully with two hands, cut swatches and trimmed threads.

As the child grows up and her motor skills, attention span, and ability to assume responsibility increase, she can participate more, learning to sew straight seams about age eleven. Occasionally a child will learn to embroider. It was quite a shock, the first time I walked into the Condori shop, to see a boy embroidering. The twelve-year-old, barely taller than the machine, was filling in colors, not just sewing seams. Other family members proudly predicted that his early prowess indicated he would surpass his father and siblings.[8]

Twenty-five percent of embroiderers surveyed learned as *operarios;* they generally do not come from embroidering families. Some went on to have their own shops, but others work as *operarios* in other shops, usually providing surplus or casual labor. For most *operarios,* apprenticeship is a long-term process, from several months to a year, so the initial learning experience is a serious episode in the future embroiderer's career.[9] Only a few people are now working as *operarios,* and most of them are still apprentices. For example, Santos Checca is the only non-family member in the Condori shop. Paid a piece rate, he must work quickly, assembling *polleras* and applying trim. Thirty years old when we spoke, he had been an accomplished weaver in his hometown, Sibayo (fifteen miles upriver from Chivay). Now he was trying embroidery with the goal of earning more. As of our interview, he had only been sewing for a month and was undecided about staying with the job because it demanded a rapid pace and long hours. Of all the people with whom I ever spoke, he was the only one who said a workshop was like a factory (*fábrica*).

"Learning alone" for apprentices, like "working alone" for skilled embroiderers, was a matter of perception. Not one self-proclaimed autodidact I interviewed actually had purchased a machine and taught him- or herself without help. Learning always had occurred in a skilled embroiderer's shop. Imitation does not suffice as a learning method. Parents and other artisans lay out basic guidelines and correct errors. For the working *operario,* each error means a reduction in pay, which provides an incentive to learn quickly. For the shop owner, as well, errors cost materials and time.

Susana Bernal developed her own method to teach beginners. Although *operarios* quickly learned to sew straight seams, they often had difficulty making the transition to the tightly curved embroidery stitching. Annoyed with the time and thread wasted on hundreds of tiny bad stitches, Susana decided to let apprentices practice with an unthreaded needle on paper. Only if they successfully sewed in a circle with the feed dog down and drew basic patterns without ripping up the paper did they advance to threaded needle on fabric.

"Apprenticeship," therefore, encompasses many different types of learning experiences. When I asked embroiderers how long it took to learn to embroider, their answers ranged widely, from one week to two years. I initially attributed the discrepancies to individual differences in ability to master skills but soon realized that differences also inhere in the varied tasks themselves, expectations about accomplishments, and goals in using those skills.

The production system is flexible, even idiosyncratic. In the Condori workshop, an adult male *operario* learned alongside the owner's twelve-year-old. In *bordados*' heyday in the 1970s, the Supo-Casaperalta shop had sixteen *operarios,* with apprentices coming and going constantly. In today's moribund economy, few shops can take on unskilled apprentices, especially the smallest ones, for an individual owner has little time to train helpers.

Learning, in general, and apprenticeship, in particular, are rarely analyzed in literature on the Andes.[10] The learner's active role demands further attention. In learning to weave, for example, children's mimicry predominates over parents' oral instruction (Franquemont and Franquemont 1987; Medlin 1986). Assumptions about the "automatic" nature of social reproduction disguise the immense quantity of knowledge, as well as the amount of practice, required to master craft activities. At the other extreme, discussions of workshops as factories-in-the-making, based on the "guild" model, sometimes presume that the novice masters tasks in a strict sequence and that upward mobility is his goal. In urban La Paz, Bolivia, concludes Hans Buechler, apprentices in various trades have "the ultimate objective of becoming an independent producer" (1989:37). In Caylloma embroidery shops, even when apprentices become *operarios* quickly by acquiring adequate skills, establishing an independent shop is not necessarily their goal. Rather, embroidery is more often a temporary supplement to, or substitute for, other ways of earning a living, such as farming their own plots, getting hired locally as a day laborer, migrating to the coast for the harvest, weaving, and marketing.

In the *bordado* system, family labor predominates. Unlike a guild system, it does not feature specific, named levels of skill, like "journeyman," through which the apprentice must advance. Attaining technical skill is not the only factor in success. Embroiderers who excel in artistry and creativity are not always the most financially successful, for they may produce few garments. In fact, one of the oldest embroiderers is one of the least skilled. After embroidering for more than thirty years, this elderly man continues to work when health permits, producing garments with uneven designs, skimpy amounts of thread, and cheap materials. As his eyesight worsened, the quality of his work declined, but because he prices garments accordingly, he stays in business, serving the many women who cannot afford luxurious garments.

"I Don't Work, I Just Help My Family": Gendered Tasks and the Social Value of Labor

Fieldwork brings joy when encountering unexpected contradictions on a daily basis makes you rethink your position. One day I found Gerardo Vilcasán at home in Coporaque, cheerfully embroidering flowers on a vest. Only the day before I had seen him in his patio, shoveling mud to make adobe bricks. It jarred me to see him doing two such distinct jobs, but he was apparently quite at ease with both. The contradiction, I decided, lay in my preconceptions about sewing. In the United States, sewing is generally a female task. Only certain narrow aspects fit the profile of a male activity. Tailoring, designing, and cutting have long been male-dominated trades in the garment industry, but home sewing is women's province, associated with necessity and poverty—"making" as "making do." In Caylloma, however, both men and women are involved in embroidering women's clothes. Nonetheless, they perform some different tasks.

The gendered division of labor in embroidery has practical and ideological facets; some relate to women's bodies, some to artistic expression, and all influence the value imputed to gendered tasks. Men usually draw the designs and, in turn, prize this activity, evaluating it higher than women do. Drawing, associated with skill and artistry, brings prestige to an individual artist, which attracts more business and allows him to command higher prices. Drawing is labor, however, not just design. In some respects it plays a minor role, for it takes only a small amount of the total time spent making a garment. But because men often view drawing as the most important step, for them it stands for the entire production process. When they say "men embroider" they tend to mean "men draw the designs."

While the gendered ranking of tasks influences the overall production-and-exchange process, other factors may matter more to the consumer. No matter how ardently they desire the latest fashions, most women also care about cost and quality, the timely completion of a commissioned garment or ensemble, and the proper fit of each garment. Responsibility for these aspects of production tends to fall to women.

Influencing women's varied attitudes toward embroidery, it emerged, are questions of control. Women contest men's control (or claims to control), to some extent, by promoting the importance of their tasks, performing tasks usually done by men, and even running their own shops. The amount of time that men and women invest in the total process also varies. The surveys clearly show that in most shops, women do more productive work: they perform a wider variety of tasks on a regular basis and put in more hours for more weeks of the year. The amount of each worker's productive labor, his or her control over the production process, and his or her share of the earnings are all different matters. The kinds of tasks and the amount of time spent on them depend on family relations, individual preferences for embroidery tasks, and other activities both in and out of the shop. Some tasks are more compatible with embroidering than others. Drawing may be more compatible with men's other duties or, more likely, with their perception of their duties. Once several garments are prepared, an individual artisan can quickly draw designs on all of them, leaving the color-filling and garment completion for other workers. Thus, men can draw a lot in a little time. Women tend to spend more time in the shops and, when they leave, to stay away for shorter periods. They usually go for a few days, such as to fairs, but sometimes have longer absences during school vacations to visit distant relatives or take the children to Arequipa. Men, on the other hand, tend to work in the shops more sporadically, for shorter, more intense periods; when they go away, they stay gone longer, perhaps spending several months working in mining, agriculture, or schoolteaching.

My *compadres* Juan Condori and Nilda Bernal, an embroidering couple, offer an example. While Juan was away working in the Caylloma mine, Nilda stayed involved in embroidery. Nilda does not draw. She cut and began assembling several garments and filled colors on others Juan had drawn. When he returned to Coporaque several months later, she had a stack of garments ready for him to draw. Juan quickly became involved with the district council, and his civic duties kept him from sewing. Nilda became so concerned about meeting promised deadlines for garments-in-progress that she once urged him to get up at dawn to complete a commission. Although Nilda relied on Juan's skills at drawing, she kept every other aspect of the business running.

All married couples have different relationships, but a woman's flexibility to perform embroidery tasks depends heavily on kinship relations—with her husband, but even more so with her siblings and in-laws. It is a contradiction, and one that causes considerable tension, that married women have the network and contacts to be good traders but less free time for travel. Child care consumes women's time, but women who have fewer children are not necessarily freer to travel; rather, they may be more restricted because they lack older children to look after the younger ones in their absence. Nilda turned to older female relatives for child care; she partly reciprocated by selling her mother-in-law's goods as well as her own.

Although more women are now doing the "male" activity of drawing, "women's" tasks have barely penetrated the male domain. In Arequipa, the "Chivay Chino" and his wife, Natividad, both work at embroidery, in particular, making luxury fiesta garments. Beyond specializing in fine drawing, he cultivates the mystique of the artiste, "working alone." Natividad takes an active role in fitting garments as well as assembling and attaching trim. In their downtown workshop, she showed me several *corpiños* (vests) to fit different size women's torsos. The *corpiño,* she insisted, was "the basic, the essential" thing; fit was everything. She had taken classes in *corte y confección* (cutting and sewing). Such classes are often promoted by women's groups and NGOs to help women obtain supposedly marketable skills. Improving her skills, Natividad believed, had given their business an edge because women increasingly demand *corpiños* that fit their bodies.

Cutting, shaping, and sizing garments are tasks that affect production and exchange in ways primarily linked to women. The work requires a familiarity with the female body that differs from the aesthetics of exterior appearance. This kind of intimate, somatic, kinesthetic knowledge comes from wearing *polleras,* so women's personal experience enables them to contribute uniquely to *pollera* production. As both users and producers, women may be the harshest critics of other women's taste in *bordados.* Fitting garments is largely a female task, often done at home, and one that only a few embroidery shops take time to do. After purchasing a garment, customers often must take in the *corpiño* side seams, and they routinely hand-sew the waistband on the *pollera* and snaps on the blouse collar and cuffs. The kind of bodily knowledge involved in measuring and fitting remains private knowledge for each woman and gendered knowledge among all women. Women know the female body in ways that men do not, and the intimate contact of fitting remains an arena of privacy where men should not become involved (except when males wear *polleras* as Witites).

Given that women sometimes do all the tasks, why do men say they are the embroiderers? How do the tasks of production intersect with the overall relations of production? And how does control over embroidery production intersect with gender and status? To a certain extent, male control over embroidery involves control over women: control over women's images and control over women's labor. Many of the men who said that they were owners were the same ones who said that men embroider or that they worked alone. Thus, they downplayed the women's contributions, treating female tasks as domestic labor. This is not strictly a male distortion, for women often concur in this characterization, stating that they are "just helping their families."

By stressing the importance of design and of the individual artist, men associate themselves with the realm of fashion. Caylloma identity, in part, depends on identification with a specific community and its dress style. As men seek to create a certain look among "their" women, promoting ethnic images is not only a question of cultural aesthetics but one of influence over female behavior. Men become designers, directing fashion as a way to control the display of women's bodies. Simultaneously covered from head to foot by garments, yet lavishly embellished with embroidery, the clothed female body seems a billboard advertising the male designer's accomplishments.

As a male domain, however, drawing also implies a complicated relationship between control and freedom. Men are not only the primary artists in their workshops; as owners and managers of the shops, men presumably direct the labor of all workers. Because men are outside the home and the shop more often than women, however, even on a daily basis their contributions are less constant; it cannot be assumed that they regularly exercise control. Women, working daily in home-shops and kiosks, stay involved in a wider variety of productive tasks and, at the same time, fulfill reproductive duties. Rare indeed is the woman who claims drawing for her skill and/or identifies herself as the *dueño.* Nevertheless, women's participation in embroidery, as a profession and a style of family organization, remains the backbone that enables its continued development as a viable livelihood for Cayllominos.

Conclusion

In the total system of Caylloma *bordado* production and exchange, productive practices have symbolic dimensions, structured by gendered and ethnic representation. Ideologies of work are gendered in ways that permeate the economic system. Noncapitalist systems have been assigned an implicitly gendered status within theoretical literature that associates femaleness with domestic economy; Marilyn Strathern (1988) terms this "the gender of the gift." In the Colca Valley, however, the association between female and domestic does not withstand scrutiny. There, capitalist and noncapitalist systems are intertwined, and the barriers between public and private domains, and between production and reproduction, are far from sharp. Within the petty commodity production form, both men and women are occupied by multiple productive tasks and sometimes share labor among different productive units, whether workshops or families. Likewise, the production of garments intended for sale is the norm, not the exception, for both men and women. Nevertheless, an association of femaleness with noncapitalist domesticity lingers in the ideology that child care, "helping" the family, and skill transmission are reproductive activities.

Many workshops are independent nuclear family units, but relationships of competition and cooperation cut across other family and social relationships. Competition between workshops is an undeniable reality, so every artisan should know his or her customers' preferences as well as the technical and financial sides of the business. Competition also occurs within workshops, because relations of production are structured by gender, kinship, and generation as well as by technical skill. Cooperation, on the other hand, forcefully unites each workshop so that it can compete against other shops; at the same time, cooperation between workshops occurs in ways influenced by kinship. Finally, cooperation and competition occur between producers and consumers, who share knowledge of clothing consumption patterns but often disagree about price.

Labor and its organization are at the heart of embroidery production. More embroidery businesses succeed or fail because of labor than because of technical skill and capital. Labor is consistently undervalued, and women's labor in particular is often treated as "help." Sustained struggle for the family's benefit is part of an overall productive ideology within which kinship masks exploitation even as it factors into workshop success. Intensive labor is necessary to generate earnings, even if they are not profits, and the prestige that accompanies a thriving business. Labor time and labor costs are not reckoned in family shops in the same way as in a capitalist wage-labor system. Rather, when almost no money is paid to workers, the cost of labor is not monetary but social.

In some workshops, workers are exploited by the owners, including their own relatives. Low or no pay; long hours, especially during fiesta season; muscle strain from sewing; and little or no opportunity to advance all characterize the embroidery profession, especially for junior artisans and apprentice *operarios*. Most owners work alongside their workers, however, actively participating in self-exploitation. The conception of work itself includes this need for self-exploitation. For small workshops with limited capital, intensification of labor is the main route to increased productivity.

The gendered dynamics of Caylloma's social economy are apparent in the workshop system. In family workshops, private life is inseparable from the public dimensions of exchange spaces. As we saw in the case of Susana and Leonardo, families opt for multiple production and exchange spaces not only so they can reach more customers, but so they can balance making *bordados* and raising children. Productive labor, associated with the tasks required to make embroidered garments, overlaps with reproductive tasks, including socializing children into the workshop lifestyle and teaching them embroidery skills. Although men and women perform different tasks, what is more important is their qualitative assessment of them. As making objects intersects with teaching and learning about them, Caylloma families both strengthen and challenge the processes of making gendered difference.

8

Trading Places: Exchange, Identity, and the Commoditization of Cloth

Nilda Sells a Vest

One April afternoon in Coporaque, Nilda Bernal took an order for a black vest from my friend. While Patricia Jurewicz and I were riding the bus from Arequipa to the Colca Valley for Holy Week (Semana Santa) of 1992, we had discussed buying embroideries. A textile designer from the United States, then living in Arequipa, Jurewicz was intrigued by *bordados.* She wanted an embroidered hat, of course, but also another, unique garment. She could buy garments in Chivay market or commission them from a workshop, I explained; each had its pros and cons. My *compadres* Nilda and Juan frequently accept commissions. When we reached Coporaque and visited them, Patricia discussed having them embroider a vest (*corpiño*) for her. After six years in the *bordado* business, Nilda had developed a good sense about customers' tastes and desires. Patricia, as a professional designer, was hardly a typical tourist. Her garment should exemplify the best in *bordados* and should be one she might actually wear. Nilda suggested a half-dozen garments and colors. Nothing did the trick. Then she got a look in her eye. What about black?

She pulled out an unfinished black vest, which fit Patricia well. Nilda and Juan agreed to finish it by applying the necessary embroidery, sewing the shoulder seams, and perfecting the fit. They would trim it with fiesta colors and designs, although the black *corpiño* had been destined for mourning wear (*luto*). It took several weeks to complete, but the finished product satisfied everyone. Alongside the central band of figures were framing bands using multiple designs, all finely drawn. The garment was outstanding—higher quality than anything that could be purchased ready-made (Figure 36).

"Black" became a topic of discussion, prompted by the commission. Nilda had been puzzled, she admitted, by the foreign taste for the "dark," "sad" (*oscuro, triste*) color. But now she too was "*antojando*" black, she said—developing an eye or taste for it. Only the day before, Patricia and I had observed the Good Friday ritual use of black, so Patricia knew "black" meant "mourning" in Caylloma, but she also saw black as a U.S. wardrobe basic.

In creating the commissioned garment, Nilda, Juan, Patricia, and I were all involved in trading places. Their home became a salesroom; domestic space became commercial. Their traditional roles as artisans who make garments on commission were maintained, but modified by interacting with a foreign tourist. Their interactions with Patricia were initiated by me, as friend and *comadre*, but a direct relationship also surfaced among the three of them as fellow designers and as sellers and buyer. The garment, while entirely traditional in its designs, figures, construction, and technique, was nonetheless a novelty in the way it combined festival and mourning styles. I learned how tourist sales in Caylloma have spurred changes in design by observing genuine tourists *in situ* in Chivay's market and stores, but even more by conversing about tourism with artisans, such as Nilda, who occupy the trading places of Caylloma.

"Trading places" conceptually encompasses goods for other goods, money, or services, and, more broadly, ideas, identities, and categories. In those trading places, artisans' multiple means of circulating and obtaining *bordados* are framed by the market.[1] In this chapter, I examine exchange as a set of practices that produce identities and occur within families, households, and workshops. These practices are closely related to production, for the line between exchanging and making is blurry (Chapter 7). Trading places are both physical places where exchanges are carried out, such as Chivay market, and social spaces where changes in identity and social relations occur, such as from artisans to vendors.

Gender structures practices of exchange largely through kinship. *Bordados* are often produced and exchanged by the same person or members of the same family. Does gender influence who sells an embroidered object differently than who makes it? What is the relationship between artisans and vendors? As a vendor travels, she or he becomes familiar with different

36 VEST EMBROIDERED BY JUAN CONDORI AND NILDA BERNAL

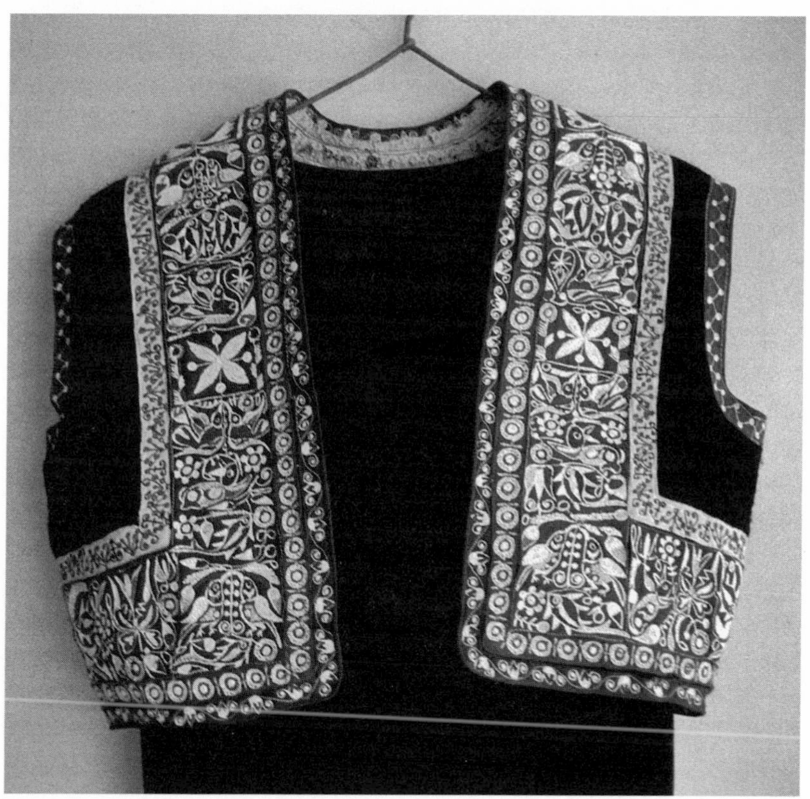

exchange settings and transaction patterns. She often uses ethnic clothes to gain leverage in commercial transactions in both rural and urban settings, thus trading on her ethnic identity. I am especially concerned with the links formed thereby between the marketing of objects and the marketing of ethnicity itself. Trading places encompasses the idea of the capitalist Indian: the ethnic artisan who promotes and advocates his or her own product and thus simultaneously reauthenticates and folklorizes her identity.

Black cloth and clothes offer an ideal window for analyzing exchange and identity. "Black" circulates between the realm of death and funerals, and the dominion of tourist fashion. My attendance at All Souls' Day and Good Friday ceremonies sparked my understanding of more general exchange of cloth and clothes in the different spaces. Through diverse social networks, women and men market *bordados* in Caylloma and Arequipa, and increasing tourism has unique implications for economy, identity, and ethnicity. In particular, the simultaneous marketing of objects and identities juxtaposes sacred and secular uses of cloth and drives ritual objects to become commoditized.[2]

Most enterprises that sell *bordados* are small-scale, and they interact with many customers, middlemen, and suppliers; vendors participate in an economy with many informal characteristics. The urban-rural networks that sustain both city and country dwellers have points of intersection in Chivay market kiosks, regional and provincial fairs, and the informal street markets of Arequipa—everywhere an artisan must travel to buy and sell, wheel and deal, and keep the ball of commerce rolling. Yet trading places are only partial solutions; each trade and each place only sharpens the contradictions and conflicts in Cayllomino vendors' lives.

Just the Same but Black: Mourning Rituals, Tourism, and Fashion

When Nilda took Patricia's *corpiño* order, she drew on her substantial knowledge of color, taste, custom, and economy. Patricia, the buyer, has a degree in design from a U.S. university and studied fashion in New York; she probably has more appreciation of *bordados* than the typical tourist. But like other domestic and foreign tourists to the Colca Valley, she sought the rare, precious, and beautiful, and looked to an artisan to provide it. Tourists venture forth from Arequipa in search of natural wonders and cultural exoticism: towering snow-capped peaks, scenic vistas, condors, vicuñas, picturesque colonial villages, native inhabitants. The characteristic, colorful, embroidered clothes seem suitable "authentic" mementos. Shopping in Chivay market, tourists often buy the garments on display. Tourists from the United States and Europe are more likely to view black clothes as fashion statements. Sometimes, vendors told me, tourists say the colors are too bright and ask for similar clothes in another color.

Just the same. But black.

Few tourists realize, however, that people in the Colca Valley associate black with death. Black clothes are worn for Catholic mourning rituals (Spanish *luto*): funerals, All Souls' Day, and Good Friday.[3] Black garments are occasionally displayed for sale, but those garments have sacred connotations and their use is largely divorced from fashion. Some artisans and vendors, however, now stock black garments to meet the tourist demand. In the production and exchange of black cloth and clothes, this change has altered ritual cloth and its sacred character by turning it into a secular commodity.

The black cloth and clothes made and used in rituals in the Colca Valley are sometimes handwoven and usually embroidered. The sacredness embodied in cloth objects, through multiple uses and transformation under the impact of international market penetration, is played out in different practices. The "sacred textiles" I discuss here are mostly new objects made for ritual uses in contemporary society, rather than the ancient textiles usually considered heirlooms. In Caylloma, families keep a few antique objects in ritual bundles. While some mourning textiles may be one hundred years old or more, very few if any are pre-Hispanic or colonial relics. In other parts of the Andes, relic textiles have received the lion's share of scholarly and public attention for their religious, political, and economic significance, especially after entering the international art market.[4] My concerns with sacredness relate to the market somewhat differently.

In Caylloma, several special kinds of textiles are made for ritual uses, but they are also commodities. The finished products are bought and sold. Many potentially sacred cloths, like all other cloths, are readily available for sale in the market. Commoditization of objects both precedes and follows sale to tourists, with many detours also comprising the sacralization-and-secularization process. Some potentially sacred cloths are appropriated for fashionable tourist clothes and so are never used in ritual contexts.

The increasing secularization of sacred textiles cannot be attributed to "outside influences" alone. Local artisans also initiate change. Cayllomino artisans make all embroidered garments explicitly for sale, and their primary consumers are local people, not tourists. Commoditization refers most broadly to capitalist exchange: buying and selling in the marketplace. What happens when a thing is transformed into an object of desire and an object of consumption? Commoditization goes hand in hand with changes in identity; the marketing of image and ethnicity is a component of the successful sale of objects.

Black Clothes and Mourning

One day I ran into Felícitas Bernal in Coporaque, soon after I returned following several years' absence. Her white straw hat had a black hatband, but none of her other garments was black. The band, she said, was for her mother, who had died the previous year. This small incident made me aware that even tiny amounts of black signify mourning; subsequently, when I met a woman wearing black, I knew her family had suffered a loss and I expressed appropriate condolences.

Mourning customs in many societies prescribe one color to indicate mourning, who should wear clothes of that color, and for how long. In European Catholic tradition, the use of black for mourning dates to the Middle Ages; it is still common in many Latin American and Mediterranean countries (Hollander 1978:372–374; Freedman 1986).[5] The contemporary use of black mourning clothes in Peru seems to be a Spanish colonial legacy, but it cannot be ascertained when the tradition was established. In many South American rural communities, black is customary daily dress and not particularly associated with mourning.[6] In the Colca Valley, the association between black and mourning largely holds sway.[7]

Caylloma garments made in mourning style are: for women, the shawl (*phullu*), skirt (*pollera*), jacket (*saco*), and vest (*corpiño*); for men, the poncho. Extremely similar in form and design to daily and festival garments, mourning garments differ primarily in color and fabric. They are black, but never plain black. All feature small amounts of white, blue, and dark green. Shawls and ponchos have thin color stripes. Polychrome embroidered borders also employ the blue-and-white scheme. The ground fabric of shawls and ponchos is usually handwoven of alpaca or synthetic yarn, whereas vests and skirts use *bayeta* or commercial synthetic fabrics. While similar mourning garments are used throughout the valley, their details vary by village, as do those of daily dress. The Cabanaconde *phullu* is larger than the

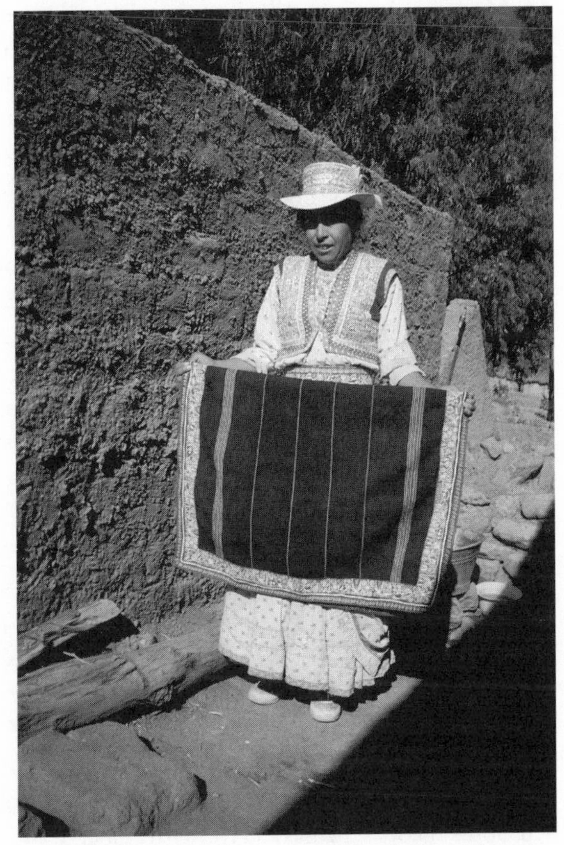

37 NILDA BERNAL HOLDS A BLACK SHAWL EMBROIDERED BY HER AND JUAN CONDORI. PHOTOGRAPH BY PATRICIA JUREWICZ.

Chivay version. Cabanaconde mourning *polleras* are trimmed with rickrack, as are nonmourning skirts, but the trim is blue. Chivay-style mourning *polleras* use blue or dark green applied yarn.

A shawl (*phullu*) that Nilda and Juan were embroidering as a commission had the typical layout and colors of Caylloma mourning shawls (Figure 37). After obtaining the woven shawl elsewhere, a local woman brought it to them to embroider the border.[8] The handwoven piece is mainly black with several narrow bands of white and blue woven stripes. All edges are trimmed with a wide blue commercial-cloth border, on which the characteristic birds and flowers are embroidered. Only the drawing (outlining), in white, had been done when I saw it; Nilda would finish the *phullu* by augmenting the figures with blue.

Men usually wear only one mourning garment, a poncho roughly five feet square. It resembles the *phullu:* black with white, blue, and occasionally dark green stripes. Mourning ponchos, like daily wear, are handwoven of alpaca or synthetic yarn and feature next-to-no embroidery, typically a narrow embroidered neck-binding with a simple, one-color swirl. Men's regular daily ponchos are the same size and are usually pink with green stripes or tan with pink stripes.

People wear black mourning clothes for all funerals, mourning by immediate family members of the deceased for one year, a memorial mass observed at the end of that year, All Saints' and All Souls' Days, and Good Friday. Although women in mourning should wear black for a year, they rarely wear all black garments for that long; more often, a few months after the funeral they reduce the number from the total outfit to a few garments. The occasions when I most closely observed black clothes in use were All Souls' Day and Good Friday.

All Souls' Day

> *More than anything else I wished I belonged to one of these living, celebrated families, lush as plants, with bones in the ground for roots. I wanted . . . one of those calcium ancestors to decorate as my own.* — BARBARA KINGSOLVER (1990:165)

Observed throughout Latin America, All Saints' (Todos Santos) and All Souls' (Todas Almas) Days, November 1 and 2, are often called the Days of the Dead.[9] Stemming from the European Catholic heritage, these ceremonies commemorating the dead focus on the physical remains in the cemetery, which are reminders of their continued presence. In the Colca Valley, families visit the village cemetery to offer prayers for the souls of deceased relatives, install crosses over new graves, and clean and decorate existing crosses and graves, often with wreaths (*coronas*) of fresh or paper flowers (Paerregaard 1987). In Peru, many of these customs are carried out in both rural communities and cities.

In 1991 I was privileged to participate in these ceremonies in Coporaque. People who died during the preceding year receive the most attention. One of them was Marcelina Terán, the elderly mother of Agripina Bernal, my friend and neighbor. I often stop at Agripina's small store to buy bread and sundries and to chat. On All Saints, November 1, I arrived in Coporaque on the bus from Arequipa via Chivay. After unloading my gear in my room, I crossed the street to her store. Finding the store closed but an adjoining gate open, I called out a greeting and entered the patio. In the house compound's back room were Agripina and twenty people I scarcely recognized. These relatives had come from Arequipa and elsewhere to commemorate her mother. At her invitation, I returned and shared a meal with them later that day, and accompanied them to the cemetery the next day.

The ceremonies meant more to me than observing the families' actions. My friends and *compadres* knew that I had lost my husband two years before, when we were living far from Peru. During those two days, as we spent time together, Agripina explained the mourning customs carried out by her family and others around us. I also shared Todas Almas with my *compadres* and close friends, especially Nilda and her children. The experience was saturated with conflicting emotions, as I shared the sensations of loss and memory. This was my first opportunity to commemorate publicly the loss of my husband with people who were his friends and *compadres* in Coporaque. When I arrived for fieldwork six months before, we had privately discussed our feelings about this loss. My *compadre* Epifanio wanted to ask the priest from Chivay to hold a special mass for John. Somehow we never had this mass. The time we spent in the cemetery was our first, and only, public expression of shared loss—an expression that convinced me they were family.

All Souls dawned a gloomy day; it never ceased to threaten rain. On this day, everyone spends the whole afternoon and evening in the cemetery, on the outskirts of Coporaque. I gathered with Agripina's family at her home and spent an hour talking and preparing flowers and wreaths to take to the cemetery. Beginning about noon, families all over town began the ten-minute walk to the cemetery, where they would decorate graves until 2 P.M., when the priest from Chivay would arrive and deliver prayers. Several days ahead, the immediate family of the recently deceased installs a cement tomb cover and a cross, usually metal, on the grave. On the day itself, they decorate it and pay respects. The elaborate commemorative rituals include orations in Spanish and Quechua by *cantores* ("reciters"; see Ráez 1993:283), prayers said in Spanish by the priest, and offerings left on the tomb.

As we convened in the cemetery near her mother's grave, Agripina and her aunts and uncles discussed and rearranged the wreath on the cross until they agreed it looked proper. At Agripina's behest, I photographed her mother's tomb and gave most of the images to her and to relatives who requested mementos of their farewell to their elderly relative. Reluctant to intrude on personal grief, I shot no other photographs.

In the cemetery, women wear a black shawl (*phullu*) around their shoulders (Figure 38). Agripina wore a fairly elaborate shawl and *pollera,* but her aunts wore black shawls with a skirt or with plain tan pants. Agripina's shawl was on loan from her mother-in-law. Agripina is from Coporaque and her husband, Dionisio, is from Cabanaconde. She often signified her association with his community through clothes, wearing a Cabana-style *pollera* almost daily. The relationship signaled by the *phullu* is not just with the community-at-large, however, but with her mother-in-law directly. Such loans are temporary exchanges, frequently occurring within and between families, which may become more permanent as gifts or through inheritance.

38 In the Coporaque cemetery, women wear black shawls and *polleras.*

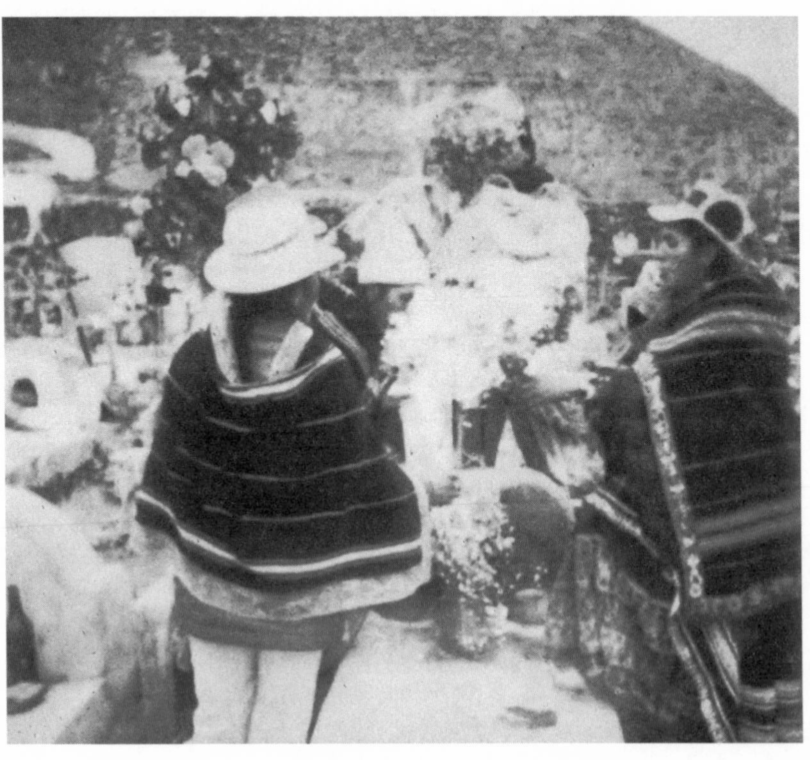

A similar but smaller cloth used in the cemetery is also called "*phullu*." On this black cloth, spread on Marcelina Terán's tomb, relatives and friends placed offerings. All around the cemetery, a similar ceremony was repeated. Each family places a different offering on its tomb, typically a small pile of grain (corn, quinoa, or barley) or bread in animal and human shapes.[10] One relative records each person's contribution. That night, everyone who made an offering attends a feast at the sponsoring relative's home. The offerings are given to the *cantores* or, some say, taken by spirits.

After Father Rafael arrived, he said a lengthy service for the entire assembled village group, then offered individual prayers for those on his list, the departed relatives for whom families had requested prayers in advance. He noted a few additions. "John Treacy," Epifanio called out. The priest walked around the cemetery, stopping at graves and saying words of benediction. To say the prayer for John, he needed to know where his grave was. This disturbed Epifanio, who began to cry out, "Where is his soul? Where are his remains?" (*¿Dónde está su alma?*) John is buried in Madison, Wisconsin. For the physical location, Epifanio chose his own mother's grave. After Father Rafael prayed and sprinkled holy water, John's friends and I said our own brief prayer. They seemed reassured by performing this small deed, which would remind them of the days they had spent with John. I was grateful they put their thoughts into action, and that I shared it with them.

For the rest of the cool, cloudy afternoon, I made my way around the cemetery with friends and *compadres*, learning where their family graves were located. The day before, I was unsure what to wear, wondering if it would be appropriate to borrow some mourning garments, and then finally deciding against it. As the chilly air penetrated my jacket, Nilda bundled me up in a thick woolen shawl. People had brought drink as well as decorations and, as day became evening, consumed considerable amounts of alcohol. After a thoroughly drunken man tripped on a grave, went sprawling, and fell into my *ahijada* Enadi and knocked her down, Nilda pronounced it time to go. I bid farewell to Agripina and her relatives, who were heartily drinking and weeping, weeping and drinking. With Nilda and her daughters, I walked slowly to their home.

Remembering the dead is a participatory experience in Latin American communities. Its collective character merges with personal experience, as I learned that afternoon. All the people of Coporaque trouped to the cemetery, and together created a sense of family, lineage, and community by attending to their "calcium ancestors." While the bones in the ground were their roots, it was the living families, with all their branches, who were "lush as plants," as Kingsolver (1990:165) phrased it. All Souls plays a pivotal role in her novel of Hispanic New Mexico. Codi, the novel's protagonist, believes she has no ancestors in a small community. By sharing funerary ceremonies with friends, she learns that she does. Through participation, she moves from feeling excluded from the heritage of the dead to knowing she belongs to a "living, celebrated family." My ancestors were laid to rest in the United States, Chile, Sweden, Argentina, Spain, France, and other countries unknown to me. None of my grandparents is still living, and my mother's father was the only grandparent I knew; he died when I was four. My husband's death was vigorously commemorated in the United States, in Washington, D.C., where he briefly lived and where he died, and in Madison where we lived together for six years and where he is buried. The prayers we said on Epifanio's mother's grave endowed John with a physical place among the village ancestors. The tears I shed for my husband's soul will bind me forever to Coporaque. Epifanio's kindness in requesting that special prayer cemented our *compadrazgo* and endeared him to me always.

Good Friday

In Latin America, Catholics wear black clothes on Good Friday (Viernes Santo, moveable date), a day of mourning for the death of Christ, and the end of Lent. In Catholic churches, a special service is held; it is the only day mass is not said. In Caylloma, people wear the same black clothes they use for personal and family mourning. The village of Yanque has an elaborate Good Friday service in its seventeenth-century Franciscan church, which Patricia Jurewicz and I attended in April 1992 at the invitation of the nuns who serve there. Also present were several hundred Yanqueños and six Peruvian tourists.

On Friday evening, Patricia and I entered the vast, candle-lit, stone church and took our seats in a pew. Men and women in black slowly filtered into the church, filling the pews and then sitting on the floor. The black clothes seemed to recede into the dim interior. The altar was draped in plain black cloth. Such cloths also form part of the paschal mourning tradition. Other communities, such as Coporaque, have elaborately woven black cloths for this purpose.[11] The hour-long ceremony includes a sermon by the priest and readings by parishioners. Then everyone focuses on the central activity: the removal of the life-size effigy of Christ from the crucifix. The figure in Yanque's church has articulated limbs. A group of men, members of the *cofradía* (church's lay confraternity), removes the figure from the cross; as they do so, its arms bend at the shoulders. Then more parishioners come forward and wash the effigy, using cotton balls and alcohol, and the men place it in a glass coffin. Still wearing black ponchos, the devotees carry the coffin on a bier through the dark streets, traversing a set course. Finally, they return the coffin to the church.

That evening, the atmosphere in the Yanque church was eerily somber. On the altar, dozens of huge candles, some three meters high, illuminated the image of Christ with compelling, flickering flames, but the church as a whole was dim. Although hundreds of people were there, the darkness of their dress accentuated that of the church and created a sense of absence as much as presence. It was a chilling and impressive experience, diminished only by the presence of tourists snapping flash photographs.

Yanque's Good Friday service has become known outside Caylloma and now attracts tourists. The life-size articulated Christ is apparently unique. The rituals, although central to Cayllominos' experiences, are being altered and commoditized. María Luisa Lobo, a Peruvian filmmaker, not only profiled the ceremonies in a documentary (1988) but encouraged several modifications to the procedures and the participants' costume. For example, she suggested that small children, dressed like angels in white dresses with metal wings, take part in the procession; they now do so routinely.[12] In the church in 1992, a group of Peruvian tourists occupied the front row of pews. They had traveled by van in a packaged tour especially to see the service. Commemorating the event by snapping flash photographs throughout the service, they participated in the ongoing commoditization of ritual and of Cayllominos' life experiences.

Commemorative clothes and ceremonies, as these three cases have shown, are tightly linked. Although Cayllominos commemorate the dead and the ancestors twice a year, we should not forget that death is a somber, omnipresent reality in a nation at war, as Peru was during the years I lived there. That presence pervades human consciousness throughout the year, although the ceremonies crystallize it only twice. Objects are the embodiment of memory. In the context of mourning rituals, black garments provide a physical prompt that encourages the living to remember the dead and, by fulfilling their obligations to the dead, to strengthen their bonds to the living.

Objects that embody memories of the dead are often glossed as "heirlooms." If "heirloom" means a valued, ancient object that was handed down within a family, then most black clothes used in mourning rituals are not heirlooms. I interpret "heirloom," instead, as an object that embodies memory and contains meaning about the past, no matter what its age. This interpretation treats "heirloom" as a type of object, similar to other mnemonic devices. What is handed down need not be one specific object; rather, the continuity is in the idea of the past, the meanings that the past holds, and the knowledge to create an object of the type that embodies such memories. Through repeated, multiple uses of such objects, the ideas invested in them are retained, even in the absence of one particular object in which those ideas are continuously embodied (Hallam and Hockey 2001). For example, a woman attending Todos Santos rituals should use a mourning shawl which conforms to a recognizable type: black with white and blue. The shawl need not be the same one she used last year or even identical to the shawls other women use this year. What matters is that mourning clothes resemble each other today and resemble those of the past in certain condensed aspects of color and/or design. A small emblem, such as Felícitas's hatband, may replace larger ones. The single garment or element assumes the function of synecdoche that the whole ensemble normally fulfills but expresses that function in even more condensed form: a part of a part stands for the whole. The uses and meanings of mourning clothes are similar to those of other mnemonic devices and discourses that encourage both ongoing habituation and connection with the past and the ancestors, but they are more narrowly configured within the broader domain of Caylloma textile traditions.

Exchange Spaces, Tourism, and the Sale of Ritual Attire

Selling Embroidery, Selling Ethnicity

Anyone can enter a home-shop or Chivay market, speak with a vendor, and purchase a garment with cash in one transaction or commission one.[13] Most vendors sell primarily from home, from Chivay market, or both, and they travel infrequently. A few depend heavily on travel, taking goods from Chivay to other Colca Valley communities and/or to weekly fairs in rural Caylloma and neighboring provinces. While a few successful vendors make a living primarily from selling rather than making *bordados,* others told me that today "there is no business" (*no hay negocio*). Because the occupation of vendor relates to other occupations and identities, numerous cooperative strategies intersect within a competitive environment. Vendors who earn a living from sales must deploy these strategies in different sales venues, but the business aspect of selling *bordados* must also accommodate other aspects of daily experience.

"Time," "help," and "knowing" are major considerations for vendors. Becoming known, making a name for oneself, and promoting one's art and business are all part of the selling game. Successful individuals who are more entrepreneurial and aggressive than their peers often attribute their success to such personality traits. Men more than women offer such explanations. Despite the appeal of a go-getter ideology, other factors are more likely to have a positive impact. Having a larger family business in which artisans delegate many tasks leaves them "time" to travel and sell, and provides the "help" which frees up that time. They "know" the ins-and-outs of embroidery—making higher-quality garments; using materials efficiently; and innovating new colors, motifs, and objects for different markets. Finally, they sell other people's works on consignment or commission. Vendors do compete with each other for shares of the closed market among Caylloma's female consumers, but they also stress the importance of looking outward, such as by expanding markets through tourism, NGOs, and cooperatives and by promoting sales through publicity. The successful vendor judiciously combines these skills, having learned over the years how to balance opportunity, risk, security, and social interaction.

The majority of vendors rely on a few standard garments for the bulk of sales. Most vendors sell all the embroidered garments, although a few specialize in hats. In answering my surveys, they agreed that the best-sellers are second-quality garments, especially those which wear out fastest, the *camisa* (blouse) and *corpiño* (vest), often sold as a matched set, so they try to keep these in stock. Smaller items also cost less to make, in both materials and time, than *polleras*. The backbone of the *bordado* business is the vendors who rely on higher-volume sales. Most vendors are also artisans and produce similar-quality garments in the mid-price range, thereby remaining competitive with fellow vendors without getting a reputation for undercutting.

Three businesses exemplify different strategies. In their workshop, for many years Susana Bernal and Leonardo Mejía usually sewed intensively together for several days before a fiesta, and then Leonardo traveled and sold in the sponsoring town while Susana stayed with their children. They sometimes traveled together to sell at a distant fair. After Leonardo became a schoolteacher, however, more *bordado* work fell to Susana. She owed her success in part to "help" from family and neighbors, which enabled sales, as well as production, in the family shop. In addition, after many years in the *bordado* business, customers know Susana and her extended family. Others' knowledge of Susana, not only her knowledge of the business, assured customers' return. Susana's sales style is not aggressive, and her solid reputation is based on reliability and quality goods. During Leonardo's absence, she expanded her opportunities to sell by traveling to more fairs, often alone; she enlarged the stock in her kiosk; and she created small, innovative, tourist-oriented items, which she sold in Chivay market or, using intermediaries, in Arequipa tourist stores.

Rosalía Valera employs a different strategy for her business in Coporaque. This workshop produces middle-of-the-road goods and accepts few commissions. Rather than maintain a Chivay kiosk, she sells on the road, spending the vast majority of her time trading at regional fairs. Well known as an aggressive salesperson, she relentlessly promotes her own goods, often at the expense of others (Chapter 3). Furthermore, Rosalía herself no longer embroiders; her adult daughter and a male *operario* do all the construction and embroidery in her shop, and she also sells embroideries made by Juan and Nilda, her son and daughter-in-law. Having two regular staffers and ready access to a second shop gives Rosalía more opportunity to travel and goods to sell. In addition, she sells more than embroideries. She buys agricultural produce from other farmers in Coporaque and sells it at the higher-altitude fairs. Rosalía also extends credit to customers using the "fifty-fifty" system. A customer pays down half the selling price; the next week, Rosalía collects the balance due. Instead of cash, she also accepts payment in wool, fleece, meat, and grain; all have established but fluctuating monetary equivalents.

Nilda Bernal takes a third approach: her sales are dependent both on *bordado* production and her mother-in-law's activities. Although Nilda and Juan sell their *bordados* out of their home-shop, she also works as a traveling vendor. During 1992, while Juan worked at the Caylloma mine and after my goddaughter Enadi started school, Nilda began to travel occasionally to other towns and the regional fairs. For example, one weekend she went to a holiday fair in Tisco, a town fifteen miles upriver. Some of the *bordados* she sold were made by her and Juan; others were from Rosalía's shop, on which her mother-in-law paid a small sales commission. Taking their younger daughter, Lorena, with her, she usually left Enadi with her own mother or Rosalía.

Middlepersons and merchants, indispensable to *bordado* use and popularity, are linchpins of rural economy. *Bordado* artisans who produce small amounts rarely keep a Chivay market kiosk, but often seek more outlets for their products. Vendors try to diversify their offerings. Rosalía, for example, as a broker of goods and cash, has become a regular player in the region's economic networks. Centered in Coporaque, she moves through Chivay to the regional fairs but carries out few of her activities in and around Chivay market. Several merchants centered in Chivay, however, have larger-volume businesses. Melitón Cutipa and his wife, in their sixties in the early 1990s, have had a market stand for more than twenty years. Cutipa primarily sells *bordados* but also sells industrially manufactured clothes and materials for *bordados.* From artisans, he takes complete garments on consignment or buys outright. For example, he sells hats—both white Chivay-style and embroidered Cabana-style—made by various artisans, taking a small percentage of the retail sale price as a commission. Because consumers know appropriate prices, Cutipa cannot raise them, so the artisan absorbs the cost of his service.

Of the few large merchants in Caylloma, the major retail stores are all in Chivay; none is primarily devoted to textile crafts. Eleuterio Mamani has the largest general store, which occupies a sizeable corner of the plaza across from Chivay market. In his truck, he or his driver travels to other communities, supplying tiny shops in with sundries, kerosene, and alcohol. His store carries only a few embroidered items but several shelves of cloth and other materials.

Bordados use about fifty different materials; the only ones produced locally are sheep-wool fabric (*bayeta*) and alpaca yarn and fiber. Several businesses in Caylloma supply the fabrics imported from outside the province, the region, and the nation to the artisans, and some of those also sell finished embroideries. Ten such vendors are in Chivay market. Froylán Quinto and his wife own the largest fabric store in Caylloma, located in Chivay, four blocks from the market. They carry a wide variety of fabrics, trims, and yarns used for *bordados,* but no finished garments. They also rent musical instruments, so one may find a drum sitting on a bolt of velvet. Not only does Quinto regularly stock several hundred fabrics, his prices tend to be lower than those of small vendors, and he extends credit to regular customers. Some artisans travel to obtain materials, but several claimed that Quinto's prices are the same as in Arequipa, so combined with the credit, they find no advantage to buying in Arequipa (except wholesale).

Beyond Caylloma, larger forces shape the small-scale social exchanges. NGO involvement in marketing is largely channeled through cooperatives which challenge the alpaca cartel's domination, with only a few Chivay-based groups providing loans to embroiderers. Nevertheless, such organizations apply their programs through the microlevel exchange relationships. Kin usually provided the vital "time" and "help," with a few key relatives and/or *compadres* doing the lion's share to keep the system moving. Crucial players are often relatives in Lima and Arequipa, and more than one-quarter of the artisans surveyed have a relative abroad, sometimes in the United States.

Cabanaconde hats provide a concrete example. Artisans embroider directly onto a purchased wool felt hat. Only one brand, Arrogui, is considered suitable, as its felt is both high quality and malleable enough for embroidering on the machine. And only the Arrogui factory in Lima makes these hats; the main Caylloma supplier is Juan Tejada of Cabanaconde. Tejada's cousin, who works at the factory, ships several dozen to Arequipa several times a year. Tejada brings them to Caylloma, where he sells them outright to embroiderers or commissions artisans to embroider hats, which he distributes to Chivay market kiosks and stores or sells "direct," meaning from his home, in Cabanaconde. He usually embroiders other garments rather than hats. When I visited his home, he had fifteen finished hats on hand—three times more than other vendors. The previous year, he exulted, a Japanese tourist bought fifty hats from him!

Tejada's multiple roles as embroiderer, vendor, and middleman are far from unusual. Social networks increase access to labor and materials; at least one family member in a shop usually travels to Arequipa or Juliaca and brings materials to Caylloma. While this saves money on materials, it also incorporates other aspects of exchange. Artisans who buy materials in Juliaca cannot sell the highly localized Caylloma *bordados* there, but they can trade produce, including maize, other grains, and fruit, grown in Caylloma.

Closer to home, some *bordado* sale venues are outside the province and even outside the department of Arequipa. These are weekly regional fairs in highland locations several hours from Chivay. Some vendors go to all four: Chalyuta on Monday; Ichuhuayco, Tuesday; Chichas, Friday; and Chalhuanca, Saturday. Chalhuanca, in the department of Apurímac, is the farthest from Chivay, requiring a two-night stay, so fewer Caylloma vendors go there. Modesta Condori, a woman in her midtwenties, works in her father's Chivay shop with her brothers and husband. While Modesta travels four or five days a week, her husband sews and cares for their young daughter. She does not mind traveling to Chalhuanca, where she was born there and has relatives; her family moved to Chivay in the 1970s when her father worked for MACON. On days without fairs, she stays in Chivay and sells from a sidewalk stand outside the market.

Even vendors like Modesta Condori and Rosalía Valera, who travel constantly and do not have kiosks, remain connected to the Chivay merchants to obtain materials; more-distant sources are sometimes impractical or unreliable. Especially during peak season, Carnival, in the rush to finish and deliver garments, speed trumps cost. Convenience and credit prompt artisans to obtain materials from Quinto's store. Many vendors keep afloat or weather dry spells through credit and loans. Artisans also try to reduce costs by using their materials prudently, which feeds into their attempts to enter new markets and/or expand sales through intensification and diversification. Small garments, accessories, and doll clothes, which use remnants, improve the return on expenditures for fabric. Branching out into souvenirs, artisans diversify their markets.

As artisans face the future, most apparently want to continue. Two survey questions concerned preferences and plans: Do you intend to keep embroidering? What work, if any, would you rather do? Only a handful anticipate leaving embroidery soon. Most want to continue embroidering and selling but are looking toward a different arena, such as expanding from selling out of their home to renting a kiosk, or from kiosk to opening a store.

Selling regular amounts on a daily basis, accessing the usual markets, obtaining materials, and delivering completed orders to customers are all factors in running a successful embroidery business. Success depends largely on an individual's ability to maintain simultaneous relationships with others in several exchange networks. To promote the long-term continuity of her business, she must sometimes subordinate immediate goals to the ongoing participation in such networks. For example, although Nilda Bernal hoped to travel more and sell her own *bordados,* until her children were older, she needed to coordinate sales with her mother-in-law. Looking within family is only one route to maintaining multiple strategies. Entering credit and consignment arrangements is another. Equally important is looking outward and diversifying sales opportunities. Such ventures entail taking risks by obtaining loans through NGOs, innovating new products, and locating new sales venues—all of which may mean negotiating the domain of tourism.

Tourism, Identity, and the Promotion of Ethnicity

> *To have a souvenir of the exotic is to possess both a specimen and a trophy; on the one hand, the object must be marked as exterior and foreign, on the other it must be marked as arising directly out of an immediate experience of its possessor. It is thus placed within an intimate distance; space is transformed into interiority, into "personal" space. . . .*
>
> — SUSAN STEWART (1984:147)

Around Coporaque, the mayor was known as "the Tourist" ("el Turista"). Ricardo Ramos did not live in the village but came and went as he pleased, people said; arriving just as fiestas began, he left once they were over. One day my friend Leonardo Mejía surprised me by saying, "He's like you." As I wondered how I resembled a native, male, political authority, he continued, "He's a tourist."

Was I a tourist or not? This was not the first time a Cayllomino had said so. "I'm not a tourist, I'm an anthropologist!" I would protest. Living and studying in Coporaque surely did not belong in the same category as sight-seeing. However much it went against the grain, I finally had to concede their point. I am a foreigner, came and went frequently, and apparently had money without working. Finding myself classified together with the mayor as a tourist, even jokingly, gave me pause. Mayor Ramos owned a print shop in Arequipa, which was apparently his primary means of support. He drove around the valley in a pickup truck. He owned lands in Coporaque, and other family members had land in Chivay, where they were active in politics. The fact that he did not live permanently in Coporaque left him wide open to teasing about being a tourist.

My foreignness included my distinctly nonlocal tastes and preferences about clothes—tastes which I never dislodged completely. Vendors, assuming other *gringos* had similar tastes, often asked me how to increase sales to tourists. These conversations made me more aware of changes in embroidered garments and other objects intended to accommodate tourists' desires. The few times I observed "authentic" tourists in Chivay market and stores, I rarely spoke with them. My aversion to tourists, no matter how important to defining my identity as an anthropologist, did not noticeably alter most Cayllominos' opinions.

Through individual transactions with vendors, tourists buy garments, usually in the same sales venues where Cayllominos shop. In the city of

Arequipa, some stores are geared toward tourists, and others specialize in providing garments for migrants. When tourists travel to the Colca Valley, though, they are buying more than souvenirs. They are consuming ethnicity itself. Thus tourism is affecting the identities of the artisans who make *bordados* and the vendors who sell them. Vendors of embroidered clothes clearly have a stake in the marketing of ethnicity, but specific occurrences in the market, shops, and fairs form part of a broader pattern. These exchanges are another aspect of trading places. Identities are exchanged and transformed as ethnicity becomes commoditized and Indian identity becomes a good that can be sold—as often noted for North America (Meyer and Royer, eds. 2001; Phillips and Steiner, eds. 1999).

Processes of transformation and commoditization further complicate the discourse about national, regional, and racial identities that is sold in the global marketplace to attract foreign tourists to Caylloma and other parts of Peru. An image of the Colca Valley as an archaic survival is promoted both in guidebooks and academic discourses on pre-Columbian and colonial topics. The commoditization of the image goes hand in hand with the commoditization of objects that outsiders consider part of it. Tourists buy objects; local ceremonies draw tourists. Even dead bodies are promoted as attractions. The archaized image is both reinforced and contradicted by the modern media that present it, including high-tech formats.[14] Caylloma's "Indians" constitute the indigenous Other for white, urban Arequipa in the interest of attracting tourists as well as in regional self-identification. Tourism in Arequipa usually includes a day-trip to the valley, featuring the Canyon of the Condors, but excludes the department's other rural areas. The exoticism of the locale is accented through descriptions of an "unspoiled" valley that abounds in natural wonders, with one of the principal Andean condor habitats in South America, adjacent to a large nature preserve where vicuñas roam.[15]

Tourism to the valley, sparked by MACON, rose steadily in the 1970s–1980s. MACON's development-expansion program, initiated by the Arequipa Chamber of Commerce and the Majes Authority (AUTODEMA), received financial support from the Peruvian national tourism agency, FOPTUR (de Romaña, Blassi, and Blassi 1987:195–196). One initiative expanded lodgings by converting MACON workers' former housing into a tourist inn (ibid.), but little investment was made in local infrastructure. Over the next ten years, tourism to Peru in general plummeted, reaching its nadir during my fieldwork years, 1991–1993. Terrorism and cholera fueled negative U.S. State Department travel advisories and relentless bad international press. While the overall decline affected Arequipa and the Colca Valley, closing hotels, restaurants, and travel agencies, Arequipa's continued reputation as one of the safest parts of the country brought tourists who skipped Lima and even Cusco.[16]

All travel to the Colca Valley begins in the city of Arequipa. Tourists may choose a high-priced tour, of which there are only a few, or make their own arrangements for a bus or the *colectivo.* Backpacking, ecotourist types enjoy roughing it in the rugged valley. Not only does the high altitude cause discomfort, but there are few amenities and no luxury hotels or tasty regional cuisine. The area's appeal is the exotic and the picturesque, providing Gringo Trail war stories of crowded buses, lumpy beds, and real craft bargains.

In two years of fieldwork, I saw perhaps one hundred foreign tourists in the valley and twice that many Peruvian tourists. During my weeks of intensive surveying in Chivay market, the few couples or small groups who wandered around were quite conspicuous. All the vendors eyed them with interest but rarely called out to them, knowing that they would buy a few items from one or two stands. Apparently unaware of fiesta days, except for Semana Santa, tourists often arrived on normal weekdays when business was slow and quickly descended to the Canyon.

Tourism in the city of Arequipa centers on its Spanish colonial heritage, especially during the week around Founders' Day (August 15), when a large folklore festival, Festidanza, is held on the city fairgrounds. Other tourist activities occur year-round: tours to local scenic spots and shows of "typical Andean" music and dances. Folkloric events in the city often include Colca Valley groups; for example, my *compadre* Epifanio and his band accompanied a Coporaque school team that danced in Festidanza. Not all urban performances are folklore staged for tourists. Festivals for the patron saints of Caylloma villages are usually held in Arequipa neighborhoods inaccessible to tourists and not publicized to them. Such fiestas, although smaller than in home communities, have *mayordomos,* as well as more general sponsorship by the migrant association (Asociación Provincial de Caylloma), and are not sponsored by tour agencies.

Craft souvenirs are available in Arequipa at several shops on and around the Plaza de Armas, as well as six blocks away in the Fundo de Fierro, a gallery of twenty shops adjoining San Francisco Church. Several Fundo shops sell Caylloma embroideries, usually made in valley workshops, and one is devoted to alpaca crafts woven by members of ADECALC (Asociación de Criadores de Alpaca de Caylloma), a herders' and artisans' group in Callalli. In addition, the "Chivay Chino" and several other artisans make garments and dance costumes for Cayllominos' use (Chapter 3). Migrants and urban dance teams buy, or sometimes rent, garments to perform in the city or back home. Walking through downtown Arequipa one day, I was surprised to encounter a Caylloma-style embroidered costume on a mannequin in a huge, new shop window. This display marked the new location of Kepicentro, the largest costume-rental business, which is not a workshop. Formerly shoe-horned into a tiny shop on a narrow side street, it had become one of few occupants in a new commercial center, spacious but inordinately overpriced, built as part of the city's modernization campaign. The costume was neither accurate nor complete, featuring a blouse and hat never worn with Caylloma *polleras.* Intrigued, I stepped inside. The walls were festooned with "Latin American" costumes, such as a bullfighter's outfit, and with *polleras* from Caylloma and Cusco, all rubbing elbows with disguises of Mickey Mouse, Bugs Bunny, and other imported icons. Although the commercialization of *polleras* in this novel way seemed incongruous, such transformations are in fact consistent with the folklorization stemming from generations of urban migration. Questions of authenticity in Arequipa's performative domains were entangled with marketing strategies in both urban and rural sales venues.

Authenticity and innovation shape artisans' and vendors' creation of new objects and quest for new markets. Vendors must keep their eye on the objects themselves in order to appeal to the customers. Color is a significant factor. Hot pink and lime green, colors beloved by local customers, scream "Gaudy!" and affront the North American aesthetic. Black, however, is a color tourists desire. Black clothes are a significant part of *bordado* sales altered by tourism. Objects formerly intended for purposes of mourning and commemoration, now made and marketed for secular rather than sacred contexts, intertwine in the trading places of Caylloma. To Caylloma artisans, the foreign taste was far from obvious. So ingrained was the association of black with mourning that it masked aesthetic considerations. "Why do *gringos* dress so sad?" asked Nilda Bernal.

Taste results from such thorough cultural conditioning that very few people see it as such. "I would just wear it more," one says, or "I have lots of black clothes." The visual preferences that dominate aesthetic choice, naturalized through a process of habituation, are gradually made part of "distinction" (Bourdieu 1984): the selective apparatus people employ when they choose among alternatives in dress and other cultural features. In western fashion, black has been well established for at least a century but enjoyed a substantial vogue in high art and fashion as early as the Renaissance (Schneider 1978; see also Harvey 1995 and Hollander 1978). What John Tierney calls "the black fetish" in New York might hold sway because black is practical, elegant, unnatural, or even satanic (1994:32–34). Its very austerity lends it the allure of power.

Tourists to Caylloma request black clothes which resemble traditional clothes but feature brightly colored embroidery. While Caylloma artisans continue to produce the "authentic" black mourning clothes, to meet tourist demand, they now produce modified garments, which I term "hybrid" mourning-tourist clothes. On black backgrounds, instead of blue embroidery, hybrid garments feature the polychrome embroidery of daily wear, which contrasts handsomely to the dark ground. One such hybrid garment is the vest Juan and Nilda made for Patricia.

The fabrics used in black clothes have changed as well. "Natural" fabrics might seem more "authentic" local elements and synthetics cheap substitutes that are foisted onto tourists, but this is not the case (see Schneider 1994 and Tolen 1995). Claiming to prefer "natural" fibers and dyes, tourists may associate black with undyed alpaca yarn. Such yarn, usually confined to ponchos, carrying cloths, and shawls, is rarely found in *bordados.* Black fabric used in Caylloma is not always handwoven and is as likely to be imported as locally produced. Imported and luxury fabrics are now widely used in dark colors and black. Most black yarn, except in Callalli and higher-altitude communities, is synthetic, usually factory-dyed acrylic. True black undyed wool or fiber is rare. The "black" *bayeta* (sheep wool) fabric in *polleras* may be undyed dark brown or overdyed medium brown.[17] Other black fabrics have crossed into Caylloma from other ethnic groups. Some are luxury fabrics used for special-occasion clothes by elite white Arequipeños. For example, the artisan Hugo Vilcape made his wife a *pollera* of dark blue velvet printed with metallic designs—a fabric brought to Cabanaconde, he said proudly, by a cousin who lives in the United States.

While Cayllominos' recent use of black cloth for fiestas apparently contradicts its preferred use for mourning, this paradox highlights the exaggerated duality between "secular" and "sacred" practices. Black clothes do not exclusively connote mourning for Cayllominos. They have additional uses in ritual as well as outside the sacred realm.

One way that sacred and secular blur is through clothes used by widows, especially the elderly, who often continue to wear black after the mourning period ends. Associated with senior age status, their black clothes become acceptable daily wear. More often than black exclusively, old women wear other dark or muted colors. Second, for practical reasons, women of any age also use mourning clothes as daily wear. Susana Bernal acquired a black *bayeta* mourning-style *pollera* after her mother died. One day three years later, when I noticed she was wearing it, I became alarmed that a relative had died. No one had; rather, it was winter, and Susana wore the wool skirt for warmth. Third, practical utility is a social value, which Cayllominos do not take for granted. Yarn and fabric matter not only for aesthetic and economic reasons. Alpaca, if properly spun and woven, is much stronger and more durable than synthetic yarn; an alpaca poncho will sustain heavy use for many years. Farmers deploy many textiles in agriculture. A "mourning" poncho also makes a suitable ground cloth on which to collect produce in the fields. In a farming society, objects too must earn their living, performing their service in the mundane, as well as the sacred, realm. Seeing a mourning poncho on the ground during harvest made me consider the numerous gray areas in contextual usage of "sacred" cloth. If a ritual poncho can be pressed into service for the most mundane activity, what gives the object its sacred quality? The meaning of black cloth has become unmoored from mourning. Recall Nilda's recent "eye for black."

While brightly colored *bordados* still rule, black is gaining ground. In Chivay market and artisans' workshops, black clothes long constituted a small percentage of those made, displayed, and sold.[18] Sales were low in the early 1990s, when fewer people bought *bordados;* as sales slowly increased over time, so did the percentage of black garments. The relationship between artisans' expectations of tourists and actual sales is complex. Selling more black clothes could deplete the supply of "authentic" black items, but the more likely effects of tourist demand are to spur production and create issues of quality. An increase in lower-quality, lower-priced items, a familiar process in craft "development," is often lamented as the epitome of the loss of authenticity. But just as frequently, artisans also create higher-quality, higher-priced items, such as Patricia's vest, for more affluent or discriminating buyers.

Increased tourism, such as Caylloma experienced in the mid-1990s, may alter more radically the types of objects produced. Even if authenticity is what tourists want to purchase, sometimes their knowledge of "authentic native costume" is less than expert, such as their preference for "natural" fibers now rarely used.

Still and all, black objects constitute less than half of the total sold. Caylloma garments appeal to tourists not only as garments but as souvenirs to display. At U.S.$35–$50, Cabanaconde-style embroidered hats are expensive by local standards; Cabaneños buy them infrequently, but they fall within most tourists' reach. When choosing between a hat and a *pollera* at the same price, the tourist often prefers the souvenir which will look attractive hanging on a wall to the one which will be packed away.[19]

A recent phenomenon, apart from color, is the development of a few retail establishments in Caylloma that actively cater to tourists. They carry a much higher percentage of novelty items, which Cayllominos do not use. Livia Sullca's shop is, hands down, the stellar establishment in this domain. Having built her career as the only Chivay vendor specializing in tourist art, Sullca works hard on the displays and wants to attract more tourists. She asked me to take photographs, featuring her ten-year-old daughter modeling *polleras,* which she would make into postcards/advertisements. Jenny was wearing typical daily wear: pants and a T-shirt, this one bearing a 7-Up advertisement.[20] "Go put on your *polleras*!" insisted her mother. Normally, she wears them only for festivals and school dance performances. Because her hair is only shoulder length, long braids had been made of black yarn and sewn into her hat. Once fully outfitted, she posed holding several heart-shaped bags (Figure 39).

Within Sullca's wonderland of embroidered souvenirs, Colca Valley dolls are the primary specialty. She does sell traditional garments, which she and commissioned artisans make. What Livia particularly enjoys is making and selling tiny things. She has created new styles of bag, purse, belt pouch, and backpack (*ch'uspa, bolsa, kanguro, mochila*). Increasingly, all of these use black background fabric. Nonetheless, dolls dominate her store, in six or eight different styles, 30–80 cm high.

"Barbie" is the star. The pert plastic doll wears traditional Caylloma-style *bordados,* modified to fit the miniature form, but sewing-machine embroidered the same way as full-size *polleras.* This popular item sells for U.S.$10. Since the unclothed doll costs about U.S.$.50 (wholesale), almost all Sullca's expenditure is for the mini-*bordados.* Barbie (Mattel Corporation) dolls are marketed globally. Mattel itself has produced various "ethnic" Barbies, but the one it calls "Native American Barbie," for example, does not present the dress of any specific tribe but reflects outsiders' interpretations of Native American identity (Lord 1994:186). Genuine Barbies are sold throughout Latin America, where blondes outsell all other hair colors (ibid.:195–196). Mattel sets prices lower than in the United States because it sees the Latin American market as soft (ibid.:196), but the dolls are still pricey. Most plastic fashion dolls in Peru are bootlegs, called "Barbi" in Spanish but produced in Asia for a fraction of the cost.[21]

Sullca has appropriated the ultimate emblem of the hegemony of fashion and has transformed the chorus-girl silhouette into the woman of substance enveloped in the voluminous local costume. The bootleg Barbie dressed in authentic ethnic garb speaks not only of the commercialization of Caylloma *bordados.* Miniature souvenir representations of female body image also signify the condensation of ethnicity within gender. Because femaleness is the dominant symbol of Indianness, signified by the comparative paucity of male ethnic dress, Barbie is the ideal symbol for this relationship. For years, Sullca made no Colca "Kens"; no one would buy male dolls, she claimed, because they lack *bordados.* During my visit in 2000, however, I found that she was selling Witite dolls: Ken dressed "*de polleras.*"

More broadly, both the overall commercialization and the specializa-

39 LIVIA SULLCA'S STORE, CHIVAY; HER DAUGHTER JENNY MODELS *POLLERAS.*

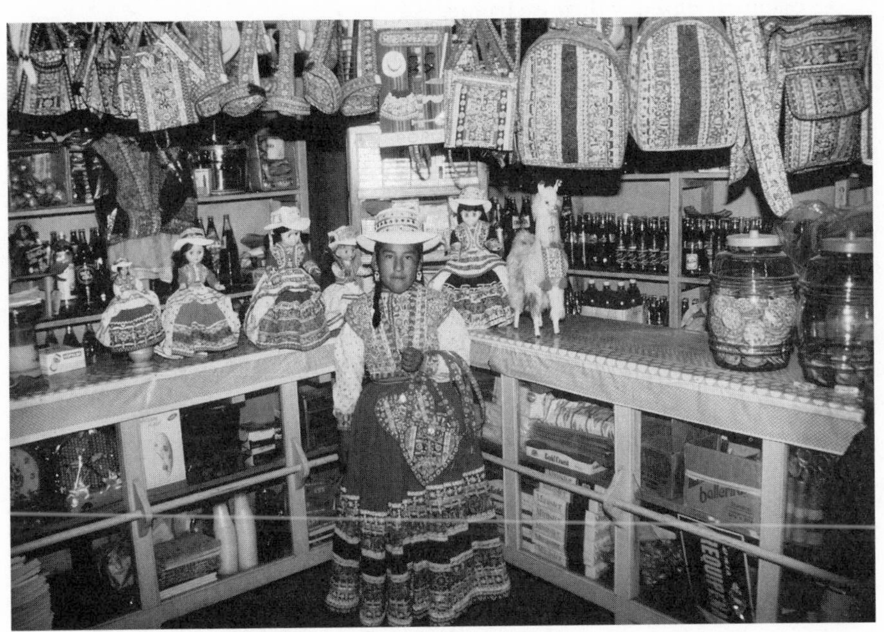

tion in different commodities tell us much about changes in exchange relations, as Colloredo (1999), Meisch (2002), and Orlove and Rutz (1989) have explored. As marketing, economy, class, and ethnicity intertwine in *bordado* sales, their articulation prompts us to rethink categories. When I began studying commerce in Caylloma, I suspected that class and ethnicity would closely correlate in marketing arrangements. It seemed logical to postulate that production and exchange would be divided between artisans who make handmade crafts and who are primarily Indian, and merchants, who are primarily *mestizo.* Because Andean communities are well known for their highly developed systems of reciprocal economic and kinship relations, their participation in capitalist society has often been viewed as part of a dual economy. In this model, *mestizos* are the merchants and capitalists, and in those roles, they exploit Indians, who are not capitalists. In practice, however, class and ethnic divisions were far from neat. My study presents little data about "traditional Andean" relations of barter and noncapitalist exchange, although they operate in Caylloma. Family members make garments for and obtain them from relatives: a godmother provide clothes for the godchild she is baptizing; a mother-in-law lends, then ultimately gives, a *pollera.* I have chosen not to detail the "traditional Andean" exchanges, in large part, to emphasize that *bordados* are a business: over and over, in market, workshop, and home, it impressed me, how thoroughly commercialized is their exchange.

Economic success in Peru is often accompanied by social whitening, but in Caylloma this is not always the case. No single class or ethnicity can adequately encompass artisans, vendors, or merchants because they are in constant movement. Most artisans are vendors at some time in their careers and may go on to become merchants. Their identities do not fit neatly bounded categories because ethnicity is relational and situational. The blurring of boundaries has ideological ramifications. To posit strict divisions between artisans and merchants would reinforce preconceptions that Indians are not capitalists. To review just one case, Rosalía Valera, a woman who was once an artisan, is now a successful vendor at the same time as she wears *polleras,* lives on her land as a peasant farmer, and participates in community religious festivals. Is Rosalía an Indian? Or does her economic activity make her a *mestiza*? Does a change in occupation compel a change in ethnic identity?

The Caylloma situation suggests that we should reconsider the role of Indian identity *in* marketing to encompass identification *as* marketing.

Cayllominos are apparently buying into the hegemonic discourse that renders Indian identity exotic; they seem to be folklorizing themselves to market identity. The sale of souvenirs like Barbie dolls, by appropriating notable visual qualities of Caylloma women, markets their identity as a commodity. Does this mean Cayllominos are selling off, or selling out, identity? Perhaps, instead, by selling it they are keeping it.

Caylloma *bordados* embellish many subjects and objects: bodies and representations of them. Embroidery is an object saturated with local cultural value which has been transformed into an object of desire and an object of consumption. The meanings of *bordados* have been altered through circulation in diverse "regimes of value" (Appadurai 1986), in which associations attached to objects are constantly challenged and altered. In analyzing such attachments and detachments, Annette Weiner posits that exchange moves society because an object is not only attached to current values, but it acts as a kind of reinvestment, endowing contemporary society with the worth of the past; she terms this "the paradox of keeping-while-giving" (1992: 6–9). Caylloma vendors are apparently "giving" the representation of their "indigenous" identity to consumers when they sell *bordados* to tourists. Yet these objects must be distinguished from the "inalienable possessions" of which Weiner writes, for many are made expressly to be alienated. The alienation of object and that of culture are not the same, however. As Cayllominos participate in capitalist economy, they are challenging a dominant paradigm that relegates their goods, and themselves, to a noncapitalist sphere: They are not giving, but taking; they are selling-while-keeping as they avail themselves of the benefits of the market.

For Caylloma's Indian capitalists, Indianness is part of what propels them to become capitalists. To be capitalists, they must be Indians, and to be Indians, they must be capitalists, because what they are selling is Indian identity. Andean exchange does not exist outside the sphere of capitalist exchange. Although Cayllominos participate in an intricate web of reciprocity, Indian identity depends on capitalism.

Conclusion

Caylloma cloth has a dazzling variety of forms and uses. I have long found it difficult to reconcile that coy plastic Barbies inhabit the same cultural universe as austere alpaca ponchos. Both objects are used in secular contexts, but in my western cosmogram they would never comfortably coexist. In fact, I drove them apart with labels: "sacred," "secular"; "mundane," "ritual"; "authentic," "tourist." Reconsidering the meanings of ritual objects and commodities made me realize that it was necessary to address shifts in meaning through analyzing the interpenetrating nature of categories and the transformation of the same object in different contexts.

Examining the objects in the social economy where they are consumed renders borders suspect. Sale of embroidered garments is part of daily life for Caylloma's artisans; loss of relatives to illness and death is part of the mundane world as well. Yet Catholic religious practice and local tradition exhort Cayllominos to separate a time and place for commemoration of personal and communal loss—a space constituted, in part, by black fabric with which people surround their bodies and which they place in churches and cemeteries. The authenticity of their experience and the objects that represent it need not be discounted by tourism. Authenticity shapes the marketing of ethnicity not only to tourists but to Cayllominos themselves. Many commercial establishments are simultaneously workshops and stores that create and modify ethnic clothes and sell them to the authentic, native consumers. As culture brokers, artisans and vendors promote ethnicity as a cultural good and, at the same time, as one that will earn money. In all these trading places, vendors and artisans may change roles many times daily and for longer terms.

As Indianness relates to market sales, ethnicity has become commoditized. Ethnic identity has been reified and promoted as a thing that is marketable and consumable: for instrumental uses in sale itself, as clothes reaffirm and exaggerate Indian appearance, and in the broader realm of folklorization, as a segment of national culture is promoted for foreign and national tourists to consume. Cayllominos risk folklorizing themselves and de-authenticating their identity. As people move away, returning to the valley only for ceremonial occasions, they are sometimes mockingly called tourists and their authenticity as natives is questioned by relatives who have remained in the home communities.

The production and use of black clothing in Caylloma simultaneously continue along traditional paths and are rerouted by tourist desires. Cayllominos continue to commemorate the dead, observing the responsibilities that the living have to the dead and to each other. In doing so, they involve fabric in a communal experience that is made salient at specific times each year. The observation of Catholic rites and customs is an important part of village life. Tenderness toward the dead helps make life possible for the living in Caylloma's harsh environment. Participating in those events and attending ceremonies in churches, I too traded places. Although I was incorporated into the community, part of me remained a tourist. Coporaque is my home only in an episodic way, but sharing moving experiences with friends and *compadres* is the way I learned about the bonds expressed through black.

"Black" is more than a color that "symbolizes" different cultural values. Black creates boundaries, demarcating ritual space around bodies among Cayllominos. Black also creates communication, establishing shared, though conflictual, grounds for discourse between Caylloma artisan vendors and tourists. For this new buyer, black is not sad; it speaks not of loss, but of finding; it signifies the novelty of experience. Once the tourist purchases her memento, she participates in a new phase of the cycle, resacralizing the souvenir as an untouchable object to be admired. She will remove it once again from the realm of the mundane, tucking it away in the reliquary of a closet, hanging it on the wall as artwork, or donning it as fancy dress for a cocktail party. In the eyes of others, longing for the unreachable artifact enhances its value. For the owner, the object of desire becomes an emblem of her exclusivity and, at the same time, of her membership in the secular cult of multicultural connoisseurship.

Conclusion

Why Women Wear *Polleras*

The women of Caylloma don *polleras* to work in cornfields and to dance in fiestas. They make *polleras* in workshops with husbands, sons, and daughters, and they sell finished garments to neighbors, friends, and strangers. From infancy to death, the cloth walls called *polleras* are cultural homes that Caylloma's women inhabit. The process of making and wearing *polleras,* in which many Cayllominos engage, is part and parcel of what creates their gendered identities. Women wear *polleras* because they are women, and women become women by wearing *polleras.*

In writing primarily about women's clothes, I have apparently privileged gender over ethnicity. Yet for Cayllominas, gender cannot be separated from ethnicity. Their choice to use the garments called *polleras* depends on their racial and ethnic identity as "indigenous" people, "peasants," and people of Caylloma. The social space of identification with the place of Caylloma cannot be separated, in Peruvian idiom, from the space of Indianness. White women do not dress "*de polleras*"; "*blancas*" and "*criollas*" dress "*de vestido.*" The politics of belonging dictates that wearing a distinct style of dress—the *polleras* called *bordados*—expresses identification with a collectivity, which is explicitly an ethnic presence. Inclusion in one community of practice means exclusion from another.

Two apparently contradictory answers provide a key to class as related to ethnicity and belonging. Why do women wear *polleras*? "To show they have more money," said one woman; "so they'll think I don't have money," claimed another. *Bordados* are elaborate assemblages in which men and women invest time, energy, and money. The price of *polleras* is high, in both monetary and social terms. Investing in these fancy cloth confections must be considered in a long-term strategy of resource allocation—a strategy in which prestige, style, and taste are chips with which to play the local game of social advancement.

Women stated simply, "I wear *polleras* because I like them." They may refer to the entire ensemble, a specific garment, or the chance to change clothes on occasion. The heightened awareness of the visual domain among artisans and consumers means that specific kinds of garments mean different things; a luxurious first-quality velvet skirt is a far cry from a workaday *bayeta* model. It also means Caylloma women wear *polleras* not just because they are Cayllominas but because they are individuals who value style.

When Cayllominas don elaborate *bordados* for festivals, we may be tempted to view their expenditures as conspicuous consumption. However, *bordados* have characteristics particular to their production in Caylloma. Expenditures by community members on embroidered clothes are an investment in localized cultural capital. Women wear *polleras* because their relatives, friends, and neighbors are the producers, and these are the people from whom they desire to purchase beautiful things.

Finally, the "why" of women's use of *polleras* can only be understood by considering the "how" and "why" of instances when they do not use them—the reasons, such as racism against indigenous people, that women gave for not wearing them. Why *women* wear *polleras* also gained more pointed meaning when contrasted with why *men* wear them. Women wear *polleras* because men do not wear them—because *polleras* are women's clothes, a defining feature of femaleness and a way to establish gendered boundaries.

Of course, we cannot forget that men wear *polleras* too, but they do so on bounded, ritual occasions which serve to reinforce the notion that, at bottom, *polleras* are women's clothes.

I have taken the position that wearing *polleras* is a positive aspect of Caylloma social practice. *Bordados* embody resistance, which has always proceeded through appropriation. Rather than retreating from the modern world into the comfortable traditional home of *polleras,* Caylloma's women deploy *polleras* as political and economic instruments to help them achieve their goals. Women wear *polleras* because clothes condense power. This power depends on symbols to express values and goals; those symbols are effective only in a total economy that incorporates political goals and material objects, merging them into a unified, yet uneasily balanced domain of representation.

How to Finish a *Pollera*

This study is about ambiguity, in terms of how categories are constituted: categories which in the academy we call gender, ethnicity, and dress, and, in some very particular and peculiar ways, the intellectual project we call ethnography. The work is concerned with representation in a number of ways. The subject of the book is clothes, but the subject is also the genre —how anthropologists conceive and develop certain types of representational approaches and procedures. In all these ways, then, the book is about practice—what happens?—and about experience—how does what happens affect us?

This book is about gender, and in saying so I acknowledge that in most respects my approach to gender is solidly mainstream. I mostly worked with, and mostly wrote about, women, and until recently most anthropological works about gender primarily have been about *women.* I did not start out to write much about masculinity, and I do not often overtly pinpoint it here. Still and all, I write about *gender.* From my inclusion and discussion of seemingly small events and everyday occurrences—a man makes adobes one day, and embroiders little birds the next—to more isolated, ritualized performances—a man shoves his neighbor and tries to start a fistfight one day, and puts on a *pollera* and dances around disguised as a woman the next—this project explores contradictions and ambiguities in categories and identities, male and female, masculine and feminine.

Nowhere are the ambiguities of gender as a Euro-American and as a

Latin American category more apparent than in the subject matter I have chosen: embroidery. Ambivalence haunted my decision to focus on embroidery, to treat *bordados* as the quintessential form of Caylloma clothing. In discussing false borders in the introduction, I juxtaposed my expectations about the aftermath of a bombing event in Chivay to life as usual that I found when I went there—life that included, and sometimes depended on, embroidery. Such experiences led me to question my own, and Caylloma people's, connection with the tough realities of daily life, and pushed me to ponder the meaning of the feminine, frivolous, and superficial "embroidery" compared to the harsh, violent, and deep-seated climate of "war." Once I concluded that to dismiss embroidery would mean not only to collaborate in the trivialization of a culturally meaningful form but to render a disservice to the men and women who created it, I was forced to confront the reasons for such negative valuations and to probe the positive value of creativity in troubled times.

This book about gender, then, is *a* book, one book, one product, out of a constellation of possibilities that the rich material I gathered might have become. Creating this book—not some other one, but this particular work—and making my decisions and sticking to them about what kind of creative project was appropriate for me as an anthropologist who lived in a foreign country in deeply troubled times, proceeded apace with my evaluations of how Caylloma's artisans made such decisions and acted based on those decisions. Through many brief incidents, as well as longer, more thought-out and felt-out episodes, my learning about clothing in Caylloma unrolled. The fact that creativity was imperiled in wartime contained contradictions and ambiguities, and made me constantly rethink my position. Like the tiny stitches that attached designs to materials, these nagging doubts were not distractions to be dismissed—they were substantial and not just superficial. In fact, the distinctions between substance and superfice were precisely the false borders that I had to transgress in order to resolve the quandaries of the symbolic economy concept that guided the research from the outset. The tensions that underlie their creation made these emblems—*bordados,* gender, ethnicity—emphatically ambiguous. Yet the subject of the book is not ambiguous; there is no question of this author hedging or waffling. The subject of the book is ambiguity—facing head-on and staring down the contradictions, imbalances of power, and inadequacies of resources that characterize real life for real people in Peru today.

In the mid-1930s, a woman who is now recognized as one of America's most distinguished "native anthropologists" returned to her home community in her new roles of ethnographer and folklorist. Approaching childhood buddies, beloved aunts and uncles, and local ne'er-do-wells who loved to tell tall tales, Zora Neale Hurston explained that she had come to collect folk tales. "'What you mean, Zora . . . them big old lies we tell . . . ?'" demanded one of the storytellers. "'You come to the right place if lies is what you want. Ah'm gointer lie up a nation!'" (Hurston 1990: 8, 19).

My position as a storyteller among storytellers depends on honesty: assessing my position as ethnographer, as stranger and friend, as widow, *comadre, gringa, chilena*. But it does not depend on truth. I cannot verify that any of the information I have reported here is true. Like the storytellers who promised Hurston they would honestly deliver lies, as an ethnographer I must take the position that my job is not to tie up loose ends but to embroider—sometimes in ways like those of Caylloma people, sometimes by devices of my own choosing—within the borders of the ambiguous emblem that we call ethnography. I hope that I have helped the reader see how the object—*bordados*—can be a subject, and to understand that by looking at the surface—by embroidering on the truth—we can also enrich our view of substance.

As I conclude this book, once again I am packing up my stuff. Preparing for a trip to Peru, I am surrounded by suitcases and boxes, bags and trunks of things in my Rhode Island home, where *bordados* still enrich my person and decorate my space. A Cabana hat sits on a shelf in the foyer, and a tourist's passport case loops around my bedroom doorknob. From my desk, I pick up a tiny bag with black background and see green-yellow-and-pink hummingbirds flit around the flowers crowding its surface. Holding this miniature object and admiring this embroidered scene, my fingers miss the touch of other stitches and my mind hears again the voice of my *comadre* Nilda admitting she too has developed a taste for black. And walking through the streets of Providence, my feet recall other walks in other landscapes; I seem to hear my neighbor Dionisio recommend sleeping out in the *campo* to breathe good air, and the passionately artistic Marcial proclaim that embroidery is like painting a landscape.

Throughout this ethnography, I have struggled to retain a focus on the daily lives of ordinary people and to employ this narrow focus in service of an effort to understand as well the broader forces that shape their lives. Adhering to its primary role as an ethnography of the body, this book became a many-stranded braid that serves as an ethnography of rural life, a regional and historical ethnography, and a personal and biographical ethnography. The stories moved from my taking a walk and picking beans, which immersed us in the daily realm of subsistence agriculture in the Colca Valley, to the complex journey of a doll that becomes a souvenir representing the valley to the world. They show how Caylloma's inhabitants live in the province on their own terms and how they are connected with areas as seemingly distant as the United States. And from my tale about commissioning a *pollera* as it helped me to understand the meaning of color and design for Cayllominos, to the episode about the thwarted *tuna* vendor who could not instrumentally deploy her ethnic garb one day because the urban war rudely intervened, this ethnography has moved from the physical body to the temporal body. It chronicles the lives of many individuals whose paths crossed mine, not only during two fieldwork years in troubled times, but in the decade since the war's official end.

Throughout the book, I also have explored the relationship between theory and method in performing ethnography. The book is about gender and representation not just as subject matter. Gender had meaning as representation and performance as well, in terms of how I worked with people in Caylloma, how I personally and professionally understood the means and meanings of clothing the body, and how I generated the written product that is this text. Theoretical perspectives about gender certainly informed what and how I observed about the practices of other people. As I hunted and gathered among those perspectives, the conviction became ever stronger that my personal experience was central, not peripheral, to that understanding. Knowing why women wear *polleras* meant intruding into kitchens, workshops, lives; querying about marriage, birth, death; trying those *polleras* on for size. Being accepted into a "women's circle" or sphere because of my gender was but a window into the larger issue of coming to terms with the existing cultural constructions of gender in Caylloma: How did those constructions influence how women there perceived me? How was my "freedom" as female—to come and go in Caylloma, to be a traveler as others were—culturally structured on their terms? How did Cayllominos perceive the garment of culture—as it fit them and as it fit me?

Rosalind Morris (1995:547) stated that "ethnographies are . . . about performing gender." To reprise, and perhaps distort, her statement, I believe that gender in part is about performing ethnography. Performing gender-as-ethnography, for this anthropologist, meant learning by doing things that Caylloma women did. It also meant, for years after I moved back to the United States from Peru, continuing to adhere to principles of action and performance in creating the ethnographic product. While a certain sensibility came from my cultural encoding into gendered practices of emotional openness, at the same time I struggled with academic standards and rules of evidence. My stay in Peru convinced me firmly, and I can't say it often enough, that I'm a *gringa* through and through. Perhaps it is a paradox that being a Latina has made me more sensitive than ever to this *gringaización*. As ten-year-old Norma Vilcasán did not hesitate to point out to me, the skirt I was wearing was nothing like a *pollera;* unembroidered, it was not finished. And, as Rosalía Valera made me aware, there's *polleras* and then there's *polleras;* my tastes in *bordado* style would never be shared by everyone. The garment of Caylloma culture fits imperfectly, loose here, tight there. The life of Cayllominas is not my life, and their clothes are not my clothes.

In 1944 the artist Arshile Gorky created an oil painting on canvas titled "How My Mother's Embroidered Apron Unfolds in My Life" (now in the collection of the Seattle Art Museum). Gorky drew on his Armenian roots, deriving the work from abstract Armenian shapes in his mother's apron, which he saw in a photograph (Ash 1995). In an article analyzing this work, John Ash reproduces the painting but not that photograph. We do not see the visual source of the bold, distorted, convoluted, distended, and disturbed shapes and colors that Gorky wrought from memory and distress, but Ash gives us some of Gorky's words. His mother had died twenty-five years earlier, after the Ottoman government expelled their family from Armenia. But artists are driven, Ash correctly noted, "by memory and sense impressions of hallucinatory vividness." Years later, Gorky wrote, "'My Mother told me stories while I pressed my face into her long apron with my eyes closed. . . . All my life her stories and her embroidery kept unraveling pictures in my memory'" (Ash 1995:79, 121). So too the stories and embroidery of Caylloma people have impressed and unraveled the images that compose this ethnography. My story is their story, if only in fragmented ways, and their clothes have had a turn in shaping our embroidered lives.

Notes

Introduction: False Borders, Embroidered Lives

1. Chávez (1987) has written one of the few studies about Arequipa's urban vendors; Carpio (1990) and Durand (1979) analyze late-twentieth-century employment and development trends in Arequipa. The literature on Peruvian internal migration and the informal sector concentrates on Lima (Bunster and Chaney 1985; Degregori, Blondet, and Lynch 1986; de Soto 1989, 2002; Driant 1991; Golte and Adams 1986; Scott 1994).
2. Among the extensive analyses of agricultural production in Colca Valley communities are Denevan (2001), Gelles (2000), Guillet (1992), and Treacy (1989, 1994a). Studies of pastoralism are scarce, but see Gómez (1985) and Markowitz (1992). Denevan, ed. (1986 and 1988) include studies by anthropologists, geographers, and historians. To date, single-community ethnographic studies of the Colca Valley have far outpaced attempts to grasp the region as a whole. Manrique's (1985) treatment of Caylloma Province stresses pre-twentieth-century history. Migration out of Caylloma has occurred for many centuries. On migrants in Peru, see Paerregaard (1997), and in the United States, see the film *Transnational Fiesta* (Gelles and Martínez 1993).
3. Caylloma is a province in the department of Arequipa; the province contains a town of the same name. The province is the department's largest in size and second largest in population after the province of Arequipa (Cook 1982). Still, the city of Arequipa clearly dominates. It had about 586,000 inhabitants, or 83 percent of the department's population (706,580), according to the 1981 census. Only 5.6 percent, 39,431 people, lived in Caylloma. A 1987 count placed the department's population at 884,200 (Censo Nacional del Perú, cited in Stoner 1989; also Gallard and Vallier 1988:54–57), but more recent estimates give 1 million for the city of Arequipa alone. Cook (1982) provides a historical study of Colca Valley demography.
4. From 1991 to 1993, not one drop of rain fell in the city of Arequipa. The severe drought affected not only agriculture but the energy system. With hydroelectric power unreliable (and illogical in a region averaging 350 sunny days annually) and the diesel-fueled backup system prohibitively expensive, by mid-1992 blackouts governed almost all activities. Not only did poor neighborhoods have more blackouts than others, but most houses there are not wired so hot cables are tapped from streetlights, which caused accidental electrocutions.

5. On the war in Peru, Poole and Rénique (1992) offer a useful guide to the contemporary situation in historical context; see also Cameron and Mauceri, eds. (1997); Starn (1999); and Tulchin and Bland (1994).
6. In the 1980s through 1990s, Sendero and MRTA were the two most active insurgent movements in Peru; see Degregori (1990); Gorriti (1990, 1999); Kirk (1993); McClintock (1989); Palmer, ed. (1992); P. Stern (1995); and S. Stern, ed. (1998).
7. On the 1990 elections and Fujimori's appeal, see Degregori and Grompone (1991) and Oliart (1998). Fujimori was re-elected in 1995; when he ran again in 2000, the election's procedures and outcome were so widely disputed that he was forced to resign. Since Alejandro Toledo's election in 2000, corruption and fiscal irregularities in the Fujimori administration have been openly investigated (Burt 2000; Crabtree and Thomas, eds. 1998; Dargent 2001; Ugarteche 2002).
8. Influential works on the political economy of objects and meanings include Appadurai (1986); Baudrillard (1981 [1972]); Marcus and Myers, eds. (1995); and Weiner (1992).
9. Both the armed forces and insurgent groups flagrantly violated human rights (Americas Watch 1992; Basombrío 1998; de la Jara 2002; Muñoz 1998; Vargas 1992; Youngers and Burt 2000).
10. In "Deep Play," Clifford Geertz (1973) wrote about solidarity through a shared escape from violence in a Balinese community. My experience made me feel a greater rift from people on the street because I could retreat to a place of safety unavailable to them at that moment. Increasingly, anthropologists are probing the dilemmas of living in nations at war; essays in Nordstrom and Robben, eds. (1995) provide helpful comments, especially Feldman (1995) and Green (1995); also see Nelson (1999).
11. I use "popular" here as a translation for *popular,* pertaining to the working or lower classes, rather than to refer to "popular culture," which in the United States connotes low-brow mass-media entertainments. My use of the term draws on formulations by Néstor García Canclini (1995:4–5), who identifies the popular with inequality in power relations that both promote and restrict access to the market in "symbolic goods"; see also Phillips and Steiner, eds. (1999) and Rowe and Schelling (1991: 9–12). Lauer (1982, 1989), Mendoza (2000), Poole (1990, 1994), Romero (2001), Stastny (1984), and investigators in Cánepa, ed. (2001) comment on contemporary Peruvian popular cultural productions.
12. Habitus forms through generative schemes which are "the product of the work of inculcation and appropriation necessary in order for those products of collective history, the objective structures, . . . to succeed in reproducing themselves" (Bourdieu 1977:85). To understand asymmetries of power, we must explain how the reproduction of domination proceeds through habitus. My approach, however, maximizes the dynamic potential of habitus, giving more weight to human agency and emphasizing productive more than reproductive strategies.
13. Kondo (1990) has analyzed how the person develops through the work he or she does in Japanese family-run small factories. My use of "person" resonates with her idea of the "crafted self."

14. I sketch the *bordado* workshop system in Femenías (1996 [1991]). For Otavalo, Ecuador, Meisch (1987b) pioneered analysis of family workshops, and Colloredo-Mansfeld (1999) addresses class issues for weavers fully embedded in global capitalism; see also Rowe, ed. (1998) on Ecuador in general.
15. Markowitz (1992) offers data on weaving in high-altitude Caylloma communities and Conklin (1996) analyzes textiles from Inka burials, but otherwise little has been published. On Andean weaving more generally, see Chapter 3, n. 2.
16. In Peru until recently, studies of race largely centered on indigenous people. Attention to African and Afro-Peruvian identity and blackness is increasing; see Chambers (1999) on colonial Arequipa; also Aguirre et al. (2000), Callirgos (1993), Hünefeldt (1994), Manrique (1999), and Santa Cruz (1995). Today "*indio*" (Indian) remains a powerful epithet, with only derogatory connotations. It is not a term of self-identification by indigenous groups. Relationships among ethnic groups, indigenous groups, and national polities are discussed in Chapter 2.
17. On women's political participation in popular sectors in Peru, see Blondet (1999), Kirk (1993), Miloslavich (1993), and Vargas (1995).
18. Distinguishing sharply between "invented" and "customary" traditions, Hobsbawm (1992 [1983]) presents "invented" as nearly synonymous with "imposed" by colonial rulers. I extend to "customary" tradition the analytic scrutiny he generated for "invented" tradition.
19. As a generic term, I prefer "clothes" and also use "dress," which Barnes and Eicher (1992) advocate as the most general category. See also Hendrickson (1996) and Hollander (1978, 1994), as well as Barthes (1983) and Lipovetsky (1994) on "fashion."
20. I use "gender" in the broad sense for areas of male, female, heterosexual, homosexual, transsexual, and/or transgendered practices and ideologies, encompassing and not distinguishing between "gender" and "sex." My work builds on analyses of the discursive dimensions of gender constructedness, drawing on anti-essentialist trends in anthropology and other disciplines, which have moved the analysis of sex and gender away from attachment to preconceptions of "biology" and "nature." A detailed discussion of anthropology's substantial contributions to the analysis of gender is outside the scope of this book; see di Leonardo (1991); Kulick (1998); Moore (1988, 1994); Morris (1995); and Ortner and Whitehead, eds. (1981). Anthropological analyses of sexuality are fewer, but consult Kulick (2000) and Weston (1993a, 1993b).
21. Foucault (1978) explains how perceptions of sex identity have been based in regulatory discourse marking the surfaces of bodies; see also Butler (1993) and Morris (1995:568).
22. Initial work in Chivay market, which revealed about two hundred vendors, with more than fifty selling and making embroidered clothes, helped me decide to focus on *bordados,* and I designed and implemented appropriate surveys. In order to contextualize the embroidery vendors, I left the scope broad enough to include businesses that make and sell other garments used in conjunction with *bordados,* especially hats, and garment variants made for tourists.

23. My claim that "I speak Quechua, but the kind they speak in Ecuador" generated responses including polite indifference, remedial instruction, and mirth. The fact that I could not say "I" (*noqa* not *ñuka*) or count "one" (*hoq* not *shuj*) was ample proof to Cayllominos that whatever it was I was speaking, it certainly was not Quechua. Peruvian Quechua and Ecuadorian Quichua are, I concluded, different languages, not dialects. On the Quechua variants of Coporaque (Caylloma) and Cotahuasi (in a neighboring province, La Unión), see Kindberg and Kindberg (1985) and Buckingham and Kindberg (1987).

1. Traveling

1. People in the valley also keep chickens, guinea pigs, sheep, and cows; in higher-altitude villages and ranches, they keep llama and alpaca herds; see Gómez (1985), Markowitz (1992), and Webber (1988, 1993).
2. Upon marriage, women add their husband's patronym to their own and drop the matronyms: Maximiliana's surname is Terán de Malcohuaccha. In practice, however, a married woman usually calls herself, and is called, by her birth patronym: Maximiliana Terán. Children of either sex take the patronym as their primary surname, followed by the matronym, yielding, for example, Carlos Malcohuaccha Terán, but in practice, Carlos Malcohuaccha.
3. On farming in the Colca Valley, see Denevan (2001); Denevan, ed. (1986, 1988); Gallard and Vallier (1988); Gelles (1990, 1994, 1995, 2000); Guillet (1992); Hurley (1978); Paerregaard (1992, 1994); Swen (1986); and Treacy (1989, 1994a, 1994b).
4. Valley farmers grow barley specifically for sale to the Cervecería del Sur, a large brewery in Arequipa.
5. Respiratory ailments are among the most common health complaints (Stoner 1989).
6. Caylloma's colonial history has been explored by Benavides (1987, 1988a, 1988b, 1990), Gelles (1990, 1995, 2000), Málaga (1977), Manrique (1985), Pease (1977), and Wernke (2003), among others.
7. On widowhood and its effects on fieldwork, little has been written, but see Freedman (1986). Renato Rosaldo (1989) movingly recounts his grief and rage after his first wife, Michele Zimbalist Rosaldo, died during fieldwork in the Philippines.
8. The nested geo-political structure is: *municipio* (municipality), roughly equivalent to a U.S. incorporated township, headed by an *alcalde municipal* (municipal mayor); *distrito* (district), encompassing the *municipio* and adjacent *anexos* (annexes, i.e., villages and hamlets), headed by the *gobernador* (governor); *provincia* (province), similar to a county, headed by the *alcalde provincial* (provincial mayor); then the *departamento* (department), like a state, headed by the *prefecto* (prefect).
9. *Tía* and *tío* (Spanish), literally "aunt" and "uncle," are used in this area by both Quechua- and Spanish-speaking people as terms of respect for persons senior to the speaker, regardless of familial relationship.
10. On *compadrazgo* in Caylloma, see Gelles (1990:114–116; 2000:40) and Guillet (1992:120); in Cusco, Allen (1988:88–91); and in Puno, Zorn (2003). *Compadrazgo* also has

been an abusive institution because *mestizo* landlords and merchants became *padrinos* to dozens of children in peasant communities, thereby enforcing patron-clientelism and assuring access to a large unpaid labor force.

11. The *compadrazgo* relationship cemented a personal bond. Because Flora was pregnant with Lucía most of the time she worked with me, it seemed inevitable for me to become kin to that baby.
12. *Mayordomo* (fiesta sponsor) is the highest position (*cargo*) in a community's civil-religious hierarchy; see Chapter 5.
13. On domestic architecture in Coporaque and other communities, see Llosa and Benavides (1994). Guillet (1992:117–118) describes the house compound's relationship to the household in Lari. On provisioning households in the pastoral zone, see Markowitz (1992).
14. I refer to the spoken languages. Nilda completed elementary school, so she writes some Spanish; written Quechua is rarely taught in Peru, despite recent activism and government projects (García 2000b).
15. On mountain rituals, see Gelles (1990:166–208; 1994:236; 2000:75–97 and passim), Gelles and Martínez (1993), and Valderrama and Escalante (1988, 1997). Within the voluminous literature on Andean mountain cultural ecology, Murra's (1972, 1980 [1955]) works are seminal and Lehmann, ed. (1982); Masuda, Shimada, and Morris (1985); and Mayer (2001) provide indispensable guides.
16. Treacy (1989:404–429, App. 2) lists several hundred plants native to Coporaque; see also de Romaña, Blassi, and Blassi (1987:67–72, 80–81). Below Cabanaconde, more trees grow, including native *queñua*. Forestation projects have been sponsored by an NGO, FAO-Holanda.
17. *Tuna* (*Opuntia ficus-indica*) is also the host for cochineal, which is marketed globally for its red or purple dye (Treacy 1989:429; also Gelles 1990:107, 132 n. 56; 2000:37, 48–49; de Romaña, Blassi, and Blassi 1987:80).
18. Overheating also split Ampato's glacial ice, revealing pre-Hispanic burials. One body so uncovered was nicknamed the "Ice Maiden of the Andes" (Reinhard 1996; also Fine-Dare 2002; Gelles 2000:78–81).
19. Treacy (1989:64–69; 1994a:60–62) and de Romaña, Blassi, and Blassi (1987) address geomorphology.
20. On water politics, see Gelles (1990, 1994, 1995, 2000), Guillet (1992, 1994), Paerregaard (1994), and Treacy (1989, 1994a, 1994b). On the MACON project's impact, see Benavides (1983), Gelles (1990, 2000), Hurley (1978), Larico (1987), and Swen (1986).
21. This scrutiny (with multiple origins, including the civil rights movement, the women's movement, and postcolonialism) continues to alter anthropology; see Abu-Lughod (1991); Marcus (1998); Marcus and Fischer (1986); Rosaldo (1989); Sanjek, ed. (1990); and Van Maanen, ed. (1995). Departing from the controversial anthology *Writing Culture* (Clifford and Marcus, eds. 1986), essays in *Women Writing Culture* (Behar and Gordon, eds. 1995) elaborated and challenged many characterizations in it.

22. While a female academic, rejecting an attitude of subordination, may identify herself and affirm her status as female, even to specify a "marked" identity as "other," such as "woman anthropologist," can make it seem demeaned, lesser than the unmarked (Callaway 1992:29); on other identity qualifiers, see Femenías (2002d), García (2000a), Narayan (1997), and Zavella (1997).
23. Strathern (1987), Stacey (1988), and Abu-Lughod (1990) comment eloquently on feminist ethnography's conflictive possibilities. Among the many analyses of intersections and differences between multiple feminisms and anthropologies, see Gordon (1999) on the academy and di Leonardo (1991) on how an anthropology of women led to an anthropology of gender. See also Golde, ed. (1986 [1970]); Moore (1988, 1994); Sanday and Goodenough, eds. (1990); Behar (1993); Bell, Caplan, and Karim, eds. (1993); Visweswaran (1994); Wolf, ed. (1995); Lamphere, Ragoné, and Zavella, eds. (1997); and Lather (2001).
24. Personal concerns and voice have a long history. A primary pioneering work is *Return to Laughter* (Bowen 1964 [1954]), Laura Bohannon's pseudonymous ethnographic novel. Since male academics recently began to use personal voice, they have applied the term "experimental ethnography" to such works (M. Wolf 1992:50; Behar 1995:4; and D. Wolf 1995). Even to categorize ethnography as either conventional (i.e., realist) or experimental, however, impedes understanding of the numerous, early feminist contributions to innovative ethnographic writing (Gordon 1995: 431).

2. *Fabricating Ethnic Frontiers: Identity in a Region at the Crossroads*

1. Political boundaries differ from cultural and ethnic boundaries. North of the Colca River and west of Cabanaconde, in an area called *adentro,* "inside" the valley, are several communities which are politically not part of Caylloma but of Castilla, the neighboring province. Their cultural practices are similar to those of Cayllominos, including the *pollera* styles worn, and they have close kin ties with Cayllominos. Their own provincial capital, Aplao, is five days away, whereas Chivay is only two.
2. Llama caravans still make the trek but in greatly diminished numbers; see Casaverde (1977) and Paerregaard (1991a).
3. Many of the laborers who built roads and railroads were press-ganged, sparking widespread resistance (Kapsoli 1984; Manrique 1985).
4. The *haciendas* consisting of agricultural lands in the valley itself were fairly small. The largest holdings were alpaca *estancias* in the *puna,* such as those owned by the Riveras of Yanque, which were broken up or appropriated during Agrarian Reform of the 1960s (Benavides 1988b; Markowitz 1992; Mauricio de Romaña, personal communication 1992). Guillet (1992:31) insists that there were no *haciendas* in the Colca Valley, so villagers were neither scrambling for land nor indebted to *hacendados* (owners). But, via the presence of *haciendas* in Caylloma, in the herding areas outside the valley, villagers did incur such debts.
5. Each region, headed by its own president, was generally larger than an existing de-

partment but sometimes its equivalent. Within Región Arequipa, the Colca Valley was designated a "Micro-región." The regions' autonomy, always limited, ended after the 1992 *autogolpe,* when Fujimori disbanded them.

6. Within the widespread attention to the multiple meanings of race and ethnicity, Harrison (1995) provides a thorough review. Also see Harris (1995) and Mörner (1970), as well as Appelbaum, Macpherson, and Rosemblatt, eds. (2003); Domínguez, ed. (1994); Graham, ed. (1990); and Hale (1986) on historical roots of racialized ethnic categories.
7. Part of the problem is with customary usage and translation. The noun "indigene" sounds stilted and awkward in English; it is not an equal counterpart to the Spanish "*indígena,*" which is at home in the vernacular. The other potential synonym, "native," is accompanied by a load of colonialist baggage that is even greater in English than in Spanish.
8. She traces this process solely in Cusco without considering the implications of that region's anomaly.
9. In a masterful historical review of ethnic categorization in the Andes, Harris notes that the ethnicity of *mestizo* "is in a way antiethnic, defined in terms of what it is not," while Indian "implies a bounded group . . ." (1995:373).
10. Scholarly attention to contemporary ethnic politics and the relationship of indigenous people to citizenship and the state in Latin America has mushroomed in recent years. Influential general works include Alvarez, Dagnino, and Escobar, eds. (1998); Arnson, ed. (1999); Brysk (2000); Domínguez and Lowenthal, eds. (1996); Langer, ed., with Muñoz (2003); Maybury-Lewis (1997); Maybury-Lewis, ed. (2002); Stavenhagen (1996); and Warren and Jackson, eds. (2002); on Mesoamerica and Central America, Campbell (1994); Cojtí Cuxil (1996); Collier, with Quaratiello (1994); Field (1996, 1999); Gould (1998); Rubin (1997); Stephen and Collier (1997); and Warren (1998a, 1998b); and on South America, Ramos (1998); Rappaport (1994, 1996); and Turner (1995).
11. Guillet reported that in Lari, people say, "We are all equal" (1992:40); I never heard anyone in a Colca Valley community say that.
12. Despite widespread debate, the relationship between "*misti*" and "*mestizo*" is an insoluble puzzle. Some believe "*misti*" is a Quechua word or a Quechuized pronunciation of "*mestizo*"; others distinguish between them by noting the abusive connotation of "*misti*"; and still others maintain that "*misti*" is corrupted from the English "mister" (Arguedas 1985 [1941]; Fuenzalida et al. 1970). In Arequipa, Misti Volcano and the Mistiano nickname further complicate the matter.
13. "Poncho" is also slang for "condom."

3. *Clothing the Body: Visual Domain and Cultural Process*

1. The "social life of things" is a concept developed by Appadurai (1986).
2. Many scholars have analyzed the relationship between contemporary and pre-Hispanic handwoven Andean garments; see my review essay (Femenías 1987). For a

solid introduction, begin with Rowe (1977) and consult Cereceda (1986); Femenías, ed. (1987); Rowe, ed. (1986, 1998); Rowe and Cohen (2002); Schevill, Berlo, and Dwyer, eds. (1996); Seibold (1990, 1992, 1995); and Zorn (1995, 1997b, 2004).

3. Sports matches, which occur at least weekly throughout a season, are a regular part of Cayllominos' lives in Arequipa. While the APC features soccer, as Paerregaard (n.d.) has stressed, it is also a broader social force that both supports and challenges regional culture through staging cultural events like dances.

4. Suni makes more *polleras* than any other embroiderer in the city, where there are several other *bordado* workshops. Girls sometimes commission *polleras* from urban artisans to dance in hometown fiestas. For many years, Suni operated one of the largest workshops in Chivay. After relocating to Arequipa, he found considerable demand for *polleras* there, too. He now keeps two workshops—one in his home in a poor neighborhood and another in downtown Arequipa, near the central market.

5. Seibold (1995:321–322) discusses attempts to enforce this law in Cusco. Elites sometimes dissociate ethnic clothes from authenticity and appropriate them for mimicry or disguise. For example, in 1993 the Alianza Francesa of Arequipa, an exclusive cultural center and school, presented a "folk" dance show. Upper-class white urban boys and girls as young as four danced to *huaynos* while dressed in the style of indigenous people of Chinchero, Cusco, and to Afro-Peruvian rhythms in tight ruffled clothes.

6. On black clothes and death rituals, see Chapter 8.

7. *Polleras* are sold as "finished" once the embroidery is completed; the customer applies a waistband; see Chapter 7.

8. True to the vagaries of fashion, lime green soon became hot in the United States. "Don't be a fashion victim—learn to wear lime green in spring" trumpeted a *New York Post* headline, and the article quoted *Vogue*'s fashion news director: "'Lime green **is** *the* color this season'" (Kling 1996:39, emphases in original).

9. Definitions are from Cusihuamán's Quechua-Spanish dictionary (1976:117): "*forraje, pasto verde; q'achu q'omer, verde claro; . . . q'achu ch'uñu, chuño fresco, recién helado*"; on "*q'achu*" as forage, see Treacy (1994a:191). In Cusco weavings, green indicates fertility (Seibold 1995).

10. Many natural phenomena are not depicted on *bordados:* mountains, condors, vicuñas (except in the national *escudo*), corn or other crops, cows, sheep, and alpacas or llamas. People and buildings are likewise absent. I saw one man's vest, made by Fermín Huaypuna in Chivay, that featured a large condor; it was commissioned by a foreigner. Recently, wall hangings called paintings, featuring condors, have been developed for tourists.

11. The lack of evidence counters outsiders' assumptions and claims. A Peruvian art historian who has documented the area's colonial patrimony told me people copied from the churches (Francisco Stastny, personal communication 1986). For illustrations and discussion of motifs on colonial buildings, see Stastny (1987), especially a rosette and a Lari house lintel with birds, rosettes, and a cross (142), and vizcachas on a house in Yanque (143).

12. Cabanaconde artists derided Chivay designs, saying they have mistakes, or are big, stretched out, or, again, just plain ugly (Melitón Picha and Juan Tejada, interviews, Cabanaconde, February 25, 1993). Embroidery with two threads, Tejada insisted, "comes out uglier."
13. Since 2000, many more artisans are producing hats; see Chapter 8.
14. "Merino" is a breed of sheep that the Spanish introduced in the sixteenth century (Orlove 1977), but in Caylloma today, *merino* refers to a synthetic yarn also used for weaving. All yarn, "natural" or synthetic, is called *lana* (Spanish, "wool"; see Tolen 1995 and Zorn 1995). Yarn spun from sheep wool is distinguished as *lana de oveja* (Spanish, "sheep").
15. For a discussion of how anthropologists have used dress in fieldwork, see Femenías (1997a:269–280).

4. *Addressing History: Representation and the Embodiment of Memory*

1. The Shippee-Johnson Peruvian Expedition, sponsored by the Peruvian government and the National Geographic Society, conducted aerial photographic reconnaissance of much of Peru and photographed extensively on the ground; see Shippee (1932a, 1932b, 1933, 1934) and Denevan (1993), Engle (1999), and Femenías (1993). In captions on file in the American Museum of Natural History, less than 1 percent of the people depicted are named.
2. On the church construction and alterations, see Gutiérrez, Esteras, and Málaga (1986:38–40, 100–104) and Tord (1983:117–122).
3. A *gobernador,* the head of a *distrito* (district), is appointed by the prefect of the department.
4. Some antique weavings are stored in bundles for ritual, rather than daily, use; see Chapter 8.
5. On anonymity and naming of "non-Western" artists, see Babcock (1993); Hail, ed. (2000); Hedlund (1989); and Steiner (1994).
6. Couples often marry after they have children together.
7. One meaning of the direct translation, "baize," is a commercial "coarse woolen stuff, with a long nap, sometimes frizzed on one side, without wale, now often dyed green and used to cover tables" (*Webster's Seventh Unabridged*), especially pool tables. This is quite different from Peruvian highland *bayeta,* despite the fabrics' shared European origin.
8. In the eighteenth century, *jerga* was rough stuff, not necessarily patterned, produced in *obrajes* (Jacobsen 1993:35).
9. In Chivay, "*venta*" (sale) means both monetary and nonmonetary exchanges: *venta para plata* (sale for money) and *cambio* (exchange) or *venta en cambio* (sale for exchange). The term "*trueque*" (barter) is seldom heard. Also see Casaverde (1977), Markowitz (1992), and Paerregaard (1991a).
10. "*Sastre*" is the common term for "tailor." "*Costurero,*" something like "seamster," a person who sews, parallels the more usual female "*costurera*" (seamstress).

11. The "Tahuantinsuyo," a pro-Indian political and cultural movement, was especially active in the southern highlands in the 1920s; see Femenías (1999) and Kapsoli (1977, 1984).
12. Jacobsen (1993:168–173) discusses late-nineteenth- through early-twentieth-century imports, including sewing machines, into southern Peru; see also Bauer (2001); Krüggeler (1997); and Orlove, ed. (1997).
13. By the 1920s, nationally produced goods outsold imports in the southern highlands. Peru's cotton textile mills, although located in Lima, were owned by powerful foreign enterprises, especially W. R. Grace and Duncan Fox (Jacobsen 1993:173; Thorp and Bertram 1978:33, 119–120, 129–130).
14. On *gente decente* in this period, see Parker (1998:24–28) for Lima, and de la Cadena (2000:44–85) for Cusco.
15. *Casimir*, in the Peruvian textile industry, does not mean "cashmere," but a fabric for men's suiting similar to worsted. It is still made industrially by large woolen-goods factories in Arequipa.
16. In addition to my own research in Coporaque and Chivay, I draw on that of Benavides (1988b) on Yanque, Gelles (2000) on Cabanaconde, and Paerregaard (1991b) on Tapay. A similar tripartite filial schema in Sonqo, Cusco, is discussed by Allen (1988). The similarity of such stories in different parts of the southern highlands, especially the tripartite structure—in which each brother corresponds to a major sphere of social power (church, capital, state)—lends an aura of the archetypal imaginary.
17. I found no female authorities in my reviews of hundreds of documents signed by Coporaque authorities (of the municipality and district) and of registers of authorities for selected years of the early twentieth century. Women held only one religious *cargo*, called *voto* or *de voto*, promising service to particular saints.
18. Luisa, who was in her seventies when I interviewed her in 1993, died in 1996; her husband died in the 1970s. For a detailed version of her narrative, see Femenías (1997a:357–360).
19. Eudumila Cáceres died in 1999; her home was sold and, in 2000, was the Chivay headquarters of Alejandro Toledo's presidential campaign.

5. Dancing in Disguise: Transvestism and Festivals as Performance

1. "Witite" is spelled many different ways in different sources: Witite, Wittite, Wititi, Huitite, etc. I spell the term "Witite" throughout for the sake of consistency. Lira's Quechua-Spanish dictionary gives *witi, witiy,* and *wititítiy,* "to equivocate or err; to disappoint or let down; to snap or crack [like a whip]; error or fallacy"; "to convulse [as] fish or worms out of their medium; to revolve"; and *witikk,* "one who beats or cracks a whip, or one who is beaten" (1944:1165; 1982:336). Three Aymara-Spanish dictionaries also list Witite or possibly related terms: Ayala (1988:197) gives *wititi,* "buffoon (fool)"; Deza (1989:77), *huitiña,* "to walk alone"; Bertonio (1956 [1612]:389), *vititha,* "to walk hurriedly, to walk like small children or birds." The term is common in local Colca Valley Spanish; "*wititear*" means to dance the Witite dance. All translations from Spanish to English are my own.

Scholars who discuss the Witite's presence in valley fiestas include Bernal (1983), Gelles (1990), Hurley (1978), Ráez (1993), Stoner (1989), and Valderrama and Escalante (1988, 1997).

2. Within the recent dramatic expansion of literature on cross-dressing, scholars increasingly address diverse nondualistic gender embodiments. Many studies associate transvestism with homosexuality (Bullough and Bullough 1993; Bullough, Bullough, and Elias, eds. 1997; Ekins 1997; Ekins and King, eds. 1996); among those which stress distinctions from and relationships to nonheterosexual identities and behaviors, Epstein and Straub (1991), Garber (1992), Kulick (1998), Nanda (2000), Newton (1979), Parker (1999), Prieur (1998), and Sifuentes-Jáuregui (2002) are especially useful. Instances of males cross-dressing in female garb in Andean festivals are analyzed by Harris (2000) and Harvey (1991, 1994b).
3. On the annual fiesta cycle and related rituals, see Benavides (1988b); Bernal (1983); Gelles (1990, 2000); Pease, ed. (1977); and Treacy (1989a, 1994). Valderrama and Escalante (1988:136–137) and Ráez (1993:261) provide festival calendars. Many Latin American religious traditions include fiestas; see Abercrombie (1998); Beezley, Martin, and French, eds. (1994); Bettelheim, ed. (1993); Brandes (1988); and Guss (2000).
4. My findings on gender in fiestas challenge literature which emphasizes "women's. roles" in marriage. Some authors endow marriage with paramount importance for women more than for men; they maintain that wives "help" their husbands with *cargos* or "co-sponsor" political and religious responsibilities. For example, in Yura, Bolivia, Rasnake (1988:66–67) claims that "all kuraqkuna [community/ayllu authority] posts are assumed by the couple, and not just by the man." Complementarity-based interpretations, in stressing that women assume the responsibilities as wives, make a serious mistake by overprivileging marriage, which is only one kind of social tie, and neglecting others, thus failing to address the full extent of female sociality. Abercrombie (1998); Allen (1988); Cancián (1965); Chance and Taylor (1985); Isbell (1985 [1978]); and Meyers and Hopkins, eds. (1988) analyze *cargo* systems.
5. I observed Carnival celebrations in several Colca Valley communities during my 1991–1993 fieldwork and in 1986. This description is based mostly on the Carnival I observed in the village of Coporaque in 1992, with additional information based on my observations in other communities. Detailed treatments of Carnival in Latin America include: for Mexico, Brandes (1988); Bolivia, Abercrombie (1992) and Buechler (1980); Brazil, DaMatta (1991); and the Caribbean, Aching (2002), Cowley (1996), and Scher (2003). I also draw on meanings of the carnivalesque discussed by Bakhtin (1984), Limón (1997), and Russo (1986).
6. Valderrama and Escalante (1988:167–174) offer a detailed description of these events in Yanque.
7. This interpretation of Carnival is proposed by Rasnake (1988:242); see also Turino (1993).
8. Another exception is the occasional village assembly. Chivay also has more daily traffic than other communities.
9. Although I have never seen females use slings, they do in some parts of Peru, espe-

cially during Carnival, as in Macusani, Puno (Zorn 1982; Elayne Zorn, personal communication 1997), and Cusco (Sallnow 1988:137). "Slinging" (*warakada* in Hispanicized Quechua) also means "lightning strike" (Valderrama and Escalante 1988). Storms in general imply male sexuality and fertility; lightning as the destructive side of storms' natural power may be traced to Inka concepts of power and domination embedded in Illapa, an impressive cosmological force which took the form of thunder and lightning (Silverblatt 1988:178).

10. Other versions of this story tell that local men disguised themselves to escape soldiers who invaded the area, sometimes Spaniards during the sixteenth-century Spanish conquest, other times Chileans in the nineteenth-century War of the Pacific. In Yanque in the 1980s, some claimed (perhaps apocryphally) that the custom of men wearing *polleras* originated only in the 1950s based on Manuel Rivera, "a powerful *misti* who had committed a murder and escaped his jailers dressed in women's clothes" (Maria Benavides, personal communication 1994).
11. Archaeological evidence indicates that the Inkas were present in the Colca Valley (Treacy 1989, 1994a; Wernke 2002, 2003). Pease (1977:140) points out that it is more likely that an Inka representative (*panaka*-mate), rather than the Inka himself, entered into this marriage. See also Manrique (1985:34) and Valderrama and Escalante (1997).
12. In 1993, Dionisio was in his midthirties. A native of the village of Cabanaconde, he had lived for five years with his wife, Agripina, and their young son in Coporaque, her hometown.
13. The Laymi of Bolivia speak of "marriage by capture"; although marriage or cohabitation usually proceeds according to the couple's mutual consent, the Aymara term "speaks of the man 'stealing' the woman from her home (*warmi suwaña*)" (Harris 2000:156, 187).
14. The accounts may relate to the virilocal postmarital residence patterns in Colca Valley communities; the woman leaves her paternal home and enters that of her husband and in-laws. Spanish folk and literary traditions include transvestite, homoerotic, and robber bridegroom tales (Gossy 1998; Goytisolo 1977; Perry 1990, 1999; Velasco 2000; Zayas y Sotomayor 1983).
15. Bernal uses the term *pelea danzando.* I deliberately translate this term as "dancing fight" rather than "ritual battle," the usual term in literature on Andean expressions of conflict. As Benjamin Orlove (1994:133–134) has thoroughly and convincingly argued, both "ritual" and "battle" are "Western" concepts, which not only may be at odds with the ways that diverse Andean actors think of the events, but have been applied indiscriminately by scholars to diverse kinds of events. Often called *tinku* or *tinkuy,* such fights occur frequently in the Andes, often in association with Carnival. For references on "ritual battles," see Sallnow (1987:136–142 nn. 18 and 20) and Orlove (1994:147).
16. Numerous questions remain about the alleged ban, including the identity of the victim(s), whether they were state authorities or peasants, the association between the ban on this ritual practice and other cultural practices throughout Peru, and at-

titudes toward fiestas and dancing fights nationwide. On Cabanaconde, see Gelles (2000:129–130), and for a compelling fictional treatment, see Arguedas (1985 [1941], 1988 [1941]).

17. Ritualized, culturally specific instances of gendered cross-dressing, often analyzed by anthropologists as "third gender" (Herdt 1994) roles, usually involve men who do not physically or culturally fit into traditional male roles, bodies, or dress and who assume a feminized persona as a lifestyle or career (see Herdt 1994:62–67, 70–71). Among these roles, Native American cases, often called "berdache" (Jacobs, Thomas, and Lang, eds. 1997; Lang 1998; and Roscoe 1991, 1994), and the South Asian *hijra* (Nanda 1994, 1999 [1990]) have been the subject of substantial scholarly attention.
18. On contemporary issues concerning masculinity, homosexuality, and gay activism in Peru, see Arboleda (1995), Bossio (1995), Cáceres (1996), Fuller (1997), Halperin (1990), Murray (1995a, 1995b), and Ugarteche (1993, 1997). For perspectives on diverse sexualities elsewhere in Latin America, consult, among others, Balderston and Guy, eds. (1997); Bergmann and Smith, eds. (1995); Bliss (2001); Carrier (1995); Chávez-Silverman and Hernández, eds. (2000); Chiñas (1995); Foster (1997); Foster and Reis, eds. (1996); Green (1999); Higgins and Coen (2000); Lancaster (1992); Molloy and Irwin, eds. (1998); Parker (1999); Parker et al., eds. (1992); Taylor and Villegas, eds. (1994); and Wilson (1995).

6. Marching and Meaning: Ethnic Symbols and Gendered Demonstrations

1. Even among the elite, in the early 1990s there were no women judges and very few women attorneys. In 1995, 10.8 percent of Peru's congressional representatives were women (Craske 1999, cited in Molyneux 2001:226).
2. In the 1980s, more women from popular sectors began to enter electoral politics, previously restricted to upper-class, urban whites (Barrig 1994, 1998; Blondet 1990, 1991; Vargas 1989; Villar 1994). The 2000 presidential campaign had the first female candidate. It takes tremendous courage even to declare candidacy. Elected officials and candidates are among the most frequent victims of assassination. In 1992, Sendero brutally murdered María Elena (Malena) Moyano, assistant mayor of Villa El Salvador, Lima's largest working-class neighborhood. Attackers shot and killed her, then dynamited her body (Barrig 1994:171–172; 1998:119–121; Miloslavich 1993; Vargas 1992). During the 1993 municipal election campaign, more than one hundred candidates were assassinated nationwide. Americas Watch (1992) details anti-female human rights violations. Women were also active in Sendero (Andreas 1985; Balbi and Callirgos 1992; Coral 1998; Kirk 1993). Other useful guides to gendered politics in late-twentieth-century Peru include Anderson (1998); Blondet (1995, 1999); Bourque and Warren (1980); Harvey (1989); Macassi and Olea, eds. (2000); and Vargas (1995).
3. Scholars increasingly attend to correspondences and conflicts among autonomy, women's interests, feminist thought, and social movements. See Markowitz (2001)

on southern Peru, including Caylloma. On Latin America, see Alvarez (1998); Besse (1996); Craske (1999); Deere and León (1987); Dore and Molyneux, eds. (2000); Fowler-Salamini and Vaughan, eds. (1994); González and Kampwirth, eds. (2001); Jaquette, ed. (1989, 1994); Jaquette and Wolchik, eds. (1998); Kirkwood (1988); Lavrin (1995); Miller (1991); Molyneux (2000); Radcliffe and Westwood (1993); Rosemblatt (2000); Stephen (1997), and Deutsch's (1991) review essay. More generally, consult these influential works: Fraser (1989); Kaplan (1997); Molyneux (2001); Mouffe (1993); Pateman (1989); and Scott and Butler, eds. (1992).

4. Recent analyses of gender that address the body politic include: in Latin America, Babb (2001), Franco (1989), Kaminsky (1993), Nelson (1999), Stephenson (1999), and Taylor (1997); in general, Butler (1993); Grosz and Probyn, eds. (1995); Jacobus, Fox Keller, and Shuttleworth, eds. (1990); and Parker et al., eds. (1992).
5. Community membership is also a primary qualification to maintain use or property rights to land, as well as to represent the community legally in positions of political authority.
6. On motherhood and maneuverability among Argentina's Madres de Plaza de Mayo, see Bouvard (1994), Fisher (1993), Navarro (1989), and Taylor (1997); and more generally, Bock and Thane, eds. (1991); Crain (1994); Gordon (1994); Koven and Michel, eds. (1993); and Ruddick (1980). Influential works on the public/private debate include Ehlstain (1981); Franco (1992); Helly and Reversby, eds. (1992); and Sassoon, ed. (1987).
7. In the 1970s–1980s, NGO-sponsored women's projects in Peru mushroomed. In 1975, eight NGOS had 32 projects for women; by 1986, twelve NGOs had 298 projects (Blondet 1991:96). One study totaled over fourteen thousand grassroots women's organizations in Peru in 1986 (FLACSO 1995, cited in Molyneux 2001:184).
8. The Caylloma case differs from the general tendency that Allen (1988:119–122) observed, that Andean women's politics is always informal, a view that can deter analysis of differences between male and female ideas about politics (Bourque and Warren 1980:150).
9. During Alan García's APRA administration (1980–1985) two thousand Clubs were founded throughout Peru (Barrig 1994:171; Radcliffe 1993).
10. Unfortunately, little has been written about Clubs in peasant communities, but see Radcliffe (1993) on Puno and Seibold (1990:57–58) on Cusco.
11. A farmers' association, APACOLCA, sponsored by the NGO DESCO, is typical; it has one post for a woman, Secretary of Feminine Affairs.
12. The Federation was founded in Cusco in the 1980s to parallel the almost exclusively male Federación del Campesino (Peasant Federation). The next branch was established in Puno. The Federations have links with the PUM, Partido Unido Mariateguista (United Mariateguist Party; Radcliffe 1993:214–216). The Federation was one of dozens of women's groups that attended the first national Women's Summit in Arequipa in 1991 (Femenías 1997a:461–462).
13. Conversations with Taco and other officers and with CAPRODA's staff members and advisors were very informative. Lisa Markowitz (2001) generously shared perspec-

tives from interviewing Federation officers. I also consulted the Federation's 1991 written platform and statutes.

14. In rural community politics, many decisions are made consensually in public assemblies. People call out their endorsement of every initiative they support, usually voting orally for more than one person. This method of selecting leaders contrasts with the democratic election by a majority; one person, one vote is an important component of the Federation's operating principles.
15. Observers had no right to speak or vote; outsider participants with the privilege to speak were typically representatives of popular organizations in Cusco and urban Arequipa.
16. On gender and citizenship in Latin America, see Alvarez (1990); Blacklock and Jenson (1998); Hola and Portugal, eds. (1997); Jelin (1990); Jelin and Hershberg, eds. (1996); and Marques-Pereira and Carrier, eds. (1996). For broader theoretical perspectives, consult Benhabib, ed. (1996); Bock, ed. (1992); Dietz (1985, 1992); Ehlstain (1983); Lister (1997); Mouffe (1993); Mouffe, ed. (1992); Pateman (1988); Phillips (1991, 1993); and Yuval-Davis and Werbner, eds. (1999).
17. Several women, including officers, told me that women must be married to join Clubs, but several members whom I met were single mothers, often quite young, and others were married but separated or abandoned.
18. Major concerns are contact with the staff, scheduling of meetings, and access to resources. Perennial problems occur regarding transport and equitable distribution of food aid, the most significant material resource that the Federation oversees.
19. In 1993, Jiménez and I spoke at her home. As president of the Cabanaconde Mothers' Club, she remained concerned about the Lower Zone's marginalization in the Federation.
20. Alcalde usually implies male, while Alcaldeza is an honorary title for his wife.
21. Another pamphlet shows a similar scene (Femenías 1997a:465–466).
22. In the Coporaque 2002 municipal election, Nilda Bernal joined the Consejo as a *vocal,* the only female member of her party's slate. (Nationwide, female participation has increased since Fujimori resigned.)

7. Making Difference: Gender and Production in a Workshop System

1. A stand (*puesto*) is usually inside and a kiosk (*quiosco*) outside the market building.
2. Theories of petty or simple commodity production (PCP, SCP) addressed shortcomings of Marxist economic theories, especially regarding the articulation of modes of production. Recognizing the inadequacy of positing two distinct sectors which occasionally engaged with each other, theorists focused on systems which combine capitalist and noncapitalist elements. Analyzing domestic production in mercantile and dependent capitalist economies, they showed how ideologies of family relatedness enabled limited capitalist development and masked exploitative practices (Scott 1986; also Brass 1986 and Cook and Binford 1990).
3. Collins (1986), Harris (1981), Moore (1988:54–64), and Yanagisako (1979) question

the universality of the "household" concept; others argue that it remains a useful analytic category if cultural distinctions are specified (Wilk and Netting 1984).

4. Earnings on unreported sales go untaxed. As the Peruvian state increasingly concerned itself with formalizing the informal sector, underreporting and tax evasion became election campaign issues in 1992. SUNAT, the National Tax and Customs Service, closed hundreds of poorly documented businesses, slapping big red CLOSED! stickers on their doors. Because this crackdown coincided with my surveying, artisans sometimes hesitated to participate; if I were from SUNAT, I could close their business.
5. My *compadre* Epifanio keeps a machine in his home. Usually working alone, he occasionally embroiders clothes for his wife or female kin but does not sell or exchange these garments outside the family. The scope of my survey omits this type of domestic production. Although many families engage in it occasionally, the percentage of *bordados* exchanged solely along kinship lines and completely outside the market is quite small. Likewise, piecework and putting-out seemed uncommon, so I did not survey people who use their own machine occasionally to assemble a garment for a shop. Additional studies of Caylloma domestic clothing production and commercial weaving are needed, which could help determine the scope of kinship exchange.
6. I did not collect "drop-out" data. Although many people stayed as *operarios* or opened their own shops, there may be thousands of ex-*operarios* or ex-embroiderers who left embroidery in the thirty years since the heyday to seek steadier work or better earnings elsewhere.
7. For example, "rules," "ritual ordeal," and "secrets" appear in titles of articles about apprenticeship (Coy, ed. 1989).
8. I observed no instances when parents kept children out of school to help in workshops, which they often do for help with herding and harvesting.
9. My apprenticeship with Susana was atypical. I requested that she teach me; she agreed as a favor, for she did not then need an unskilled *operario.* Although I wanted to become competent, I did not depend on the work for earnings and so did not have to improve rapidly. We made no arrangements for pay but continued to exchange favors as before. We both knew that my apprenticeship would be very brief and that it was highly unlikely that I would get up to speed during those few days.
10. Goody (1989) discusses apprenticeship in West Africa and presents literature linking learning, family, and work; see also Kondo (1990) and Lave (1977).

8. Trading Places: Exchange, Identity, and the Commoditization of Cloth

1. There are no book-length studies of rural town markets like Chivay. Microlevel studies of Peruvian marketing address large urban markets and the informal sector and often omit gender, notes Babb (1998 [1989]:57–60), whose work offers an exception; see also Miles and Buechler, eds. (1997) and Seligmann (2004). On highland markets in Bolivia, see Larson and Harris, eds., with Tandeter (1995) and Sikkink

(1994). The markets and the women traders of Oaxaca, Mexico, have been studied in detail by Cook and Binford (1990) and Chiñas (1976), respectively. Literature on Mesoamerican and Central American marketing (e.g., Nash, ed. 1993; Smith 1986 on Guatemala) suggests similarities to Peru. Seligmann, ed. (2001) presents global concerns.

2. My concerns with objects' cultural and economic meanings resonate with recent discussions about how they circulate, especially those concerned with the commoditization of the sacred (Appadurai 1986; Cook 1993; Geary 1986; Kopytoff 1986; Marcus and Myers, eds. 1995; Phillips and Steiner, eds. 1999; Starrett 1995; Steiner 1994; Thomas 1991; Weiner 1992). Schneider's (1978) nuanced analysis of the political economy of European colored cloth has been especially influential.
3. *Luto* (mourning) applies to the period, rituals, and clothes (Ráez 1993:268).
4. In a case that created an international legal scandal, sacred ancient textiles were not merely removed from the sacred context, but stolen from their community of origin in Coroma, Bolivia, and sold for exorbitant prices on the international art market; these items of cultural patrimony were subsequently repatriated (Bubba 1993; Healy 2001; Lobo 1991).
5. During the Crusades, Christians suppressed white as the mourning color in Europe; black replaced it to indicate funerals, graveyards, and churches (Schneider 1978:414–415, 422; Harvey 1995:44–50).
6. See Allen (1988:81) and Seibold (1995:323–325) on Cusco, and Zorn (1997b) on Taquile, Peru, and Sakaka, Bolivia.
7. Black and purple are mourning cloth colors in Tarabuco, Bolivia (Meisch 1987a).
8. Weaving and embroidery are usually done by different artisans. Using such an arrangement, which is entirely typical, I obtained a mourning-type shawl for The Textile Museum in 2002.
9. On All Souls in Cusco, see Allen (1988) and Meyerson (1990), and in Bolivia, Harris (2000). The extensive literature on Mexico includes Brandes (1988); Carmichael and Sayer (1992); Garciagodoy (1998); Nutini (1988); and Sayer, ed. (1994).
10. During this period, small face-shaped rolls called *wawas* (babies) are given to children (Harris 2000:36 n. 18). (Originally Quechua, *wawa* is now the term for "baby" in Peruvian Spanish as well.) One Arequipa bakery featured Tortuninja (Teenage Mutant Ninja Turtle) *wawas.*
11. Coporaque's enormous altar drape may date to the colonial period. After Holy Week, I saw it laid out on, and completely covering, the church steps before villagers rolled and stored it for another year. Beneath perhaps a hundred repairs and patches, the original textile is tapestry woven, probably of alpaca fiber, and shows skulls and symbols of the Passion. Little is known about Caylloma colonial textile practices, and only a handful of objects survive, mostly in churches, including "the remains of colored carpets of very large dimensions (sometimes very deteriorated) which formerly decorated them with splendor" (Stastny 1987:173).
12. For information about these changes, I thank Sister Antonia Kayser (personal communication 1992). On the reverse side of the wings, which are fashioned from food-

aid oil cans, an eagle-shaped U.S. flag surmounts the message "Gift of the people of the United States of America."

13. The language of exchange is usually Quechua, but with outsiders, it is Spanish. While doing the surveys, I met only two vendors who did not speak Spanish well, one an elderly woman from Chivay, the other a middle-aged Puneña. Because many Puneños' first language is Aymara, Spanish is their trade language. I met no vendors who spoke English or any language other than Spanish, Quechua, and Aymara. Most vendors speak enough Spanish to conduct transactions, and speaking it well greatly helps selling to tourists.
14. In the mid-1990s, several frozen bodies, probably Inka, were removed from Sabancaya glacier and displayed internationally (Fine-Dare 2002; Fowler 1996; Gelles 2000:79). *National Geographic* then substantially expanded its coverage of the Colca Valley; June 1996 brought both an article in the magazine (Reinhard 1996) and a cable TV special. Several Web sites include references to the valley: www.yachay.com; www.peru.org.pe; and www.perucultural.org.pe; they are also linked to the official Peruvian site, Red Científica Peruana, www.rcp.net.pe.
15. To encourage natural and cultural resource conservation, the Peruvian government established the Colca Authority in 1986, which created a national reserve surrounding the villages (de Romaña, Blassi, and Blassi 1987:196).
16. In all of Peru, the preeminent destination is Cusco, with Machu Picchu at one end of the "Sacred Valley of the Inkas." Travel to the Colca Valley is far more difficult. In the early 1990s, it was impossible for tourists to tour the Colca Valley and return to Arequipa in one day, as they routinely do to Cusco's Sacred Valley.
17. During 1994–1995, a fiber shortage resulted after thousands of alpacas died in a drought, even as the demand for "natural" tones was growing. Because breeding policies favor white animals, colored fiber was especially scarce, so Arequipa's textile factories dyed white fiber tan and brown (Patricia Jurewicz, personal communication 1995).
18. The data I collected from vendors did not include annual income or exact numbers of garments sold.
19. During my 2002 visit, many more artisans were embroidering hats. Another factory had begun producing different color, and cheaper, blanks; the lower price greatly improved hats' appeal to tourists.
20. "Fido Dido," a middle-class teenage character, was also used to market 7-Up in Egypt (Starrett 1995).
21. Mattel's practices in Asian factories, especially the use of child labor, have been questioned, and contrast starkly with the high price of a "real" Barbie (Press 1996).

Bibliography

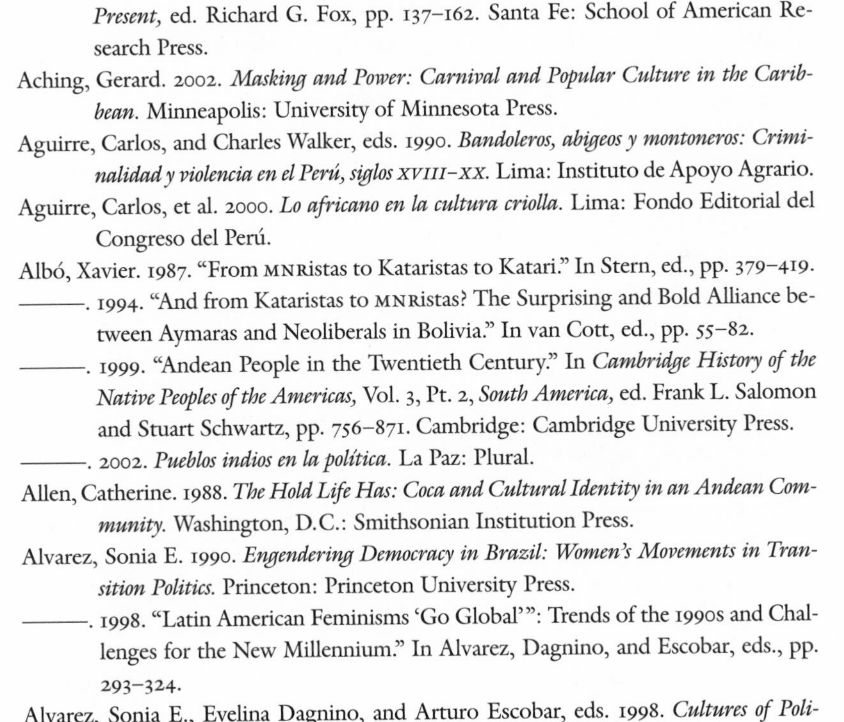

Abercrombie, Thomas A. 1991. "To Be Indian, to Be Bolivian: Ethnic and National Discourses of Identity." In Urban and Sherzer, eds., pp. 95–130.

———. 1992. "La fiesta del carnaval postcolonial en Oruro: Clase, etnicidad y nacionalismo en la danza folklórica." *Revista Andina* 10(2): 279–352.

———. 1998. *Pathways of Memory and Power: Ethnography and History among an Andean People.* Madison: University of Wisconsin Press.

Abu-Lughod, Lila. 1986. *Veiled Sentiments: Honor and Poetry in a Bedouin Society.* Berkeley: University of California Press.

———. 1990. "Can There Be Feminist Ethnography?" *Women and Performance* 5: 7–27.

———. 1991. "Writing against Culture." In *Recapturing Anthropology: Working in the Present,* ed. Richard G. Fox, pp. 137–162. Santa Fe: School of American Research Press.

Aching, Gerard. 2002. *Masking and Power: Carnival and Popular Culture in the Caribbean.* Minneapolis: University of Minnesota Press.

Aguirre, Carlos, and Charles Walker, eds. 1990. *Bandoleros, abigeos y montoneros: Criminalidad y violencia en el Perú, siglos* XVIII–XX. Lima: Instituto de Apoyo Agrario.

Aguirre, Carlos, et al. 2000. *Lo africano en la cultura criolla.* Lima: Fondo Editorial del Congreso del Perú.

Albó, Xavier. 1987. "From MNRistas to Kataristas to Katari." In Stern, ed., pp. 379–419.

———. 1994. "And from Kataristas to MNRistas? The Surprising and Bold Alliance between Aymaras and Neoliberals in Bolivia." In van Cott, ed., pp. 55–82.

———. 1999. "Andean People in the Twentieth Century." In *Cambridge History of the Native Peoples of the Americas,* Vol. 3, Pt. 2, *South America,* ed. Frank L. Salomon and Stuart Schwartz, pp. 756–871. Cambridge: Cambridge University Press.

———. 2002. *Pueblos indios en la política.* La Paz: Plural.

Allen, Catherine. 1988. *The Hold Life Has: Coca and Cultural Identity in an Andean Community.* Washington, D.C.: Smithsonian Institution Press.

Alvarez, Sonia E. 1990. *Engendering Democracy in Brazil: Women's Movements in Transition Politics.* Princeton: Princeton University Press.

———. 1998. "Latin American Feminisms 'Go Global'": Trends of the 1990s and Challenges for the New Millennium." In Alvarez, Dagnino, and Escobar, eds., pp. 293–324.

Alvarez, Sonia E., Evelina Dagnino, and Arturo Escobar, eds. 1998. *Cultures of Poli-*

tics/Politics of Cultures: Re-Visioning Latin American Social Movements. Boulder: Westview.

Americas Watch and the Women's Rights Project. 1992. *Untold Terror: Violence against Women in Peru's Armed Conflict.* New York: Human Rights Watch.

Anderson, Jeanine. 1998. "Peruvian Women and the Peruvian State." In *Women's Movements and Public Policy in Europe, Latin America, and the Caribbean: The Triangle for Empowerment,* ed. Geertje Lycklama à Nijeholt, Virginia Vargas, and Saskia Wieringa, pp. 77–96. New York: Garland.

Anderson, Ruth. 1980. *Hispanic Costume 1480–1530.* New York: Hispanic Society of America.

Andreas, Carol. 1985. *When Women Rebel: The Rise of Popular Feminism in Peru.* Westport, Conn.: L. Hill.

Appadurai, Arjun. 1986. "Introduction: Commodities and the Politics of Value." In Appadurai, ed., pp. 3–63.

———, ed. 1986. *The Social Life of Things: Commodities in Cultural Perspective.* Cambridge: Cambridge University Press.

Appelbaum, Nancy P., Anne S. Macpherson, and Karin Alejandra Rosemblatt, eds. 2003. *Race and Nation in Modern Latin America.* Chapel Hill: University of North Carolina Press.

Arboleda G., Manuel. 1995. *Social Attitudes and Sexual Variance in Lima.* In Murray et al., pp. 100–110.

Arguedas, José María. 1985 [1941]. *Yawar Fiesta.* Trans. Frances Horning Barraclough. Austin: University of Texas Press.

———. 1988 [1941]. *Yawar Fiesta.* Lima: Editorial Horizonte.

Arnson, Cynthia J., ed. 1999. *Comparative Peace Processes in Latin America.* Washington, D.C.: Woodrow Wilson Center Press; Stanford: Stanford University Press.

Ash, John. 1995. "Arshile Gorky: 'How My Mother's Embroidered Apron Unfolds in My Life,' 1944." *Artforum* (September): 78–79, 121.

Ayala Loayza, Juan Luis. 1988. *Diccionario Español-Aymara/Aymara-Español.* Lima: Editorial Juan Mejía Baca.

Babb, Florence. 1998. *Between Field and Cooking Pot: The Political Economy of Marketwomen in Peru.* Rev. ed. Austin: University of Texas Press. (Originally published 1989.)

———. 2001. *After Revolution: Mapping Gender and Cultural Politics in Neoliberal Nicaragua.* Austin: University of Texas Press.

Babcock, Barbara. 1978. "Introduction." In Babcock, ed., pp. 13–36.

———. 1993. "At Home No Women Are Storytellers." In Lavie, Narayan, and Rosaldo, eds., pp. 70–99.

———, ed. 1978. *The Reversible World: Symbolic Inversion in Art and Society.* Ithaca: Cornell University Press.

Bakhtin, Mikhail. 1984. *Rabelais and His World.* Bloomington: Indiana University Press.

Balbi, Carmen Rosa, and Juan Carlos Callirgos. 1992. "Sendero y la mujer." *Quehacer* 79.

Balderston, Daniel, and Donna J. Guy, eds. 1997. *Sex and Sexuality in Latin America.* New York: New York University Press.

Barnes, Natasha. 2000. "Body Talk: Notes on Women and Spectacle in Contemporary Trinidad Carnival." *Small Axe* 7 (March): 93–105.

Barnes, Ruth, and Joanne B. Eicher, eds. 1992. *Dress and Gender: Making and Meaning.* Oxford: Berg.

Barragán, Rosanna. 1992. "Entre polleras, lliqllas, y ñañacas: Los mestizos y la emergencia de la tercera república." In *Etnicidad, economía y simbolismo en los Andes,* ed. Silvia Arze et al., pp. 85–127. La Paz: HISBOL/IFEA.

Barrig, Maruja. 1994. "The Difficult Equilibrium between Bread and Roses: Women's Organizations and Democracy in Peru." In Jaquette, ed., pp. 151–175.

———. 1998. "Female Leadership, Citizenship, and Violence in Peru." In Jaquette and Wolchik, eds., pp. 104–124.

Barthes, Roland. 1983 [1967]. *The Fashion System.* Trans. Matthew Ward and Richard Howard. London: Jonathan Cape.

Bartra, Roger. 1987. *La jaula de la melancolía: Identidad y metamorfosis del mexicano.* Mexico City: Grijalbo.

Basombrío Iglesias, Carlos. 1998. "Sendero Luminoso and Human Rights: A Perverse Logic That Captured the Country." In Stern, ed., pp. 425–446.

———. 1999. "Peace in Peru: An Unfinished Task." In Arnson, ed., pp. 205–222.

Baudrillard, Jean. 1981 [1972]. *For a Critique of the Political Economy of the Sign.* Trans. Charles Levin. St. Louis: Telos.

Bauer, Arnold J. 2001. *Goods, Power, History: Latin America's Material Culture.* Cambridge: Cambridge University Press.

Beezley, William H., Cheryl E. Martin, and William E. French, eds. 1994. *Rituals of Rule, Rituals of Resistance: Public Celebrations and Popular Culture in Mexico.* Wilmington, Del.: Scholarly Resources Books.

Behar, Ruth. 1993. *Translated Woman: Crossing the Border with Esperanza's Story.* Boston: Beacon.

———. 1995. "Introduction: Out of Exile." In Behar and Gordon, eds., pp. 1–29.

Behar, Ruth, and Deborah A. Gordon, eds. 1995. *Women Writing Culture.* Berkeley: University of California Press.

Bell, Diane, Pat Caplan, and Wazir Jahan Karim, eds. 1993. *Gendered Fields: Women, Men, and Ethnography.* London: Routledge.

Benavides, Maria A. 1983. "Two Traditional Andean Peasant Communities under the Stress of Market Penetration: Yanque and Madrigal in the Colca Valley, Peru." Master's thesis, Institute of Latin American Studies, University of Texas, Austin.

———. 1987. "Análisis del uso de tierras registrado en las visitas de los siglos XVI y XVII a los yanquecollaguas, Arequipa, Perú." In *Pre-Hispanic Fields in the Andean Region,* ed. William M. Denevan, Kent Mathewson, and Gregory Knapp, pp. 129–146. Oxford: British Archaeological Reports International Series 359.

———. 1988a. "La división social y geográfica hanansaya/hurinsaya en el Valle de Colca y la Provincia de Caylloma." In Denevan, ed., pp. 46–53.

———. 1988b. "Grupos de poder en el Valle de Colca, siglos XVI–XX." In *Sociedad andina pasado y presente,* ed. Ramiro Matos Mendieta, pp. 151–178. Lima: Fomciencias.

———. 1990. "Tenencia de tierras agrícolas en el Valle del Colca (Caylloma, Arequipa)." *Revista Peruana de Ciencias Sociales* 2(1): 49–76.

Benhabib, Seyla, ed. 1996. *Democracy and Difference: Contesting the Boundaries of the Political.* Princeton: Princeton University Press.

Benjamin, Walter. 1968 [1931]. "Unpacking My Library: A Talk about Book Collecting." In *Illuminations,* ed. Hannah Arendt; trans. Harry Zohn, pp. 59–67. New York: Schocken.

Bentley, G. Carter. 1987. "Ethnicity and Practice." *Comparative Studies in Society and History* 29: 24–55.

Bergmann, Emilie L., and Paul Julian Smith, eds. 1995. *¿Entiendes? Queer Readings, Hispanic Writings.* Durham: Duke University Press.

Bermejo, Vladimiro. 1954. *Arequipa: Bio-bibliografía de arequipeños contemporáneos.* Arequipa: Establecimientos Gráficos La Colmena.

Bernal Málaga, Alfredo. 1983. "Danzas de las etnías collaguas y colonias: Un estudio en la Cuenca del Colca, Caylloma." Tesis de Licenciatura en Antropología, Universidad Nacional de San Agustín, Arequipa.

Bertonio, Ludovico. 1956 [1612]. *Vocabulario de la Lengua Aymara.* Facsimile ed. La Paz: Don Bosco. (Originally published by Juli: Francisco del Canto.)

Besse, Susan. 1996. *Restructuring Patriarchy: The Modernization of Gender Inequality in Brazil, 1914–1940.* Chapel Hill: University of North Carolina Press.

Bettelheim, Judith, ed. 1993. *Cuban Festivals: An Illustrated Anthology.* New York: Garland.

Blacklock, Cathy, and Jane Jenson. 1998. "Citizenship: Latin American Perspectives." *Social Policy* (summer): 127–131.

Bliss, Katherine Elaine. 2001. "The Sexual Revolution in Mexican Studies: New Perspectives on Gender, Sexuality, and Culture in Modern Mexico." *Latin American Research Review* 36(1): 247–268.

Blondet, Cecilia. 1990. "Establishing an Identity: Women Settlers in a Poor Lima Neighborhood." In Jelin, ed., pp. 12–46.

———. 1991. *Las mujeres y el poder: Una historia de Villa El Salvador.* Lima: Instituto de Estudios Peruanos.

———. 1995. "Out of the Kitchen and onto the Streets." In *The Challenge of Local Feminisms,* ed. Amritsa Basu, with the assistance of C. Elizabeth McGrory, pp. 251–275. Boulder: Westview.

———. 1999. *Percepción ciudadana sobre la participación política de la mujer.* Lima: Instituto de Estudios Peruanos.

Bock, Gisela, ed. 1992. *Beyond Equality and Difference: Citizenship and Female Subjectivity.* New York and London: Routledge.

Bock, Gisela, and Pat Thane, eds. 1991. *Maternity and Gender Policies: Women and the Rise of the European Welfare States, 1880s–1950s.* New York: Routledge.

Bossio, Enrique. 1995. "Interview with a Gay Activist." In Starn, Degregori, and Kirk, eds., pp. 477–481.

Bourdieu, Pierre. 1977. *Outline of a Theory of Practice.* Cambridge: Cambridge University Press.

———. 1984. *Distinction: A Social Critique of the Judgement of Taste.* Cambridge, Mass.: Harvard University Press.

———. 1990. *The Logic of Practice.* Trans. Richard Nice. Stanford: Stanford University Press.

Bourque, Susan, and Kay Warren. 1980. *Women of the Andes: Patriarchy and Social Change in Two Peruvian Towns.* Ann Arbor: University of Michigan Press.

Bouvard, Marguerite. 1994. *Revolutionizing Motherhood: The Mothers of the Plaza de Mayo.* Wilmington, Del.: Scholarly Resources Books.

Bowen, Elenore Smith [Laura Bohannon]. 1964 [1954]. *Return to Laughter.* New York: American Museum of Natural History/Doubleday.

Brandes, Stanley. 1988. *Power and Persuasion: Fiestas and Social Control in Rural Mexico.* Philadelphia: University of Pennsylvania Press.

Brass, Tom. 1986. "The Elementary Strictures of Kinship: Unfree Relations and the Production of Commodities." *Social Analysis* 20: 56–68.

Bridgman, Rae, Sally Cole, and Heather Howard-Bobiwash, eds. 1999. *Feminist Fields: Ethnographic Insights.* Peterborough, Ont.: Broadview.

Brysk, Alison. 2000. *From Tribal Village to Global Village: Indian Rights and International Relations in Latin America.* Stanford: Stanford University Press.

Bubba, Cristina. 1993. "Los textiles ceremoniales de Coroma." Paper presented at the Annual Meeting of the American Anthropological Association.

Buckingham, Andrew, and Eric Kindberg. 1987. *Frases útiles en la quechua de Arequipa.* N.p.: Instituto Lingüístico de Verano; Dirección Zonal de Educación de Arequipa.

Buechler, Hans. 1980. *The Masked Media: Aymara Fiestas and Social Interaction in the Bolivian Highlands.* The Hague: Mouton.

———. 1989. "Apprenticeship and Transmission of Knowledge in La Paz, Bolivia." In Coy, ed., pp. 31–50.

Bullough, Bonnie, Vern L. Bullough, and James Elias, eds. 1997. *Gender Blending.* Amherst, NY: Prometheus Books.

Bullough, Vern L., and Bonnie Bullough. 1993. *Cross Dressing, Sex, and Gender.* Philadelphia: University of Pennsylvania Press.

Bunster, Ximena, and Elsa Chaney. 1985. *Sellers and Servants: Working Women in Lima, Peru.* New York: Praeger.

Burga, Manuel, and Wilson Reátegui. 1981. *Lanas y capital mercantil en el sur: La Casa Ricketts, 1895–1935.* Lima: Instituto de Estudios Peruanos.

Burt, Jo-Marie. 1998. "Shining Path and the 'Decisive Battle' in Lima's *Barriadas:* The Case of Villa El Salvador." In Stern, ed., pp. 267–306.

———. 2000. "The Reawakening of Civil Society in Peru." *NACLA Report on the Americas* 34, no. 2 (September–October): 1–2.

Butler, Judith. 1990. *Gender Trouble: Feminism and the Subversion of Identity.* New York: Routledge.

———. 1993. *Bodies that Matter: On the Discursive Limits of "Sex."* New York: Routledge.

Cáceres, Carlos. 1996. "Male Bisexuality in Peru and the Prevention of AIDS." In *Bisexualities and AIDS: International Perspectives,* ed. Peter Aggleton, pp. 136–147. London: Taylor and Francis.

Callaway, Helen. 1992. "Ethnography and Experience: Gender Implications in Fieldwork and Texts." In *Anthropology and Autobiography,* ed. Judith Okeley, pp. 29–49. London and New York: Routledge.

Callirgos, Juan Carlos. 1993. *El racismo: La cuestión del Otro (y de uno).* Lima: DESCO, Centro de Estudios y Promoción de Desarrollo.

Cameron, Maxwell A., and Philip Mauceri, eds. 1997. *The Peruvian Labyrinth: Polity, Society, Economy.* University Park: Pennsylvania State University Press.

Campbell, Howard. 1994. *Zapotec Renaissance: Ethnic Politics and Cultural Revivalism in Southern Mexico.* Albuquerque: University of New Mexico Press.

Cancián, Frank. 1965. *Economics and Prestige in a Maya Community: The Religious Cargo System in Zinacantán.* Stanford: Stanford University Press.

Cánepa Koch, Gisela, ed. 2001. *Identidades representadas: Performance, experiencia y memoria en los Andes.* Lima: Pontificia Universidad Católica del Perú.

Cárdenas, Hugo, Norma Velásquez, Maribel Rotondo, and Edwin Alarcón. 1988. *Artesanía textil andina: Tecnología, empleo e ingresos.* Lima: Tecnología Intermedia.

Carmichael, Elizabeth, and Chloë Sayer. 1992. *The Skeleton at the Feast: The Day of the Dead in Mexico.* Austin: University of Texas Press.

Carpio Muñoz, Juan Guillermo. 1990. "Arequipa y la encrucijada del desarrollo, 1956–1988." In Neira et al., pp. 667–727.

Carrier, Joseph. 1995. De los Otros: *Intimacy and Homosexuality among Mexican Men.* New York: Columbia University Press.

Casaverde, Juvenal. 1977. "El trueque en la economía pastoril." In *Pastores de Puna: Uywamichiq Punarunakuna,* ed. Jorge Flores Ochoa, pp. 171–192. Lima: Instituto de Estudios Peruanos.

Case, Sue-Ellen, ed. 1990. *Performing Feminisms: Feminist Critical Theory and Theatre.* Baltimore: Johns Hopkins University Press.

Castañeda León, Luisa. 1981. *Traditional Dress of Peru/Vestido tradicional del Perú.* Lima: Museo de la Cultura Peruana.

Cereceda, Verónica. 1986. "The Semiology of Andean Textiles: The Talegas of Isluga." In *Anthropological History of Andean Polities,* ed. John V. Murra, Nathan Wachtel, and Jacques Revel, pp. 149–173. Cambridge: Cambridge University Press; Paris: Editions de la Maison de Sciences de l'Homme.

Chambers, Sarah C. 1999. *From Subjects to Citizens: Honor, Gender, and Politics in Arequipa, Peru, 1780–1854.* University Park: Pennsylvania State University Press.

Chance, John K., and William B. Taylor. 1985. "Cofradías and Cargos: An Historical Perspective on the Mesoamerican Civil Religious Hierarchy." *American Ethnologist* 12(1): 1–26.

Chávez O'Brien, Eleana. 1987. *El mercado laboral en la ciudad de Arequipa.* Arequipa: Fundación M. J. Bustamante de la Fuente.

Chávez-Silverman, Susana, and Librada Hernández, eds. 2000. *Reading and Writing the* Ambiente: *Queer Sexualities in Latino, Latin American, and Spanish Culture.* Madison: University of Wisconsin Press.

Chiñas, Beverly. 1976. "Zapotec *Viajeras.*" In *Markets in Oaxaca,* ed. Scott Cook and Martin Diskin, pp. 169–188. Austin: University of Texas Press.

———. 1995. "Isthmus Zapotec Attitudes toward Sex and Gender Anomalies." In Murray et al., pp. 293–302.

Clifford, James. 1988. *The Predicament of Culture: Twentieth-Century Ethnography, Literature, and Art.* Cambridge, Mass.: Harvard University Press.

———. 1990. "Notes on (Field)notes." In Sanjek, ed., pp. 47–70.

———. 1997. *Routes: Travel and Translation in the Late Twentieth Century.* Cambridge, Mass.: Harvard University Press.

Clifford, James, and George Marcus, eds. 1986. *Writing Culture: The Poetics and Politics of Ethnography.* Berkeley: University of California Press.

Cobo, Bernabé. 1979 [1653]. *History of the Inca Empire.* Trans. and ed. Roland Hamilton. Austin: University of Texas Press.

Cojtí Cuxil, Demetrio. 1996. "The Politics of Mayan Revindication." In *Maya Cultural Activism in Guatemala,* ed. Edward F. Fischer and R. McKenna Brown, pp. 19–50. Austin: University of Texas Press.

Collier, George A., with Elizabeth Lowery Quaratiello. 1994. Basta!: *Land and the Zapatista Rebellion in Chiapas.* Oakland: Food First Books.

Collins, Jane. 1986. "The Household and Relations of Production in Southern Peru." *Comparative Studies in Society and History* 28(4): 651–671.

Colloredo-Mansfeld, Rudi. 1999. *The Native Leisure Class: Consumption and Cultural Creativity in the Andes.* Chicago: University of Chicago Press.

Conklin, William J. 1996. "The Ampato Textile Offerings." In *Sacred and Ceremonial Textiles: Proceedings of the Fifth Biennial Symposium of the Textile Society of America, Chicago, Illinois, 1996,* pp. 104–110. Chicago: Textile Society of America.

Connerton, Paul. 1989. *How Societies Remember.* Cambridge: Cambridge University Press.

Cook, Noble David. 1982. *The People of the Colca Valley: A Population Study.* Dellplain Latin American Studies, 9. Boulder: Westview.

Cook, Scott. 1993. "Craft Commodity Production, Market Diversity, and Differential Rewards in Mexican Capitalism Today." In Nash, ed., pp. 59–84.

Cook, Scott, and Leigh Binford. 1990. *Obliging Need: Rural Petty Industry in Mexican Capitalism.* Austin: University of Texas Press.

Coral Cordero, Isabel. 1998. "Women in War: Impact and Responses." In Stern, ed., pp. 345–374.

Cowley, John. 1996. *Carnival, Canboulay, and Calypso: Traditions in the Making.* Cambridge: Cambridge University Press.

Coy, Michael W., ed. 1989. *Apprenticeship: From Theory to Method and Back Again.* Albany: State University of New York Press.

Crabtree, John, and Jim Thomas, eds. 1998. *Fujimori's Peru: The Political Economy.* London: University of London, Institute of Latin American Studies.

Crain, Mary. 1994. "Unruly Mothers: Gender Identities, Peasant Political Discourses, and Struggles for Social Space in the Ecuadorian Andes." *POLAR: Political and Legal Anthropology Review* 17(2): 85–97.

Craske, Nikki. 1999. *Women and Politics in Latin America*. New Brunswick, N.J.: Rutgers University Press.

Cusihuamán G., Antonio. 1976. *Diccionario Quechua: Cuzco-Collao*. Lima: Ministerio de Educación.

DaMatta, Roberto. 1991. *Carnivals, Rogues, and Heroes: An Interpretation of the Brazilian Dilemma*. Notre Dame: University of Notre Dame Press.

Dargent, Eduardo. 2001. "¿Es necesario una Comisión de la Verdad en el Perú?" *Quehacer* 129, Web version: www.desco.org/pe/qh/qh129in.htm.

Davis, Natalie Zemon. 1978. "Women on Top: Sexual Symbolic Inversion and Political Disorder in Early Modern Europe." In Babcock, ed., pp. 147–189.

de Certeau, Michel. 1984. *The Practice of Everyday Life*. Berkeley: University of California Press.

Deere, Carmen Diana, and Magdalena León de Leal. 1987. *Women in Andean Agriculture: Peasant Production and Rural Wage Employment in Colombia and Peru*. Rome: International Labour Office.

Degregori, Carlos Iván. 1990. *El surgimiento de Sendero Luminoso: Ayacucho 1969–1979*. Lima: Instituto de Estudios Peruanos.

Degregori, Carlos Iván, Cecilia Blondet, and Nicolás Lynch. 1986. *Conquistadores de un nuevo mundo: De invasores a ciudadanos en San Martín de Porres*. Lima: Instituto de Estudios Peruanos.

Degregori, Carlos Iván, and Romeo Grompone. 1991. *Demonios y redentores: Elecciones 1990, una tragedia en dos vueltas*. Lima: Instituto de Estudios Peruanos.

de la Cadena, Marisol. 1995. "'Women Are More Indian': Ethnicity and Gender in a Community Near Cuzco." In Larson and Harris, eds., with Tandeter, pp. 329–348.

———. 2000. *Indigenous Mestizos: The Politics of Race and Culture in Cuzco, Peru, 1919–1991*. Durham: Duke University Press.

de la Jara, Ernesto. 2002. "Caught in an Anti-Terrorist Web." *NACLA Report on the Americas* 35, no. 4 (January–February): 4–6, 44.

de Lauretis, Teresa, ed. 1986. *Feminist Studies/Critical Studies*. Bloomington: University of Indiana Press.

Denevan, William M. 1993. "The 1931 Shippee-Johnson Aerial Photography Expedition to Peru." *The Geographical Review* 83: 238–251.

———. 2001. *Cultivated Landscapes of Native Amazonia and the Andes*. Oxford: Oxford University Press.

———, ed. 1986. *The Cultural Ecology, Archaeology, and History of Terracing and Terrace Abandonment in the Colca Valley of Southern Peru*. Technical Report to the National Science Foundation and the National Geographic Society. Madison: University of Wisconsin, Department of Geography.

———, ed. 1988. *The Cultural Ecology, Archaeology, and History of Terracing and Terrace*

Abandonment in the Colca Valley of Southern Peru, Vol. 2. Technical Report to the National Science Foundation and the National Geographic Society. Madison: University of Wisconsin, Department of Geography.

de Romaña, Mauricio, Jaume Blassi, and Jordi Blassi. 1987. *Descubriendo el Valle del Colca/Discovering the Colca Valley.* Barcelona: Patthey e Hijos.

Desai, Gaurav. 1993. "The Invention of Invention." *Cultural Critique* 24: 119–142.

de Soto, Hernando. 1989. *The Other Path: The Invisible Revolution in the Third World.* Trans. June Abbott. New York: Harper and Row. (Originally published in Spanish as *El otro sendero.* Lima: Editorial El Barranco, 1986.)

———. 2002. *The Other Path: The Economic Answer to Terrorism.* New York: Basic Books.

Deutsch, Sandra McGee. 1991. "Gender and Sociopolitical Change in Twentieth-Century Latin America." *Hispanic American Historical Review* 71(2): 259–306.

Deza Galindo, Juan Francisco. 1989. *Nuevo Diccionario Aymara-Castellano/Castellano Aymara.* Lima: N.p.

di Leonardo, Micaela. 1991. "Introduction: Gender, Culture, and Political Economy: Feminist Anthropology in Historical Perspective." In *Gender at the Crossroads of Knowledge: Feminist Anthropology in the Postmodern Era,* ed. Micaela di Leonardo, pp. 1–48. Berkeley: University of California Press.

Dietz, Mary. 1985. "Citizenship with a Feminist Face." *Political Theory* 13(1): 19–38.

———. 1992. "Context is All: Feminism and Theories of Citizenship." In Mouffe, ed., pp. 63–85.

Domínguez, Jorge I., ed. 1994. *Race and Ethnicity in Latin America.* New York: Garland.

Domínguez, Jorge, and Abraham Lowenthal, eds. 1996. *Constructing Democratic Governance: Latin America and the Caribbean in the 1990s, Themes and Issues.* Baltimore: Johns Hopkins University Press.

Dore, Elizabeth, and Maxine Molyneux, eds. 2000. *Hidden Histories of Gender and the State in Latin America.* Durham: Duke University Press.

Driant, Jean-Claude. 1991. *Las barriadas de Lima: Historia e interpretación.* Lima: DESCO Centro de Estudios y Promoción de Desarrollo/IFEA, Instituto Frances de Estudios Andinos.

Durand, Francisco. 1979. "Movimientos sociales urbanos y problema regional (Arequipa 1967–1973)." *Allpanchis* 12: 79–108.

Eckstein, Susan. 1989. "Power and Popular Protest in Latin America." In Eckstein, ed., pp. 1–60.

———, ed. 1989. *Power and Popular Protest: Latin American Social Movements.* Berkeley: University of California Press.

Ehlstain, Jean Bethke. 1981. *Public Man, Private Woman.* Princeton: Princeton University Press.

———. 1983. "Antigone's Daughters." In *Families, Politics, and Public Policy,* ed. Irene Diamond, pp. 300–311. New York: Longman.

Ekins, Richard. 1997. *Male Femaling: A Grounded Theory Approach to Cross-Dressing and Sex-Changing.* London and New York: Routledge.

Ekins, Richard, and Dave King, eds. 1996. *Blending Genders: Social Aspects of Cross-Dressing and Sex-Changing.* London: Routledge.

El Guindi, Fadwa. 1999. *Veil: Modesty, Privacy, and Resistance.* Oxford and New York: Berg.

Engle, Frederick. 1999. "Secrets of the Colca Valley." *AIR & SPACE/Smithsonian* 14, no. 2 (June/July): 72–79.

Epstein, Julia, and Kristina Straub. 1991. "Introduction: The Guarded Body." In *Body Guards: The Cultural Politics of Gender Ambiguity,* ed. Julia Epstein and Kristina Straub, pp. 1–28. New York: Routledge.

Feldman, Allen. 1995. "Ethnographic States of Emergency." In Nordstrom and Robben, eds., pp. 224–252.

Femenías, Blenda. 1987. "Introduction." In Femenías, ed., pp. 1–8.

———. 1990. "Visions of the Andean Household: Theoretical Perspectives, Ethnographic Realities." Manuscript.

———. 1991a. "Clothing and Ethnicity in the Colca Valley: Daily Practice as Social Process." Paper presented at the 47th International Congress of Americanists, New Orleans.

———. 1991b. "Tradición y representación en el Valle del Colca, Perú." Paper presented at the Coloquio, Tradición y Modernidad en los Andes, Cochabamba, Bolivia.

———. 1993. "Photography and Clothing: The Representation of Memory in Andean Peru." Paper presented at the Annual Meeting of the American Ethnological Society and Council on Museum Anthropology, Santa Fe.

———. 1996 [1991]. "Regional Dress of the Colca Valley: A Dynamic Tradition." In Schevill, Berlo, and Dwyer, eds., pp. 179–204.

———. 1997a. "Ambiguous Emblems: Gender, Clothing, and Representation in Contemporary Peru." Ph.D. diss., Anthropology, University of Wisconsin-Madison.

———. 1997b. "From Migrants to Commuters: Traveling as a Way of Life in Arequipa, Peru." Paper presented at the 49th International Congress of Americanists, Quito, Ecuador. Also presented at the Congress of Latin Americanist Geographers Annual Meeting, Arequipa, Peru, 1997.

———. 1997c. "Masks of Defiance, Objects of Desire: Peruvian Identity as Ethnic Ritual." Paper presented at the Annual Meeting of the American Anthropological Association, Washington, D.C.

———. 1998. "Ethnic Artists and the Appropriation of Fashion: Embroidery and Identity in Caylloma, Peru." *Chungara* 30(2): 197–206.

———. 1999. "Imperial Past, National Future: How Peruvian Political Culture Reinterpreted the Incas in the 1920s." Paper presented at the Annual Meeting of the American Society for Ethnohistory, Mashantucket, Conn.

———. 2000a. "How the Mountains Create Indians: The Geography of Belonging in the Southern Andes." Paper presented at the Annual Meeting of the American Anthropological Association, San Francisco.

———. 2000b. "The War of the Wool: Commercialization and *Mestizaje* in Southern Peru, 1890–1940." Manuscript.

———. 2001. "Embroidered Landscapes: Anthropological Perspectives on Andean Art." Invited lecture, Natural History Museum of Los Angeles County.

———. 2002a. "Dancing in Disguise: Transvestism and Performance in a Peruvian Festival." Manuscript submitted to *American Ethnologist.*

———. 2002b. "The Domestication of the Body Politic: Women's Organizations in Peru." Manuscript.

———. 2002c. "Ethnic Artists and the Appropriation of Fashion: Embroidery and Identity in the Colca Valley, Peru." In *Contemporary Societies and Cultures of Latin America,* ed. Dwight Heath, pp. 266–272. Prospect Heights, Ill.: Waveland. (Originally published in *Contact, Crossover, Continuity: Proceedings of the Fourth Biennial Symposium of the Textile Society of America,* pp. 331–342. Los Angeles: Textile Society of America, 1995.)

———. 2002d. "The Gendering of Anthropology in South America." *Anthropology News* 43, no. 4 (April): 10.

———. 2004. "'Why Do Gringos Like Black?': Mourning, Tourism, and Changing Fashions in Peru." In *The Latin American Fashion Reader,* ed. Regina Root. New York: Berg.

———, ed. 1987. *Andean Aesthetics: Textiles of Peru and Bolivia.* Madison: Helen L. Allen Textile Collection and Elvehjem Museum of Art, University of Wisconsin.

Field, Les W. 1996. "State, Anti-state, and Indigenous Entities." *Journal of Latin American Anthropology* 1(2): 98–119.

———. 1999. *The Grimace of Macho Ratón: Artisans, Identity, and Nation in Late-Twentieth-Century Western Nicaragua.* Durham: Duke University Press.

Fine-Dare, Kathleen S. 2002. *Grave Injustice: The American Indian Repatriation Movement and NAGPRA.* Lincoln: University of Nebraska Press.

Fisher, Jo. 1993. *Out of the Shadows: Women, Resistance, and Politics in South America.* London: Latin American Bureau.

FLACSO. 1995. *Mujeres latinoamericanas en cifras. Tomo comparativo.* Santiago: FLACSO.

Flores Galindo, Alberto. 1977. *Arequipa y el sur andino: Ensayo de historia regional (siglos XVII–XX).* Lima: Editorial Horizonte.

———. 1987. "In Search of an Inca." In Stern, ed., pp. 193–210. Madison: University of Wisconsin Press.

———. 1988. *Tiempo de plagas.* Lima: Caballo Rojo.

Foster, David William. 1997. *Sexual Textualities: Essays on Queering Latin American Writing.* Austin: University of Texas Press.

Foster, David William, and Roberto Reis, eds. 1996. *Bodies and Biases: Sexualities in Hispanic Cultures and Literatures.* Minneapolis: University of Minnesota Press.

Foucault, Michel. 1978. *History of Sexuality, Vol. 1: An Introduction.* New York: Random House.

Fowler, Brenda. 1996. "Should Just Anybody Be Allowed to Stare?" *New York Times,* June 16, Sec. 2, p. 5.

Fowler-Salamini, Heather, and Mary Kay Vaughan, eds. 1994. *Women of the Mexican Countryside, 1850–1990: Creating Spaces, Shaping Transitions.* Tucson: University of Arizona Press.

Franco, Jean. 1989. *Plotting Women: Gender and Representation in Mexico.* New York: Columbia University Press.

———. 1992. "Going Public: Reinhabiting the Private." In *On Edge: The Crisis of Contemporary Latin American Culture,* ed. George Yúdice, Jean Franco, and Juan Flores, pp. 65–84. Minneapolis: University of Minnesota Press.

Franco, Pamela R. 2000. "The 'Unruly Woman' in Nineteenth-Century Trinidad Carnival." *Small Axe* 7 (March): 60–76.

Franquemont, Christine, and Edward Franquemont. 1987. "Learning to Weave in Chinchero." *Textile Museum Journal* 26: 55–78.

Fraser, Nancy. 1989. *Unruly Practices.* Minneapolis: University of Minnesota Press.

Freedman, Diane C. 1986. "Wife, Widow, Woman: Roles of an Anthropologist in a Transylvanian Village." In Golde, ed., pp. 333–358.

Frohlick, Susan. 1999. "'Home Has Always Been Hard for Me': Single Mothers' Narratives of Identity, Home, and Loss." In Bridgman, Cole, and Howard-Bobiwash, eds., pp. 86–102.

Fuenzalida, Fernando. 1970. "Poder, raza y etnía en el Perú contemporáneo." In Fuenzalida et al., pp. 15–86.

Fuenzalida, Fernando, Enrique Mayer, Gabriel Escobar, François Bourricaud, and José Matos Mar. 1970. *El indio y el poder en el Perú.* Lima: Instituto de Estudios Peruanos.

Fuller Osores, Norma J. 1997. *Identidades masculinas: Varones de clase media en el Perú.* Lima: Pontificia Universidad Católica del Perú.

Gallard, Patrick, and Miguel Vallier. 1988. *Arequipa: Agro y región.* Lima: Editorial Horizonte.

Garber, Marjorie. 1992. *Vested Interests: Cross-Dressing and Cultural Anxiety.* New York: Routledge, Chapman, and Hall/HarperCollins.

García, María Elena. 2000a. "Ethnographic Responsibility and the Anthropological Endeavor: Beyond Identity Discourse." *Anthropological Quarterly* 73(2): 89–101.

———. 2000b. "To Be Quechua Is to Belong: Citizenship, Identity, and Intercultural Bilingual Education Discourse in Cuzco, Peru." Ph.D. diss., Anthropology, Brown University.

García Canclini, Néstor. 1995. *Hybrid Cultures: Strategies for Entering and Leaving Modernity.* Trans. Christopher L. Chiappari and Silvia L. López. Minneapolis: University of Minnesota Press.

Garciagodoy, Juanita. 1998. *Digging the Days of the Dead: A Reading of Mexico's Días de Muertos.* Niwot: University Press of Colorado.

Gatens, Moira. 1996. *Imaginary Bodies: Ethics, Power, and Corporeality.* New York: Routledge.

Geary, Patrick. 1986. "Sacred Commodities: The Circulation of Medieval Relics." In Appadurai, ed., pp. 169–191.

Geertz, Clifford. 1973. *The Interpretation of Cultures.* New York: Harper.

Gelles, Paul. 1990. "Channels of Power, Fields of Contention: The Politics and Ideology of Irrigation in an Andean Peasant Community." Ph.D. diss., Anthropology, Harvard University.

———. 1992. "'*Caballeritos*' and *Maíz Cabanita:* Colonial Categories and Andean Ethnicity in the Quincentennial Year." Kroeber Anthropological Society Papers, pp. 14–27. Oakland: GRT Press.

———. 1994. "Channels of Power, Fields of Contention: The Politics of Irrigation and Land Recovery in an Andean Peasant Community." In Mitchell and Guillet, eds., pp. 233–274.

———. 1995. "Equilibrium and Extraction: Dual Organization in the Andes." *American Ethnologist* 22(4): 710–742.

———. 2000. *Water and Power in Highland Peru: The Cultural Politics of Irrigation and Development.* New Brunswick, N.J.: Rutgers University Press.

Gelles, Paul, and Wilton Martínez. 1993. *Transnational Fiesta.* Film distributed by University of California, Berkeley.

Golde, Peggy, ed. 1986 [1970]. *Women in the Field.* 2d ed. Berkeley: University of California Press.

Golte, Jürgen, and Norma Adams. 1986. *Los caballos de Troya de los invasores: Estrategias campesinas en la conquista de la Gran Lima.* Lima: Instituto de Estudios Peruanos.

Gómez Rodríguez, Juan. 1985. *Tecnología del pastoreo en las comunidades del Cañon del Colca.* Arequipa: Central de Crédito Cooperativo.

González, Victoria, and Karen Kampwirth, eds. 2001. *Radical Women in Latin America: Left and Right.* University Park: Pennsylvania State University Press.

Goody, Esther. 1989. "Learning, Apprenticeship, and the Division of Labor." In Coy, ed., pp. 233–256.

Gordon, Deborah. 1995. "Conclusion: Culture Writing Women: Inscribing Feminist Anthropology." In Behar and Gordon, eds., pp. 429–441.

———. 1999. "U.S. Feminist Ethnography and the Denationalizing of 'America': A Retrospective on *Women Writing Culture.*" In Bridgman, Cole, and Howard-Bobiwash, eds., pp. 54–69.

Gordon, Linda. 1994. *Pitied but Not Entitled: Single Mothers and the History of Welfare, 1890–1935.* New York: Free Press.

Gorriti, Gustavo. 1990. *Sendero Luminoso: Historia de la guerra milenaria en el Perú.* Lima: Apoyo.

———. 1999. *The Shining Path: A History of the Millenarian War in Peru.* Trans. Robin Kirk. Chapel Hill: University of North Carolina Press.

Gossy, Mary S. 1998. "Skirting the Question: Lesbians and María de Zayas." In Molloy and Irwin, eds., pp. 19–28.

Gould, Jeffrey L. 1998. *To Die in This Way: Nicaraguan Indians and the Myth of Mestizaje, 1880–1965.* Durham: Duke University Press.

Goytisolo, Juan. 1977. "El mundo erótico de María de Zayas." In *Disidencias,* pp. 63–115. Barcelona: Seix Barral.

Graham, Richard, ed. 1990. *The Idea of Race in Latin America, 1870–1940.* Austin: University of Texas Press.

Green, James M. 1999. *Beyond Carnival: Male Homosexuality in Twentieth-Century Brazil.* Chicago: University of Chicago Press.

Green, Linda. 1995. "Living in a State of Fear." In Nordstrom and Robben, eds., pp. 104–127.

Grosz, Elizabeth, and Elspeth Probyn, eds. 1995. *Sexy Bodies: The Strange Carnalities of Feminism.* New York: Routledge.

Guillet, David. 1992. *Covering Ground: Communal Water Management and the State in the Peruvian Highlands.* Ann Arbor: University of Michigan Press.

———. 1994. "Canal Irrigation and the State: The 1969 Water Law and Irrigation Systems of the Colca Valley of Southwestern Peru." In Mitchell and Guillet, eds., pp. 167–188.

Gupta, Akhil, and James Ferguson, eds. 1997. *Anthropological Locations: Boundaries and Grounds of a Field Science.* Berkeley: University of California Press.

Guss, David M. 2000. *The Festive State: Race, Ethnicity, and Nationalism as Cultural Performance.* Berkeley: University of California Press.

Gutiérrez, Ramón, Cristina Esteras, and Alejandro Málaga. 1986. *El Valle del Colca (Arequipa): Cinco siglos de arquitectura y urbanismo.* Buenos Aires: Libros de Hispanoamérica/Instituto Argentino de Investigaciones de Historia de la Arquitectura y del Urbanismo.

Hail, Barbara A., ed. 2000. *Gifts of Pride and Love: Kiowa and Comanche Cradles.* Bristol, R.I.: Haffenreffer Museum of Anthropology, Brown University.

Hale, Charles. 1986. "Political and Social Ideas in Latin America." In *Cambridge History of Latin America,* Vol. 4, ed. Leslie Bethell, pp. 383–414. Cambridge: Cambridge University Press.

———. 1997. "The Cultural Politics of Identity in Latin America." *Annual Review of Anthropology* 26: 567–590.

Hallam, Elizabeth, and Jenny Hockey. 2001. *Death, Memory and Material Culture.* Oxford: Berg.

Halperin, David M. 1990. *One Hundred Years of Homosexuality.* New York and London: Routledge.

Harris, Olivia. 1981. "Households as Natural Units." In *Of Marriage and the Market: Women's Subordination Internationally and Its Lessons,* ed. Kate Young, Carol Wolkowitz, and Roslyn McCullagh, pp. 49–67. London: Routledge and Kegan Paul.

———. 1995. "Ethnic Identity and Market Relations: Indians and Mestizos in the Andes." In Larson and Harris, eds., with Tandeter, pp. 351–390.

———. 2000. *To Make the Earth Bear Fruit: Ethnographic Essays on Fertility, Work, and Gender in Highland Bolivia.* London: University of London, Institute of Latin American Studies.

Harrison, Faye. 1995. "The Persistent Power of 'Race' and the Political Economy of Racism." *Annual Review of Anthropology* 24: 47–74.

Harvey, John. 1995. *Men in Black.* Chicago: University of Chicago Press.

Harvey, Penelope. 1989. *Género, autoridad y competencia lingüística: Participación política de la mujer en pueblos andinos.* Documento de Trabajo No. 3. Lima: Instituto de Estudios Peruanos.

———. 1991. "Mujeres que no hablan castellano: Género, poder y bilingüismo en un pueblo andino." *Allpanchis* 38: 227–260.

———. 1994a. "Domestic Violence in the Peruvian Andes." In *Sex and Violence: Issues in Representation and Experience,* ed. Penelope Harvey and Peter Gow, pp. 66–90. London: Routledge.

———. 1994b. "The Presence and Absence of Speech in the Communication of Gender." In *Bilingual Women: Anthropological Approaches to Second-Language Use,* ed. Pauline Burton, Ketaki Kushari Dyson, and Shirley Ardener, pp. 44–64. Oxford: Berg.

Healy, Kevin. 2001. *Llamas, Weaving, and Organic Chocolate.* Notre Dame: University of Notre Dame Press.

Hedlund, Ann L. 1989. "Designing among the Navajo: Ethnoaesthetics in Weaving." In *Textiles as Primary Sources,* ed. John E. Vollmer, pp. 86–93. Proceedings of the First Symposium of the Textile Society of America, Minneapolis, September 1988.

Helly, Dorothy O., and Susan M. Reversby, eds. 1992. *Gendered Domains: Rethinking Public and Private in Women's History.* Ithaca: Cornell University Press.

Hendrickson, Carol. 1995. *Weaving Identities: Construction of Dress and Self in a Highland Guatemala Town.* Austin: University of Texas Press.

Hendrickson, Hildi. 1996. "Introduction." In *Clothing and Difference: Embodied Identities in Colonial and Post-Colonial Africa,* ed. Hildi Hendrickson, pp. 1–16. Durham: Duke University Press.

Herdt, Gilbert. 1994. "Introduction: Third Sexes and Third Genders." In Herdt, ed., pp. 21–81.

———, ed. 1994. *Third Sex, Third Gender: Beyond Sexual Dimorphism in Culture and History.* New York: Zone Books.

Higgins, Michael James, and Tanya L. Coen. 2000. *Streets, Bedrooms, and Patios: The Ordinariness of Diversity in Urban Oaxaca.* Austin: University of Texas Press.

Hobsbawm, Eric. 1992. "Introduction: Inventing Traditions." In Hobsbawm and Ranger, eds., pp. 1–14.

Hobsbawm, Eric, and Terence Ranger, eds. 1992 [1983]. *The Invention of Tradition.* Canto ed. Cambridge: Cambridge University Press. (Originally published 1983.)

Hola, Eugenia, and Ana Maria Portugal, eds. 1997. *La ciudadanía: Un debate.* Santiago, Chile: Isis International.

Hollander, Anne. 1978. *Seeing through Clothes.* New York: Avon.

———. 1994. *Sex and Suits.* New York: Knopf.

hooks, bell. 1990. *Yearning: Race, Gender, and Cultural Politics.* Boston: South End Press.

Hoskins, Janet. 1998. *Biographical Objects: How Things Tell the Stories of People's Lives.* New York: Routledge.

Hughes, Robin. 1987. "Birdlife in the Colca." In de Romaña, Blassi, and Blassi, pp. 77–79.

Hünefeldt, Christine. 1994. *Paying the Price of Freedom: Family and Labor among Lima's Slaves, 1800–1854.* Berkeley: University of California Press.

Hurley, William. 1978. "Highland Peasants and Rural Development in Southern Peru: The Colca Valley and the Majes Project." Ph.D. diss., Oxford University.

Hurston, Zora Neale. 1990 [1935]. *Mules and Men.* New York: Harper and Row.

Isbell, Billie Jean. 1976. "La otra mitad esencial: Un estudio de complementaridad sexual en los Andes." *Estudios Andinos* 5: 37–56.

———. 1985. *To Defend Ourselves: Ecology and Ritual in an Andean Village.* Prospect Heights, Ill.: Waveland. (Originally published 1978.)

Jacobs, Sue-Ellen, Wesley Thomas, and Sabine Lang. 1997. *Two-Spirit People: Native American Gender Identity, Sexuality, and Spirituality.* Urbana: University of Illinois Press.

Jacobsen, Nils. 1993. *Mirages of Transition: The Peruvian Altiplano, 1780–1930.* Berkeley: University of California Press.

Jacobus, Mary, Evelyn Fox Keller, and Sally Shuttleworth, eds. 1990. *Body/Politics: Women and the Discourses of Science.* New York: Routledge.

Jaquette, Jane S. 1994. "Introduction: From Transition to Participation—Women's Movements and Democratic Politics." In Jaquette, ed., pp. 1–11.

———, ed. 1989. *The Women's Movement in Latin America: Feminism and the Transition to Democracy.* Boston: Unwin Hyman.

———, ed. 1994. *The Women's Movement in Latin America: Participation and Democracy.* 2d ed. Boulder: Westview.

Jaquette, Jane S., and Sharon L. Wolchik, eds. 1998. *Women and Democracy: Latin America and Central and Eastern Europe.* Baltimore: Johns Hopkins University Press.

Jelin, Elizabeth. 1990. "Citizenship and Identity: Final Reflections." In Jelin, ed., pp. 184–207.

———, ed. 1990. *Women and Social Change in Latin America.* London: United Nations Research Institute for Social Development/Zed Books.

Jelin, Elizabeth, and Eric Hershberg, eds. 1996. *Constructing Democracy: Human Rights, Citizenship, and Society in Latin America.* Boulder: Westview.

Kaminsky, Amy. 1993. *Reading the Body Politic: Feminist Criticism and Latin American Women Writers.* Minneapolis: University of Minnesota Press.

Kaplan, Temma. 1997. *Crazy for Democracy: Women in Grassroots Movements.* New York: Routledge.

Kapsoli, Wilfredo. 1977. *Los movimientos campesinos en el Perú.* Lima: Delva.

———. 1984. *Ayllus del sol: Anarquismo y utopía andina.* Lima: TAREA.

Kapsoli, Wilfredo, and Wilson Reátegui. 1987. *El campesinado peruano: 1919–1930.* Lima: Universidad Nacional Mayor San Marcos.

Kindberg, Eric, and Mary Lynn Kindberg. 1985. *Palabras útiles en el quechua de Caylloma, Arequipa.* N.p.: Instituto Lingüístico de Verano/Unidad de Supervisión Educativa de la Zona de Educación de Arequipa.

Kingsolver, Barbara. 1990. *Animal Dreams.* New York: HarperCollins.

Kirk, Robin. 1993. *Grabado en piedra: Las mujeres de Sendero Luminoso.* Lima: Instituto de Estudios Peruanos.

Kirkwood, Julieta. 1988. "Feministas y políticas." In *Mujeres latinoamericanas: Diez en-*

sayos y una historia colectiva, pp. 17–27. Lima: Centro de la Mujer Peruana Flora Tristán.

Kling, Cynthia. 1996. "Don't Be a Fashion Victim—Learn to Wear Lime Green in Spring." *New York Post,* May 20, p. 39.

Kondo, Dorinne. 1990. *Crafting Selves: Power, Gender, and Discourses of Identity in a Japanese Workplace.* Chicago: University of Chicago Press.

———. 1997. *About Face: Performing Race in Fashion and Theater.* New York and London: Routledge.

Kopytoff, Igor. 1986. "The Cultural Biography of Things: Commoditization as Process." In Appadurai, ed., pp. 64–91.

Koven, Seth, and Sonya Michel, eds. 1993. *Mothers of a New World: Maternalist Politics and the Origins of Welfare States.* New York: Routledge.

Krüggeler, Thomas. 1997. "Changing Consumption Patterns and Everyday Life in Two Peruvian Regions: Food, Dress, and Housing in the Central and Southern Highlands (1820–1920)." In Orlove, ed., pp. 31–66.

Krutch, Joseph Wood. 1985 [1952]. *The Desert Year.* Tucson: University of Arizona Press.

Kulick, Don. 1998. *Travesti: Sex, Gender, and Culture and Brazilian Transgendered Prostitutes.* Chicago: University of Chicago Press.

———. 2000. "Gay and Lesbian Language." *Annual Review of Anthropology* 29: 243–285.

Lamphere, Louise, Helena Ragoné, and Patricia Zavella, eds. 1997. *Situated Lives: Gender and Culture in Everyday Life.* New York: Routledge.

Lancaster, Roger N. 1992. *Life Is Hard: Machismo, Danger, and the Intimacy of Power in Nicaragua.* Berkeley: University of California Press.

Lang, Sabine. 1998. *Men as Women, Women as Men: Changing Gender in Native American Cultures.* Trans. John L. Vantine. Austin: University of Texas Press.

Langer, Erick D., ed., with Elena Muñoz. 2003. *Contemporary Indigenous Movements in Latin America.* Wilmington, Del.: Scholarly Resource Books.

Larico Cama, Margarita. 1987. "Cambios socio-culturales de la población de Chivay por influencia del Proyecto Majes." Tesis de Bachiller, Antropología, Universidad Nacional de San Agustín, Arequipa.

Larson, Brooke. 1995. "Andean Communities, Political Cultures, and Markets: The Changing Contours of a Field." In Larson and Harris, eds., with Tandeter, pp. 5–53.

Larson, Brooke, and Olivia Harris, eds., with Enrique Tandeter. 1995. *Ethnicity, Markets, and Migration in the Andes: At the Crossroads of History and Anthropology.* Durham: Duke University Press.

Lather, Patti. 2001. "Postbook: Working the Ruins of Feminist Ethnography." *Signs: Journal of Women in Culture and Society* 27, no. 1 (autumn): 199–228.

Lauer, Mirko. 1982. *Crítica de la artesanía: Plástica y sociedad en los Andes peruanos.* Lima: DESCO.

———. 1989. *La producción artesanal en América Latina.* Lima: Fundación Friedrich Ebert.

Lave, Jean. 1977. "Cognitive Consequences of Traditional Apprenticeship: Training in West Africa." *Anthropology and Education Quarterly* 8: 177–180.

Lavie, Smadar, Kirin Narayan, and Renato Rosaldo, eds. 1993. *Creativity/Anthropology.* Ithaca: Cornell University Press.

Lavrin, Asunción. 1995. *Women, Feminism, and Social Change in Argentina, Chile, and Uruguay, 1890–1940.* Lincoln: University of Nebraska Press.

Lederman, Rena. 1990. "Pretexts for Ethnography: On Reading Fieldnotes." In Sanjek, ed., pp. 71–91.

Lehmann, David, ed. 1982. *Ecology and Exchange in the Andes.* Cambridge: Cambridge University Press.

Limón, José. 1997. "Carne, Carnales, and the Carnivalesque." In Lamphere, Ragoné, and Zavella, eds., pp. 62–82.

Lipovetsky, Gilles. 1994. *The Empire of Fashion: Dressing Modern Democracy.* Trans. Catherine Porter. Princeton: Princeton University Press.

Lira, Jorge A. 1944. *Diccionario kkechuwa-español.* Tucumán: Universidad Nacional de Tucumán, Instituto de Historia, Lingüística y Folklore. Publicaciones Especiales, XII.

———. 1982. *Diccionario kkechuwa-español.* 2d ed. Bogotá: Secretaría Ejecutiva del Convenio Andrés Bello.

Lister, Ruth. 1997. *Citizenship: Feminist Perspectives.* Washington Square, N.Y.: New York University Press.

Llosa, Hector, and Maria A. Benavides. 1994. "Arquitectura y vivienda campesina en tres pueblos andinos: Yanque, Lari y Coporaque en el Valle del Río Colca, Arequipa." *Bulletin de l'Institut Français d'Etudes Andines* 23(1): 105–150.

Lobo, María Luisa. 1988. *Perú—Cuando el mundo se oscureció.* Film. Distributed by Arawak, S.A.

Lobo, Susan. 1991. "The Fabric of Life: Repatriating the Sacred Coroma Textiles." *Cultural Survival Quarterly* 15(3): 40–46.

Lord, M. J. 1994. *Forever Barbie: The Unauthorized Biography of a Real Doll.* New York: William Morrow.

Love, Thomas. 1989. "Limits to the Articulation of Modes of Production Approach: The Southwestern Peru Region." In *State, Capital, and Rural Society: Anthropological Perspectives on Political Economy in Mexico and the Andes,* ed. Benjamin S. Orlove, Michael W. Foley, and Thomas F. Love, pp. 147–180. Boulder: Westview.

———. 1999. "*Ni Chicha ni Limonada: Campiña* Traditionalism, *Mestizaje,* and the Evolution of Arequipeño Regionalism." Paper presented at the Annual Meeting of the American Anthropological Association, Chicago.

Lutz, Catherine A., and Jane L. Collins. 1993. *Reading National Geographic.* Chicago: University of Chicago Press.

Macassi, Ivonne, and Cecilia Olea, eds. 2000. *Al rescate de la utopía: Reflexiones para una agenda feminista del nuevo milenio.* Lima: Centro de la Mujer Peruana Flora Tristán.

MacLeod, Arlene Elowe. 1991. *Accommodating Protest: Working Women, the New Veiling, and Change in Cairo.* New York: Columbia University Press.

Málaga Medina, Alejandro. 1977. "Los collaguas en la historia de Arequipa en el siglo XVI." In Pease, ed., pp. 93–130.

Manrique, Nelson. 1985. *Colonialismo y pobreza campesina: Caylloma y el Valle del Colca, siglos XVI–XX*. Lima: DESCO.

———. 1988. *Yawar mayu: Sociedades y terratenientes serranas, 1879–1910*. Lima: Instituto Francés de Estudios Andinos/DESCO.

———. 1999. *La piel y la pluma: Escritos sobre literatura, etnicidad y racismo*. Lima: CIDIAG (Centro de Informe y Desarrollo Integral de Autogestión)/SUR.

Marcus, George E. 1998. *Ethnography through Thick and Thin*. Princeton: Princeton University Press.

Marcus, George, and Michael Fischer. 1986. *Anthropology as Cultural Critique: An Experimental Moment in the Human Sciences*. Chicago: University of Chicago Press.

Marcus, George E., and Fred R. Myers, eds. 1995. *The Traffic in Culture: Refiguring Art and Anthropology*. Berkeley: University of California Press.

Mariátegui, José Carlos. 1971 [1928]. *Seven Interpretive Essays on Peruvian Reality*. Austin: University of Texas Press. (Originally published as *Siete ensayos de interpretación de la realidad peruana*. Lima: Biblioteca Amauta, 1928.)

Markowitz, Lisa. 1992. "Pastoral Production and Its Discontents: Alpaca and Sheep Herding in Caylloma, Peru." Ph.D. diss., Anthropology, University of Massachusetts, Amherst.

———. 2001. "NGOs, Local Government, and Agrarian Civil Society: A Case of Evolving Collaboration from Southern Peru." *Culture and Agriculture* 23(1): 8–18.

Marques-Pereira, Bérengère, and Alain Carrier, eds. 1996. *La citoyenneté sociale des femmes au Brésil: Action collective, reproduction, informalité et domesticité*. Brussels: CELA-IS (Université Libre de Bruxelles, Centre d'études Latino-Américaines); Paris: L'Harmattan.

Martin, Biddy, and Chandra Talpade Mohanty. 1986. "Feminist Politics: What's Home Got to Do with It?" In de Lauretis, ed., pp. 191–212.

Marzal, Manuel. 1995. "Perception of the State among Peruvian Indians." In *Indigenous Perceptions of the Nation-State in Latin America*, ed. Lourdes Giordani and Marjorie Snipes. Studies in Third World Societies, no. 56. Williamsburg: College of William and Mary.

Masuda, Shozo, Izumi Shimada, and Craig Morris, eds. 1985. *Andean Ecology and Civilization: An Interdisciplinary Perspective on Andean Ecological Complementarity*. Tokyo: University of Tokyo Press.

Maybury-Lewis, David. 1997. *Indigenous Peoples, Ethnic Groups, and the State*. Boston: Allyn and Bacon.

———, ed. 2002. *The Politics of Ethnicity: Indigenous Peoples in Latin American States*. David Rockefeller Center Series on Latin American Studies. Cambridge: David Rockefeller Center for Latin American Studies, Harvard University.

Mayer, Enrique. 1970. "Mestizo e indio: El contexto social de las relaciones interétnicas." In Fuenzalida et al., pp. 87–152.

———. 2002. *The Articulated Peasant: Household Economies in the Andes*. Boulder: Westview.

McClintock, Cynthia. 1989. "Peru's Sendero Luminoso Rebellion: Origins and Trajectory." In Eckstein, ed., pp. 61–101.
Medlin, Mary Ann. 1986. "Learning to Weave in Calcha, Bolivia." In Rowe, ed., pp. 275–288.
Meisch, Lynn. 1986. "Weaving Styles in Tarabuco, Bolivia." In Rowe, ed., pp. 243–274.
———. 1987a. "The Living Textiles of Tarabuco, Bolivia." In Femenías, ed., pp. 46–59.
———. 1987b. *Otavalo: Weaving, Costume, and the Market.* Quito: Libri Mundi.
———. 2002. *Andean Entrepreneurs: Otavalo Merchants and Musicians in the Global Arena.* Austin: University of Texas Press.
Mendoza, Zoila. 1989. "La danza de 'Los Avelinos': Sus orígenes y sus múltiples significados." *Revista Andina* 7(2): 501–521.
———. 2000. *Shaping Society through Dance: Mestizo Ritual Performance in the Peruvian Andes.* Chicago: University of Chicago Press.
Meyer, Carter Jones, and Diana Royer, eds. 2001. *Selling the Indian: Commercializing and Appropriating American Indian Cultures.* Tucson: University of Arizona Press.
Meyers, Albert, and Diane Hopkins, eds. 1988. *Manipulating the Saints: Religious Brotherhoods and Social Integration in Postconquest Latin America.* Hamburg: Wayasbah.
Meyerson, Julia. 1990. *'Tambo: Life in an Andean Village.* Austin: University of Texas Press.
Miles, Ann, and Hans Buechler, eds. 1997. *Women and Economic Change: Andean Perspectives.* Arlington, Va.: American Anthropological Association.
Miller, Francesca. 1991. *Latin American Women and the Search for Social Justice.* Hanover and London: University Press of New England.
Miloslavich Túpac, Diana. 1993. *María Elena Moyano: En busca de una esperanza.* Lima: Centro de la Mujer Peruana Flora Tristán.
Mitchell, William M., and David Guillet, eds. 1994. *Irrigation at High Altitudes: The Social Organization of Water Control Systems in the Andes.* Washington, D.C.: American Anthropological Association/Society for Latin American Anthropology.
Mohanty, Chandra Talpade, Ann Russo, and Lourdes Torres. 1991. *Third World Women and the Politics of Feminism.* Bloomington: Indiana University Press.
Molloy, Sylvia, and Robert McKee Irwin, eds. 1998. *Hispanisms and Homosexualities.* Durham: Duke University Press.
Molyneux, Maxine. 2000. "Twentieth-Century State Formations in Latin America." In Dore and Molyneux, eds., pp. 33–81.
———. 2001. *Women's Movements in International Perspective: Latin America and Beyond.* London: Palgrave/Institute of Latin American Studies.
Moore, Henrietta L. 1988. *Feminism and Anthropology.* Minneapolis: University of Minnesota Press.
———. 1994. *A Passion for Difference.* Bloomington: Indiana University Press.
Mörner, Magnus, ed. 1970. *Race and Class in Latin America.* New York: Columbia University Press.

Morris, Rosalind C. 1995. "All Made Up: Performance Theory and the Anthropology of Sex and Gender." *Annual Review of Anthropology* 24: 567–592.

Mouffe, Chantal. 1993. *The Return of the Political*. London: Verso.

———, ed. 1992. *Dimensions of Radical Democracy*. London: Verso.

Muñoz, Hortensia. 1998. "Human Rights and Social Referents: The Construction of New Sensibilities." In Stern, ed., pp. 447–469.

Murra, John V. 1962. "Cloth and Its Functions in the Inca State." *American Anthropologist* 64(4): 710–727.

———. 1972. "El control vertical de un máximo de pisos ecológicos en la economía de las sociedades andinas." In *Visita de la provincia de León de Huánuco en 1562*, ed. John V. Murra, pp. 429–476. Huánuco: Universidad Nacional Hermilio Valdizán.

———. 1980 [1955]. *The Economic Organization of the Inka State*. Greenwich, Conn.: JAI Press.

———. 1989. "Cloth and Its Function in the Inka State." In Weiner and Schneider, eds., pp. 275–302.

Murray, Stephen O. 1995a. "Modern Male Homosexuality in Mexico and Peru." In Murray et al., pp. 145–149.

———. 1995b. "South American West Coast Indigenous Homosexualities." In Murray et al., pp. 279–292.

Murray, Stephen O., et al. 1995. *Latin American Male Homosexualities*. Albuquerque: University of New Mexico Press.

Myers, Fred R., ed. 2001. *The Empire of Things: Regimes of Value and Material Culture*. Santa Fe, N.M.: School of American Research Press.

Nanda, Serena. 1994. "The Hijras of India: An Alternative Sex and Gender Role in India." In Herdt, ed., pp. 373–418.

———. 1999. *Neither Man nor Woman: The Hijras of India*. 2d ed. Belmont, Calif.: Wadsworth. (Originally published 1990.)

———. 2000. *Gender Diversity: Crosscultural Variations*. Prospect Heights, Ill.: Waveland Press.

Narayan, Kirin. 1997. "How Native is a 'Native' Anthropologist?" In Lamphere, Ragoné, and Zavella, eds., pp. 23–41.

Nash, June. 1993. "Introduction: Traditional Arts and Changing Markets in Middle America." In Nash, ed., pp. 1–24.

———, ed. 1993. *Crafts in the World Market: The Impact of Global Exchange on Middle American Artisans*. Albany: State University of New York Press.

Navarro, Marysa. 1989. "The Personal Is Political: Las Madres de Plaza de Mayo." In Eckstein, ed., pp. 241–258.

Neira, Máximo, Guillermo Galdos Rodríguez, Alejandro Málaga Medina, Eusebio Quiroz Paz Soldán, and Juan Guillermo Carpio Muñoz. 1990. *Historia General de Arequipa*. Arequipa: Fundación M. J. Bustamante de la Fuente.

Nelson, Diane. 1999. *A Finger in the Wound: Body Politics in Quincentennial Guatemala*. Berkeley: University of California Press.

Nelson, Richard. 1989. *The Island Within*. New York: Random House.

Ness, Sally Ann. 1992. *Body, Movement, and Culture: Kinesthetic and Visual Symbolism in a Philippine Community*. Philadelphia: University of Pennsylvania Press.

Newton, Esther. 1979. *Mother Camp: Female Impersonators in America*. Chicago: University of Chicago Press.

———. 1993. "My Best Informant's Dress: The Erotic Equation in Fieldwork." *Cultural Anthropology* 8(1): 3–23.

Nordstrom, Carolyn, and Antonius C. G. M. Robben, eds. 1995. *Fieldwork Under Fire: Contemporary Studies of Violence and Survival*. Berkeley: University of California Press.

Nutini, Hugo G. 1988. *Todos Santos in Rural Tlaxcala: A Syncretic, Expressive, and Symbolic Analysis of the Cult of the Dead*. Princeton: Princeton University Press.

Oliart, Patricia. 1998. "Alberto Fujimori: 'The Man Peru Needed'?" In Stern, ed., pp. 411–424.

Orlove, Benjamin. 1977. *Alpacas, Sheep, and Men: The Wool Export Economy and Regional Society in Southern Peru*. New York: Academic Press.

———. 1990. "La posición de los abigeos en la sociedad regional (El bandolerismo social en el Cusco en vísperas de la Reforma Agraria)." In Aguirre and Walker, eds., pp. 277–305.

———. 1994. "Sticks and Stones: Ritual Battles and Play in the Southern Peruvian Andes." In Poole, ed., pp. 133–164.

———, ed. 1997. *The Allure of the Foreign: Imported Goods in Postcolonial Latin America*. Ann Arbor: University of Michigan Press.

Orlove, Benjamin, and Henry J. Rutz. 1989. "Thinking about Consumption: A Social Economy Approach." In *The Social Economy of Consumption*, ed. Henry J. Rutz and Benjamin Orlove, pp. 1–58. Monographs in Economic Anthropology, 6. Lanham, Md.: University Press of America/Society for Economic Anthropology.

Ortner, Sherry B., and Harriet Whitehead, eds. 1981. *Sexual Meanings: The Cultural Construction of Gender and Sexuality*. Cambridge: Cambridge University Press.

Paerregaard, Karsten. 1987. "Death Rituals and Symbols in the Andes." *Folk* 29: 23–42.

———. 1989. "Exchanging with Nature: *T'inka* in an Andean Village." *Folk* 31: 53–73.

———. 1991a. "Más allá del dinero: Trueque y economía categorial en un distrito en el Valle del Colca." Manuscript.

———. 1991b. "Power, Ethnicity, and Migration: The Rise and Fall of a Misti Family in the Colca Valley of Southern Peru." Paper presented at the 47th International Congress of Americanists, New Orleans.

———. 1992. "Complementarity and Duality: Oppositions between Agriculturists and Herders in an Andean Village." *Ethnology* 31(1): 15–26.

———. 1994. "Why Fight over Water? Power, Conflict, and Irrigation in an Andean Village." In Mitchell and Guillet, eds., pp. 189–202.

———. 1997. *Linking Separate Worlds: Urban Migrants and Rural Lives in Peru*. Oxford: Berg.

———. n.d. "The Dark Side of the Moon: Conceptual and Methodological Problems of Studying Urban Migrants and Their Native Village." Manuscript.

Palmer, David Scott, ed. 1992. *The Shining Path of Peru: A Study of Sendero Luminoso.* London: Hurst.

Parker, Andrew, Mary Russo, Doris Sommer, and Patricia Yeager, eds. 1992. *Nationalisms and Sexualities.* New York and London: Routledge.

Parker, D. S. 1998. *The Idea of the Middle Class: White-Collar Workers and Peruvian Society, 1900–1950.* University Park: Pennsylvania State University Press.

Parker, Richard. 1999. *Beneath the Equator: Cultures of Desire, Male Homosexuality, and Emerging Gay Communities in Brazil.* New York and London: Routledge.

Parker, Rozsika. 1986. *The Subversive Stitch: Embroidery and the Making of the Feminine.* London: Women's Press. Reprint of 1984 edition.

Pateman, Carole 1988. *The Sexual Contract.* Cambridge: Polity.

———. 1989. *The Disorder of Women: Democracy, Feminism and Political Theory.* Stanford: Stanford University Press.

Paz, Octavio. 1989 [1950]. *El laberinto de la soledad.* 3d ed. Mexico City: Fondo de Cultura Económica.

Pease, Franklin. 1977. "Collaguas: Una etnía del siglo XVI. Problemas iniciales." In Pease, ed., pp. 131–168.

———, ed. 1977. *Collaguas I.* Lima: Pontificia Universidad Católica.

Pelto, Pertti J., and Gretel H. Pelto. 1970. *Anthropological Research: The Structure of Inquiry.* 2d ed. London: Cambridge University Press.

Perry, Mary Elizabeth. 1990. *Gender and Disorder in Early Modern Seville.* Princeton: Princeton University Press.

———. 1999. "From Convent to Battlefield: Cross-Dressing and Gendering the Self in the New World of Imperial Spain." In *Queering Iberia: Sexualities, Cultures, and Crossings from the Middle Ages to the Renaissance,* ed. Josiah Blackmore and Gregory S. Hutcheson, pp. 394–419. Durham: Duke University Press.

Phillips, Anne 1991. *Engendering Democracy.* Cambridge: Polity Press.

———. 1993. *Democracy and Difference.* University Park: Pennsylvania State University Press.

Phillips, Ruth B., and Christopher B. Steiner, eds. 1999. *Unpacking Culture: Art and Commodity in Colonial and Postcolonial Worlds.* Berkeley: University of California Press.

Poole, Deborah. 1988. "Landscapes of Power in a Cattle-Rustling Culture of Southern Andean Peru." *Dialectical Anthropology* 12: 367–398.

———. 1990. "Accommodation and Resistance in Andean Ritual Dance." *The Drama Review* 34(2): 98–126.

———. 1994. "Performance, Domination, and Identity in the *Tierras Bravas* of Chumbivilcas (Cusco)." In Poole, ed., pp. 97–132.

———. 1997. *Vision, Race, and Modernity: A Visual Economy of the Andean Image World.* Princeton: Princeton University Press.

———, ed. 1994. *Unruly Order: Violence, Power, and Cultural Identity in the High Provinces of Southern Peru.* Boulder: Westview.

Poole, Deborah, and Gerardo Rénique. 1992. *Peru: Time of Fear*. London: Latin America Bureau.

Press, Eyal. 1996. "Barbie's Betrayal: The Toy Industry's Broken Workers." *The Nation*, December 30, pp. 10–16.

Prieur, Annick. 1998. *Mema's House: On Machos, Queens, and Transvestites*. Chicago: University of Chicago Press.

Quiroz Paz Soldán, Eusebio. 1990. "Del comercio a la industria sustitoria: 1919–1955." In Neira et al., pp. 579–665.

Radcliffe, Sarah A. 1993. "'People Have to Rise Up—Like the Great Women Fighters': The State and Peasant Women in Peru." In Radcliffe and Westwood, eds., pp. 197–218.

Radcliffe, Sarah, and Sallie Westwood. 1996. *Remaking the Nation: Place, Identity, and Politics in Latin America*. New York: Routledge.

———, eds. 1993. *"Viva": Women and Popular Protest in Latin America*. London: Routledge.

Radner, Joan N., and Susan S. Lanser. 1993. "Strategies of Coding in Women's Cultures." In *Feminist Messages: Coding in Women's Folk Culture*, ed. Joan Newlon Radner, pp. 1–30. Urbana: University of Illinois Press.

Ráez Retamozo, Manuel. 1993. "Los ciclos ceremoniales y la percepción del tiempo festivo en el Valle del Colca (Arequipa)." In Romero, ed., pp. 253–298.

Ramos, Alcida. 1998. *Indigenism: Ethnic Politics in Brazil*. Madison: University of Wisconsin Press.

Rappaport, Joanne. 1990. *The Politics of Memory: Native Historical Interpretation in the Colombian Andes*. Cambridge: Cambridge University Press.

———. 1994. *Cumbe Reborn: An Andean Ethnography of History*. Chicago: The University of Chicago Press.

———. 1996. "Introduction, Ethnicity Reconfigured: Indigenous Legislators and the Colombian Constitution of 1991." *Journal of Latin American Anthropology* 1(2): 2–17.

Rasnake, Roger. 1988. *Domination and Cultural Resistance: Authority and Power among an Andean People*. Durham: Duke University Press.

Reinhard, Johan. 1996. "Peru's Ice Maidens: Unwrapping the Secrets." *National Geographic* 189, no. 6 (June): 62–81.

Remy, María. 1994. "The Indigenous Population and the Construction of Democracy in Peru." In van Cott, ed., pp. 107–130.

Rippy, J. Fred. 1959. *British Investments in Latin America, 1822–1949: A Case Study in the Operations of Private Enterprise in Retarded Regions*. Hamden, Conn.: Archon Books.

Romero, Raúl. 2001. *Debating the Past: Music, Memory, and Identity in the Andes*. New York: Oxford University Press.

———, ed. 1993. *Música, danza y máscaras en los Andes*. Lima: Pontificia Universidad Católica/Instituto Riva-Agüero.

Rosaldo, Renato. 1989. *Culture and Truth: The Remaking of Social Analysis*. Boston: Beacon.

Rosaldo, Renato, Smadar Lavie, and Kirin Narayan. 1993. "Introduction: Creativity in Anthropology." In Lavie, Narayan, and Rosaldo, eds., pp. 1–8.

Roscoe, Will. 1991. *The Zuni Man-Woman.* Albuquerque: University of New Mexico Press.

———. 1994. "How to Become a Berdache: Toward a Unified Analysis of Gender Diversity." In Herdt, ed., pp. 329–372.

Rosemblatt, Karin Alejandra. 2000. *Gendered Compromises: Political Cultures and the State in Chile, 1920–1950.* Chapel Hill: University of North Carolina Press.

Rowe, Ann Pollard. 1977. *Warp-Patterned Weaves of the Andes.* Washington, D.C.: The Textile Museum.

———, ed. 1986. *The Junius B. Bird Conference on Andean Textiles.* Washington, D.C.: The Textile Museum.

———, ed. 1998. *Costume and Identity in Highland Ecuador.* Washington, D.C.: The Textile Museum; Seattle: University of Washington Press.

Rowe, Ann Pollard, and John Cohen. 2002. *Hidden Threads of Peru: Q'ero Textiles.* Washington, D.C.: The Textile Museum/Merrell Publishers.

Rowe, William, and Vivian Schelling. 1991. *Memory and Modernity: Popular Culture in Latin America.* London and New York: Verso.

Rubin, Jeffrey. 1997. *Decentering the Regime: Ethnicity, Radicalism, and Democracy in Juchitán, Mexico.* Durham: Duke University Press.

Ruddick, Sara. 1980. "Maternal Thinking." *Feminist Studies* 6(2).

Russo, Mary. 1986. "Female Grotesques: Carnival and Theory." In de Lauretis, ed., pp. 212–229.

Sallnow, Michael. 1987. *Pilgrims of the Andes: Regional Cults in Cusco.* Washington, D.C.: Smithsonian Institution Press.

Sanday, Peggy Reeves, and Ruth Gallagher Goodenough, eds. 1990. *Beyond the Second Sex: New Directions in the Anthropology of Gender.* Philadelphia: University of Pennsylvania Press.

Sanjek, Roger. 1994. "The Enduring Inequalities of Race." In *Race,* ed. Steven Gregory and Roger Sanjek, pp. 1–17. New Brunswick, N.J.: Rutgers University Press.

———, ed. 1990. *Fieldnotes: The Makings of Anthropology.* Ithaca, N.Y.: Cornell University Press.

Santa Cruz, Nicomedes. 1995. "Peru's African Rhythms." In Starn, Degregori, and Kirk, eds., pp. 290–291.

Sassoon, Anne Showstack, ed. 1987. *Women and the State: The Shifting Boundaries of Public and Private.* London: Unwin Hyman.

Sayer, Chloë, ed. 1994. *The Mexican Day of the Dead: An Anthology.* Boston: Shambhala Redstone.

Schechner, Richard. 1988 [1977]. *Performance Theory.* Revised and expanded edition. New York and London: Routledge.

Scher, Philip W. 2003. *Carnival and the Formation of a Caribbean Transnation.* Gainesville: University Press of Florida.

Schevill, Margot B., Janet C. Berlo, and Edward Dwyer, eds. 1996. *Textile Traditions of*

Mesoamerica and the Andes: An Anthology. Austin: University of Texas Press. (Originally published New York: Garland, 1991.)

Schneider, Jane. 1978. "Peacocks and Penguins: The Political Economy of European Cloth and Colors." *American Ethnologist* 5: 413–448.

———. 1994. "In and Out of Polyester: Desire, Disdain, and Global Fiber Competitions." *Anthropology Today* 10(4): 2–10.

Schneider, Jane, and Annette B. Weiner. 1989. "Introduction." In Weiner and Schneider, eds., pp. 1–29.

Scott, Alison MacEwen. 1986. "Towards a Rethinking of Petty Commodity Production." *Social Analysis* 20: 106–115.

———. 1994. *Divisions and Solidarities: Gender, Class, and Employment in Latin America.* New York: Routledge.

Scott, James. 1990. *Domination and the Arts of Resistance: Hidden Transcripts.* New Haven: Yale University Press.

Scott, Joan, and Judith Butler, eds. 1992. *Feminists Theorize the Political.* New York: Routledge.

Seibold, Katharine. 1990. "The Last Incas: Social Change as Reflected in the Textiles of Choquecancha, Cuzco, Peru." Ph.D. diss., Anthropology, Indiana University, Bloomington.

———. 1992. "Textiles and Cosmology in Choquecancha, Peru." In *Andean Cosmologies through Time: Persistence and Emergence,* ed. Robert V. H. Dover, Katharine E. Seibold, and John H. McDowell, pp. 166–201. Bloomington: Indiana University Press.

———. 1995. "Dressing the Part: Indigenous Costume as Political and Cultural Discourse in Peru." In *Contact, Crossover, Continuity: Proceedings of the Fourth Biennial Symposium of the Textile Society of America,* pp. 319–330. Los Angeles: Textile Society of America.

Seligmann, Linda J. 2004. *Peruvian Street Lives: Culture, Power, and Economy among Market Women of Cuzco.* Urbana: University of Illinois Press.

———, ed. 2001. *Women Traders in Cross-Cultural Perspective: Mediating Identities, Marketing Wares.* Stanford: Stanford University Press.

Shippee, Robert. 1932a. "The Great Wall of Peru and Other Aerial Photographic Studies by the Shippee-Johnson Peruvian Expedition." *Geographical Review* 22: 1–29.

———. 1932b. "Lost Valleys of Peru: Results of the Shippee-Johnson Peruvian Expedition." *Geographical Review* 22: 562–581.

———. 1933. "Air Adventures in Peru." *National Geographic* 63, no. 1 (January): 81–120.

———. 1934. "A Forgotten Valley of Peru." *National Geographic* 65, no. 1 (January): 111–132. Photographs by George Johnson.

Sifuentes-Jáuregui, Ben. 2002. *Transvestism, Masculinity, and Latin American Literature: Genders Share Flesh.* New York: Palgrave.

Sikkink, Lynn. 1994. "Household, Community, and Marketplace: Women as Managers of Exchange Relations and Resources on the Southern Altiplano of Bolivia." Ph.D. diss., Anthropology, University of Minnesota, Minneapolis.

Silverblatt, Irene. 1988. "Political Memories and Colonizing Symbols: Santiago and the Mountain Gods of Colonial Peru." In *Rethinking History and Myth,* ed. Jonathan Hill, pp. 174–194. Urbana: University of Illinois Press.

Smith, Carol. 1986. "Reconstructing the Elements of Petty Commodity Production." *Social Analysis* 20: 29–46.

Spalding, Karen. 1984. *Huarochirí: An Andean Society under Inca and Spanish Rule.* Stanford: Stanford University Press.

Stacey, Judith. 1988. "Can There Be a Feminist Ethnography?" *Women's Studies International Forum* 11(1): 21–27.

Starn, Orin. 1991. "Missing the Revolution: Anthropologists and the War in Peru." *Cultural Anthropology* 6(1): 63–91.

———. 1994. "Rethinking the Politics of Anthropology: The Case of the Andes." *Current Anthropology* 35(1): 13–38.

———. 1995. "Peasants at War: Violence and Resistance in Peru's Andes." *Cultural Anthropology* 10(4): 547–580.

———. 1999. *Nightwatch: The Politics of Protest in the Andes.* Durham: Duke University Press.

Starn, Orin, Carlos Iván Degregori, and Robin Kirk, eds. 1995. *The Peru Reader: History, Culture, Politics.* Durham: Duke University Press.

Starrett, Gregory. 1995. "The Political Economy of Religious Commodities in Cairo." *American Anthropologist* 97(1): 51–68.

Stastny, Francisco. 1984. *Las artes populares del Perú.* Lima: Edubanco.

———. 1987. "The Art of the Colca Valley." In de Romaña, Blassi, and Blassi, pp. 160–181.

Stavenhagen, Rodolfo. 1996. *Ethnic Conflicts and the Nation-State.* New York: St. Martin's Press.

Stegner, Wallace. 1992. *Where the Bluebird Sings to the Lemonade Springs: Living and Writing in the West.* New York: Penguin.

Steiner, Christopher B. 1994. *African Art in Transit.* Cambridge: Cambridge University Press.

Stephen, Lynn. 1991. *Zapotec Women.* Austin: University of Texas Press.

———. 1997. *Women and Social Movements in Latin America: Power from Below.* Austin: University of Texas Press.

Stephen, Lynn, and George A. Collier. 1997. "Reconfiguring Ethnicity, Identity, and Citizenship in the Wake of the Zapatista Rebellion." *Journal of Latin American Anthropology* 3(1): 2–13.

Stephenson, Marcia. 1999. *Gender and Modernity in Andean Bolivia.* Austin: University of Texas Press.

Stern, Peter A. 1995. *Sendero Luminoso: An Annotated Bibliography of the Shining Path Guerrilla Movement.* Albuquerque: SALALM Secretariat.

Stern, Steve. 1998. "Introduction: Beyond Enigma: An Agenda for Interpreting Shining Path and Peru, 1980–1995." In Stern, ed., pp. 1–12.

———, ed. 1987. *Resistance, Rebellion, and Consciousness in the Andean Peasant World, 18th to 20th Centuries.* Madison: University of Wisconsin Press.

———, ed. 1998. *Shining and Other Paths: War and Society in Peru, 1980–1995.* Durham: Duke University Press.

Stewart, Susan. 1984. *On Longing: Narratives of the Miniature, the Gigantic, the Souvenir, the Collection.* Baltimore: Johns Hopkins University Press.

Stoner, Bradley. 1989. "Health Care Delivery and Health Resource Utilization in a Highland Andean Community of Southern Peru." Ph.D. diss., Anthropology, Indiana University, Bloomington.

Strathern, Marilyn. 1987. "An Awkward Relationship: The Case of Feminism and Anthropology." *Signs* 12(2): 276–292.

———. 1988. *The Gender of the Gift.* Berkeley: University of California Press.

Swen, Herman. 1986. "Tuteños, chacras, alpacas y macones: La comunidad de Tuti y el Proyecto de Majes en el surandino del Perú." Master's thesis, Anthropology, University of the Netherlands.

Szeminski, Jan. 1987. "Why Kill the Spaniard? New Perspectives on Andean Revolutionary Ideology in the 18th Century." In Stern, ed., pp. 166–192.

Taylor, Diana. 1997. *Disappearing Acts: Spectacles of Gender and Nationalism in Argentina's "Dirty War."* Durham: Duke University Press.

Taylor, Diana, and Juan Villegas, eds. 1994. *Negotiating Performance: Gender, Sexuality, and Theatricality in Latin/o America.* Durham: Duke University Press.

Thomas, Nicholas. 1991. *Entangled Objects: Exchange, Material Culture, and Colonialism in the Pacific.* Cambridge: Harvard University Press.

Thorp, Rosemary, and Geoffrey Bertram. 1978. *Peru 1890–1977: Growth and Policy in an Open Economy.* London: Macmillan.

Tierney, John. 1994. "Color Blind." *New York Times Magazine,* September 18, pp. 32–34.

Tolen, Rebecca. 1995. "Wool and Synthetics: Dress, Race, and History in Chimborazo, Highland Ecuador." Ph.D. diss., Anthropology, University of Chicago.

Tord, Luis Enrique. 1983. *Templos coloniales del Colca-Arequipa.* Lima: L. E. Tord/Industrial Atlas.

Treacy, John. 1989. "The Fields of Coporaque: Agricultural Terracing and Water Management in the Colca Valley, Arequipa, Peru." Ph.D. diss., Geography, University of Wisconsin-Madison.

———. 1994a. *Las chacras de Coporaque: Andenería y riego en el Valle del Colca.* Ed. Maria A. Benavides, Blenda Femenías, and William M. Denevan. Lima: Instituto de Estudios Peruanos.

———. 1994b. "Teaching Water: Hydraulic Management and Terracing in Coporaque, the Colca Valley, Peru." In Mitchell and Guillet, eds., pp. 99–114.

Tulchin, Joseph S., and Gary Bland. 1994. *Peru in Crisis: Dictatorship or Democracy?* Woodrow Wilson Center Current Studies on Latin America. Boulder and London: Lynne Reiner.

Turino, Thomas. 1993. *Moving Away from Silence: Music of the Peruvian Altiplano and the Experience of Urban Migration.* Chicago: University of Chicago Press.

Turner, Terence. 1995. "An Indigenous People's Struggle for Socially Equitable and Ecologically Sustainable Production." *Journal of Latin American Anthropology* 1(1): 98–121.

Turner, Victor. 1974. *Dramas, Fields, and Metaphors: Symbolic Action in Human Society.* Ithaca: Cornell University Press.

Ugarteche, Oscar. 1993. *Historia, sexo y cultura en el Perú.* [Lima]: Movimiento Homosexual de Lima.

———. 1997. *India bonita, o, Del amor y otras artes: Ensayos de cultura gay en el Perú.* Lima: Movimiento Homosexual de Lima.

———. 2002. "Cleaning Up after Fujimori: Peruvian Panel Probes 'Economic Crimes' Linked to Privatization. An Interview." *NACLA Report on the Americas* 35, no. 4 (January/February): 42–43.

Ulfe, María Eugenia. 2001. "Variedades del carnaval en los Andes: Ayacucho, Apurímac y Huancavelica." In Cánepa, ed., pp. 399–436.

Urban, Greg, and Joel Sherzer. 1991. "Introduction: Indians, Nation-States, and Culture." In Urban and Sherzer, eds., pp. 1–18.

———, eds. 1991. *Nation-States and Indians in Latin America.* Austin: University of Texas Press.

Urton, Gary. 1981. *At the Crossroads of the Earth and the Sky: An Andean Cosmology.* Austin: University of Texas Press.

Valderrama, Ricardo, and Carmen Escalante. 1988. *Del Tata Mallku a la Mama Pacha: Riego, sociedad y ritos en los Andes peruanos.* Lima: DESCO.

———. 1997. *La doncella sacrificada: Mitos del Valle del Colca.* Arequipa: Universidad Nacional de San Agustín/Instituto Francés de Estudios Andinos.

van Cott, Donna, ed. 1994. *Indigenous Peoples and Democracy in Latin America.* New York: St. Martin's.

van den Berghe, Pierre, and George Primov. 1977. *Inequality in the Peruvian Andes: Class and Ethnicity in Cuzco.* Columbia: University of Missouri Press.

Van Maanen, John, ed. 1995. *Representation in Ethnography.* Thousand Oaks, Calif.: Sage.

Vargas, Virginia. 1989. *El aporte de la rebeldía de las mujeres.* Lima: Centro de la Mujer Peruana Flora Tristán.

———. 1992. "Women: Tragic Encounters with the Left." *NACLA Report on the Americas* 25, no. 5 (May): 30–34.

———. 1995. "Women's Movements in Peru: Rebellion into Action." In *Subversive Women: Women's Movements in Africa, Asia, Latin America and the Caribbean,* ed. Saskia Wieringa, pp. 73–100. London: Zed.

Vargas Llosa, Mario. 1987. "El Valle de las Maravillas/The Valley of Marvels." In de Romaña, Blassi, and Blassi, pp. 23–29.

Velasco, Sherry. 2000. *The Lieutenant Nun: Transgenderism, Lesbian Desire, and Catalina de Erauso.* Austin: University of Texas Press.

Villar Márquez, Eliana. 1994. *Por mérito propio: Mujer y política.* Lima: Centro de la Mujer Peruana Flora Tristán.

Visweswaran, Kamala. 1994. *Fictions of Feminist Ethnography.* Minneapolis: University of Minnesota Press.

Warren, Kay B. 1998a. *Indigenous Movements and Their Critics: Pan-Maya Activism in Guatemala.* Princeton: Princeton University Press.

———. 1998b. "Indigenous Movements as a Challenge to the Unified Social Movement Paradigm for Guatemala." In Alvarez, Dagnino, and Escobar, eds., pp. 165–195.

Warren, Kay B., and Jean E. Jackson, eds. 2002. *Indigenous Movements, Self-Representation, and the State in Latin America.* Austin: University of Texas Press.

Webber, Ellen Robinson. 1988. "Alfalfa and Cattle in Achoma." In Denevan, ed., pp. 91–111.

———. 1993. "Cows in the Colca: Household Cattle Raising in Achoma, Peru." Master's thesis, Geography, University of Wisconsin-Madison.

Weiner, Annette B. 1992. *Inalienable Possessions: The Paradox of Keeping-While-Giving.* Berkeley: University of California Press.

Weiner, Annette B., and Jane Schneider, eds. 1989. *Cloth and Human Experience.* Washington, D.C.: Smithsonian Institution Press/Wenner-Gren Foundation.

Weismantel, Mary. 1988. *Food, Gender, and Poverty in the Ecuadorian Andes.* Philadelphia: University of Pennsylvania Press.

———. 2001. *Cholas and Pishtacos: Stories of Race and Sex in the Andes.* Chicago: University of Chicago Press.

Wernke, Steven A. 2002. "Eco-Logistical Practice over the Longue Durée: Intermediate Elites and Hybrid Community Structures in the Colca Valley, Peru." Paper presented at the 67th Annual Meeting of the Society for American Archaeology, Denver.

———. 2003. "An Archaeo-History of Andean Community and Landscape: The Late Prehispanic and Early Colonial Colca Valley, Peru." Ph.D. diss., Anthropology, University of Wisconsin-Madison.

Weston, Kath. 1993a. "Do Clothes Make the Woman?: Gender, Performance Theory, and Lesbian Eroticism." *Genders* 17: 1–21.

———. 1993b. "Lesbian/Gay Studies in the House of Anthropology." *Annual Review of Anthropology* 22: 339–367.

Westwood, Sallie, and Sarah A. Radcliffe. 1993. "Gender, Racism, and the Politics of Identities in Latin America." In Radcliffe and Westwood, eds., pp. 1–29.

Wilk, Richard R., and Robert McC. Netting. 1984. *Households: Comparative and Historical Studies of the Domestic Group.* Berkeley: University of California Press.

Wilson, Carter. 1995. *Hidden in the Blood: A Personal Investigation of AIDS in the Yucatan.* New York: Columbia University Press.

Wolf, Diane L. 1995. "Situating Feminist Dilemmas in Fieldwork." In Wolf, ed., pp. 1–55.

———, ed. 1995. *Feminist Dilemmas in Fieldwork.* Boulder: Westview.

Wolf, Margery. 1992. *A Thrice-Told Tale: Feminism, Postmodernism, and Ethnographic Responsibility.* Stanford: Stanford University Press.

Yanagisako, Sylvia. 1979. "Family and Household: The Analysis of Domestic Groups." *Annual Review of Anthropology:* 161–205.

Yashar, Deborah. 1998. "Contesting Citizenship: Indigenous Movements and Democracy in Latin America." *Comparative Politics* 31: 23–42.

Youngers, Coletta, and Jo-Marie Burt. 2000. "Defending Rights in a Hostile Environment." *NACLA Report on the Americas* 34, no. 1 (July–August): 43–46, 53.

Yuval-Davis, Nira, and Pnina Werbner, eds. 1999. *Women, Citizenship and Difference.* London: Zed; distributed in U.S. by St. Martin's Press.

Zamosc, Leon. 1994. "Agrarian Protest and the Indian Movement in the Ecuadorian Highlands." *Latin American Research Review* 29(3): 37–68.

Zavella, Patricia. 1997. "Feminist Insider Dilemmas." In Lamphere, Ragoné, and Zavella, eds., pp. 42–61.

Zayas y Sotomayor, María de. 1983. *Parte segunda del Sarao y entretenimiento honesto [Desengaños amorosos].* Ed. Alicia Yllera. Madrid: Cátedra.

Zorn, Elayne. 1982. "Braiding in the Macusani Area of Peru." *Textile Museum Journal* 19–20: 41–54.

———. 1995. "(Re-)fashioning Identity: Late Twentieth-Century Transformations of Dress and Society in Bolivia." In *Contact, Crossover, Continuity: Proceedings of the Fourth Biennial Symposium of the Textile Society of America,* pp. 343–354. Los Angeles: Textile Society of America.

———. 1997a. "Coca, Cash, and Cloth in Highland Bolivia: The Chapare and Transformations in a 'Traditional' Andean Textile Economy." In *Coca, Cocaine, and the Bolivian Reality,* ed. Madeline Barbara Lèons and Harry Sanabria, pp. 71–98. Albany: State University of New York Press.

———. 1997b. "Marketing Diversity: Global Transformations in Cloth and Identity in Highland Peru and Bolivia." Ph.D. diss., Anthropology, Cornell University, Ithaca.

———. 2003. "'We Are Compadres with New York': Performing Transnational Kinship in Peru and the U.S." Manuscript.

———. 2004. *Weaving a Future: Tourism, Cloth, and Culture on an Andean Island.* Iowa City: University of Iowa Press.

Index

Boldface page numbers indicate pages on which illustrations appear.

Abu-Lughod, Lila, 28, 73, 75, 309n.21, 310n.23
activism, 89, 100, 218–219, 223–226, 238–240, 317n.3, 318n.6
Adriazola, Luisa, 39, 178–179, 314n.18
aesthetics, 22, 66–67, 71, 105, 108, 115, 125–140, 145, 264, 267–270, 289–291
agriculture, 3, 15, 38–43, **42**, 56, 69–70, 79, 82, **99**, 123, 129, 222–223, 244, 250, 261, 263, 291, 305n.2, 308nn.3, 4, 318n.11; *chaquitaclla,* 40; fields, 36–37, 41, 43–45, 97, 206, 222, 230, 242, 252; irrigation, 69–70, 92–93, 309n.20
Alfaro, Gerardo, 134, 208
All Saints' Day and All Souls' Day, 159, 270, 271, 274–280, 296–297
ambiguity, 16, 17–24, 76, 186, 199–202, 204–205, 214, 229, 236
American Museum of Natural History, 30, 313n.1
ancestors, 152, 156–157, 167, 177, 180–182
Andes, 64, 83–84, 87–89, 97, 99, 160, 188, 190, 193, 194, 206, 208, 247, 260, 309nn.15, 18, 316n.15; southern, 79, 80
animals: cattle, 39, 58, 84, 109, 305n.3, 308n.1; donkey, 36; fish, 131, 138; guinea pig, 58–59, 131, 308n.1; horse, 36; monkey, 131; as motifs, 131, 132, 135, 136, 312nn.10, 11; sheep, 53, 159–160, 164, 171, 176, 308n.1, 313n.14; *vizcacha,* 66, 131, 312n.11
apprenticeship, 30, 134, 243, 248, 254, 256, 258–261, 266, 320nn.7, 9, 10
architecture, **56,** 132, 139, 147–150, 253, 309n.18, 312n.11, 313n.2
Arequipa (city), 17, 33, 46, 49–50, 79–81, 99, 105, 124, 135, 147, 150, 151, 173, 267, 270, 274–275, 283, 284, 305nn.1, 3, 4, 311n.12; central market, 1, 256, 312n.4; cultural production, 186, 288, 312n.5, 321n.10; history, 81–85, 161, 169–179, 307n.16; industry, 11, 83–85, 139, 172, 290, 308n.4, 322n.17; migrants, 1–13, 47–48, 95, 116–118, 120–121, 134, 146, 165, 190, 194, 252, 284, 286–289, 312n.3; race and ethnicity, 82–83, 85, 89, 102, 146, 174–179; textile sales, 270, 282, 287, 289–290; tourism, 282, 286–289, 322n.16; travel and transportation, 38, 48, 61–65, 70, 78, 148, 163, 172, 241; White City (Ciudad Blanca), 8, 81, 85, 101; workshops, 118, 134, 173, 256, 263, 289, 312n.4
Arequipa (department and provinces), 9, 68, 80–84, 100, 151, 170, 227, 232, 233, 250, 284, 305n.3, 310nn.1, 5
Arguedas, José María, 162, 317n.16
art and artists, 3, 16, 17, 22, 23, 28–

29, 33, 103, 112, 125–140, 145–146, 152, 155–156, 258, 261, 271, 306n.11, 312n.10, 313n.12, 321n.4; anonymity, 155, 313n.5; drawing, 130–136, 145, 254, 256–257, 260, 262–265, 268, 273; gendered attitudes, 134–135, 245–246, 254–255, 258, 261–266, 312n.11; painting, 17, 130, 132–133, 312n.10; signature, 136; stone carving, 132
artisans, 13–14, 20, 29, 30, 49, 50, 54, 57, 61–63, 101, 103–106, 112, 115, 121–140, 154–158, 241–266, 267–273, 281–285, 289–296, 313nn.12, 13, 320nn.4, 5, 6, 9, 321n.8

bag (*ch'uspa*), 110, 292, **293**
beauty, 13, 14, 18–20, 23, 67–68, 78, 94, 115, 126, 151, 180. *See also* aesthetics
belt (*chumpi, faja*), **96,** 109–110, **293**
Belaúnde Terry, Fernando, 70
Benjamin, Walter, 32
Bentley, G. Carter, 92
Bernal, Eufemia, 256
Bernal Málaga, Alfredo, 194, 201, 203–206, 209, 315nn.1, 3, 316n.15
Bernal Suni, Felícitas, 119, 128, 143, 227, 255, 272
Bernal Suni, Hilario, 62, 134, 256
Bernal Suni, Susana, 30, 35, 51, 62–63, 103–108, **104,** 122, 125, 128, 134–135, 140, 141, 156–157, 241–245, 251–253, 255–258, 260, 266, 281–282, 291, 320n.9
Bernal Terán, Agripina, 85, 196, 200, 274–277, **276,** 316n.12
Bernal Terán, Candelaria, 30, 52–60, **53,** 141–142, **142,** 192
Bernal Terán, Delia, 192, 213–214
Bernal Terán, Nilda, 30, 31, 35, 52–60, 128–130, 192, 195, 263, 267–270, 273, **273,** 275, 277, 282, 285, 289–291, 304n.14, 319n.22
bird, 131, 132, 137, 138, 273, 312n.11; condor, 271, 287, 312n.10; hummingbird, 21, 68, **111,** 131, 132, **133**
blouse (*camisa*), 2, 3, 105, 109, 123, 124, 224, 233, 281, 289
body, 80, 87, 90, 92, 125, 126, 130, 144–146, 187, 198, 207–210, 229, 233–235, 254, 261–264, 293, 295, 317n.17; body politic, 219–222, 238, 318n.4; clothing the body, 18–19, 24–28, 33, 74, 94–100, 103–146, 152–153, 156–157, 174–179, 183, 220, 230, 235–239; embodiment, 34, 109, 119, 147–184, 187, 192, 194, 208–212, 279–280, 315n.2
Bolivia, 80, 82, 86, 88, 89, 95, 97, 99, 163, 178, 190, 315nn.4, 5, 316n.13, 321nn.4, 6, 7, 9; La Paz, 81, 260
bordados, 2–3, 13–15, 17–24, 28–29, 33–36, 41, 59, 94–98, 100, 118, 143, 298–304, 307n.22, 312n.10, 313n.12; characteristics, 103–115; children's, 54; history, 152–158, 162–174, 180–184; production, 243–252, 307n.14, 312n.4, 320n.5; sale and exchange, 267–271, 289–295; tailoring, 263–264. *See also* aesthetics; embroidery; *polleras*
borders, 16, 17–33, 78–102, 141, 143, 146, 187, 207, 236, 310n.2
Bourdieu, Pierre, 19, 20, 27, 290, 306n.12
British: influence on Peru, 82, 101, 168; textiles, 83, 162, 167–171, 314n.13
Butler, Judith, 26, 27, 307n.21

Cabana, Alejandro, 165, 166
Cabana, Lucrecia, 165
Cabanaconde, 57, 63, 70, 79, 90, 92–93, 109, 112, 120–123, 125, 130, 131, 132, 135–137, 155, 162, 166–167, 224, 230, 232, 255, 256, 273, 276, 284, 290, 309n.16, 310n.1, 313n.12, 314n.16, 316n.12, 317n.16, 319n.19
Cabanas ethnic polity, 79, 202

Cáceres, Alejandro, 137, 166
Cáceres, Eudumila, 150–151, 161, 163, 174, 175, 177, 179, 180, 183–184, 314n.19
Cáceres, Luis, 8, 10, 98
Cáceres family of merchants, 168–169, 177
cactus, 38, 68, 131; prickly pear, 2–3, **3**, 9, 11, 13, 68, 124, 200, 309n.17
Cacya, Wenceslao, 156, 165
Callalli, 65, 112, 120, 161, 172, 232, 289, 290
camelids, 312n.10; alpaca, 3, 11, 20, 33, 43, 63, 65, 71, 81, 84, 98, 100, 109, 139, 147, 159, 164–167, 171, 173, 272–274, 283–284, 289–291, 295, 308n.1, 321n.11, 322n.17; llama, 3, 63, 71, 147, **149**, 151, 176, 308n.1; vicuña, 66, 131, 271, 287
capital, 83–84, 154, 266; cultural, 20, 211; social, 193, 211; symbolic, 20, 106, 180
capitalism, 15, 34, 146, 167–174, 180, 244, 246, 265–266, 270, 272, 293–296, 319n.2
Carnival, 33, 103–104, 141, 190–196, 200–202, 205–206, 208–210, 285, 315nn.5, 7, 9, 316n.15. *See also* play
carrying cloth (*lliklla*), 8, **53**, 110, **160**, **197**, 199–200, 215, 290
Casaperalta, Viviana, 165–166, 173, 260
Catholic church, 43, 44, 53, 68, 90, 93, 189, 192, 206, 224, 226, 271, 272, 274, 278–280, 296, 312n.11, 321nn.5, 11
Caylloma (town), 91, 97, 170, 244, 263
Caylloma Province, 2–3, 9, 11, 13, 24, 37, 45–51, 61, 66–71, 76, 77, 100–102, 105–108, 112, 116–124, 131–132, 144–146, 217–224, 227–232, 238–239, 244–248, 250, 255, 261, 265–268, 270–271, 280–284, 287–297, 305n.3, 307n.15, 310nn.1, 4, 317n.3, 320n.5; history, 20, 79–84, 90–91, 137, 147–184, 189, 202–207, 212, 214, 305n.2, 308n.6
Cayo, Rodolfo, 130, 134, 137, 256
Cayo, Rosalvina, 134, 157, 167, 174
Cayo, Sergio, 134
Chambers, Sarah, 82, 307n.16
Checca, Santos, 259
children, 13, 15, 39, 43, 47, 112, 119–121, 143, 157, 162–165, 200, 215–217, 222–224, 238, 241–244, 251–253, 262–263, 308n.2, 309n.10, 313n.6, 320n.8
Chile, 8, 31, 48, 80, 81, 124, 139, 190, 278, 316n.10
Chivay, 2, 13–14, 33, 44–45, 49–50, 60, 68, 79, 90, 93, 97, 112, 116–117, 120, 128, 135–138, 141–142, 183–184, 203, 255, 275, 286, 301, 310n.1, 312n.10, 313n.9, 315n.8; church, 61, 147–148, 183, **251**, 313n.2; history, 147–151, **149**, 161–173, 175, 177, 180, 194; market, **3**, 11, 14, 19, 49, 50, 61–63, 78, 96, 96 fig. 9, 123, 130, 134, 137, 148, 156, 157, 165, 166, 167, 241–245, **242**, 249–253, **251**, 267–271, 280–288, 291, 307n.22, 322n.13; politics, 34, 215–219, 223, 228, 229, 231–232; rituals and festivals, 43, 194; tourism, 268, 271, 292–293; travel, 36, 38, 47, 49, 60–66, 70–71, 81, 280
Chivay Chino, 118, 173, 256, 263, 289, 312n.4
Choquehuanca, Juan de Dios, **257**
citizenship and civil rights, 12–13, 70, 100, 219, 220, 224, 226, 227–230, 233–235, 309n.21, 311n.10, 319n.16
class, 10, 12, 19, 22, 80, 84, 87, 89, 91–93, 95, 101, 109, 124, 150, 161–162, 167–184, 191, 204, 228–230, 235–237, 239, 248, 294, 312n.5, 317n.2
climate, 3, 38, 40, 60–61, 65–71, 124–125, 222–223, 305n.4, 309n.18
cloth, 79, 141–142, 243, 244, 259, 260, 321n.2; *bayeta* and *jerga*, 115, 124, 158–164, 171, 176, 179, 222, 243–244,

272, 283, 290, 291, 313nn.7, 8; history in Caylloma, 81, 90–91, 152–154, 158–162, 170–171, 177, 179; silk, 161; synthetic, 115, 158, 243, 272–274, 290–291; *tela,* 107, 158, 161–162, 164, 171, 179. *See also* cotton

clothes, 91–93, 158, 250–251, 307n.19, 312n.5; children's, 54, **120, 142,** 159, **159, 160,** 176, 292, **293**; daily use, 42, 49, 117–124, 187, 190, 199, 200, 207, 272; *de pollera* and *de vestido* styles, 94–97, 107, 122, 124, 142–143, 230, 233, 235–240; display, 20, 55, **96,** 129, 250–251, 264, 271, 283, 289, 292–293, **293**; ethnic, 79–80, 90, 94–100, 125, 150–153, 161–162, 218–221, 230, 233–239, 294–295; female, 21, 28–29, 33–34, 98, 103–125, 127–130, 140–146, 185, 187, 199–201, 207–208, 214, 218–224, 230, 233–240, 261, 263–264, 267, 276, 292–293; festival and ritual, 21, 33–34, 98, 112, 116–121, 185–214, 215–240, 267–280, 321nn.3, 7; male, 21, 28–29, 33, 80, 94, 98–100, 148, 151, 158–161, 163–164, 167, 176, 185–187, 195–202, 207–210, 218, 220, 274, 293, 314n.15; political use, 34, 90, 98–102, 207, 215–240; "Western," 35, 42, 54, 55, 64, 92, 95, 109, 116–118, 121, 126–127, 138–144, 148, 150–151, 161–162, 165, 171–179, 181–184, 216–218, 224, 230, 235–240, 292

Cobo, Bernabé, 203

coca, 91, 163

Colca River, 36–38, 44, 65, 69–70, 84, 147, 172, 310n.1

Colca Valley, 2, 18, 36–37, **41,** 44, 46–51, **53,** 57, 61–63, 68–71, 79, 84, 90–94, 106, 112, 130, 135–137, 161, 189–192, 199, 202–204, 245–246, 249, 265, 310n.1, 311nn.5, 11, 315n.5, 316n.14, 322n.15; festivals and rituals, 267, 270–280, 288, 315n.5; history, 150, 163–164, 167–175, 180, 305n.3; Inkas, 79, 85, 316n.11; political economy, 46, 48, 69–71, 172, 180, 310n.4; tourism, 270–271, 278–280, 286–295, 322nn.14, 16

Collaguas: ethnic polity, 79, 94, 202–203; Province, 83

Colloredo-Mansfeld, Rudi, 294, 307n.14

color, 21, 66, 98–99, 105, 115, 127–138, 280–281, 309n.17, 321nn.2, 5, 7, 17, 19; black, 34, 122, 267–280, **276,** 289–291, 296–297, 321nn.5, 7; green, 66–71, 127–130, 145, 272–274, 289, 312nn.8, 9; white, 121, 161, 272–274, 279–280, 283, 321n.5, 322n.17

commerce, 1–8, **3, 11,** 13, 15, 17, 34, 48, 61–63, 95, **96,** 103–105, 115, 124, 129, 136–137, 147–148, **149,** 154, 162–175, 241–245, **242,** 249–254, 263, 267–297, **293,** 320nn.1, 4, 5, 321n.4, 322nn.13, 18, 19

community, 153, 155, 156, 167, 169–170, 174–179, 182, 189–193, 195, 198–199, 205, 209, 211–212, 216, 220–224, 226–232, 235–240, 248, 249, 252, 264, 277–278, 318n.5; dress and, 2, 80, 94–100, 112, 117–118, 122–125, 126, 136, 153, 174–179, 220–224, 235–240, 264; of practice, 19, 106, 130, 144; rural settlements, 2–3, 44, 82, 169–170, 189, 193, 205, 310n.1, 318nn.5, 13; social and affective bonds, 22, 33, 37, 43, 74–77, 117–118, 122–125, 146, 167; speech community, 31–32

Condo, Luis, 205–206

Condorhuilca, Epifanio, 30, 52–60, 69, 275, 277–278, 288

Condori, Felipe, 255, 259, 260

Condori, Modesta, 284–285

Condori Valera, Juan, 30, 52–60, **120,** 123, 129, 263, 267–268, 273, 282, 290

Coporaque, 17, 35–47, **37, 53,** 63, 91, 123, 128, 135, 203, 222, 224, 272, 282–283, 286, 288, 308n.23, 309nn.13, 16, 314nn.16, 17, 316n.12; artisans, 123, 128, 135, 242, 244, 252, 253, 255, 261, 267; daily life, 35–47, 55–60; festivals and rituals, 103, 189–197, 205–207, 213, 274–278, 315n.15, 321n.11; gendered politics, 216–217, 219, 227, 319n.22; kinship, 52–55, 178
cost, 9, 11, 18, 20, 105, 108–109, 112, 115, 123–124, 136, 140, 145, 148, 161, 171, 242–243, 249, 260–262, 266, 281–285, 291–293, 322n.19
cotton, 83, 161–162, 314n.13
crafts, 12–13, 22, 61–62, 84, 258, 260, 283, 286–295; awards, 130
creativity, 16–18, 21–24, 28, 74, 115, 130–140, 145, 155, 166–167, 180–183, 261
culture, 16, 86, 187, 195, 201–202, 207, 209, 213, 306n.11; cloth compared to, 24–29; public, 219–224
Cusco, 63, 65, 81, 97, 99, 101, 163, 170, 232, 288, 289, 308n.10, 311n.8, 312nn.5, 9, 314nn.14, 16, 315n.9, 318nn.10, 12, 319n.15, 321nn.6, 9, 322n.16
custom, 33, 94, 125, 127, 144, 152–158, 171–172, 177, 179–184, 206, 316n.10
Cutipa, Melitón, 283
Cutipa Carcasi, Flora, 13, 29, 52, 116–118, 177, 309n.11

daily life, 16–17, 22, 27, 40–42, 46, 58, 94, 108, 109, 117, 152, 186–187, 190, 202, 206, 211, 222–223, 237, 239, 291
dance, 19, 33, 44, 51, 54, 98, 116–118, 121, 125, 140–141, 144, 146, 185–214, **186, 197,** 288–289, 292, 312nn.3, 5, 314n.1, 316n.15
Davis, Natalie Zemon, 185, 193, 202, 209
death, 16, 47–48, 85, 117–118, 122, 144, 152, 189, 206, 209, 212, 270–280, 296–297, 312n.6, 317n.2
de Certeau, Michel, 27, 45, 76–77
de la Cadena, Marisol, 86, 314n.14
design, 33, 34, 97–99, 104–108, 112–115, 127–140, 154–155, 244, 254, 256, 260–265, 268, 272–274, 280, 290–292; designs, embroidered, 2, 130–132, **133,** 135–138, 166–167, 172, 254; designs, woven, 132, **133**
development, 12, 15, 287, 291; urban, 1, 10–11, 81, 84–85, 147–150
discourses, 30–31, 33, 152–154, 156, 175, 180–182, 188, 202, 218–219, 222–224, 229–230
dolls, 285, 292–295, **293**

ecology, 33, 48, 80, 83, 287; cultural, 88, 309n.15; desert, 66–71
economic value, 10, 15–16, 21, 155, 247–248, 266, 295, 321n.2
economy: ethnic, 34, 154; informal sector, 15; symbolic. *See also* symbols, symbolic economy
Ecuador, 86, 88, 89, 95, 307n.14
education, 97, 119–121, 176–177, 179, 199, 226, 229, 237, 241–242, 252, 256, 262, 309n.14, 320n.8
emblems, 10, 16–24, 139, 167, 171, 178–179
embroidery, 15, 34, 57, 58, 62, 95, 105, 112, 128, 143, 145, 241–266, **242, 257,** 267–268, 271, 273, 282–285, 290, 295, 313n.12, 320n.5, 321n.8; figurative usage, 23–24, 130–140; history, 137–138, 152–158, 162–167, 170–174, 179–184
emotion, 33, 35–38, 51, 59–60, 64, 71–77, 80, 89, 123–125, 151–154, 156, 174, 181–183, 249, 274–280, 296–297
ethnicity, 16, 19, 21, 33, 34, 80, 101, 109,

124, 127, 152–153, 162, 167–184, 187–189, 198, 202–204, 208, 212–213, 218–219, 221, 227–240, 272, 280–296, 311nn.6, 10; categories, 79, 85–91, 294–295, 311nn.7, 9; Cayllomino, 11–13, 17–18, 80, 89–100, 144–146, 185–188, 192, 199, 202, 210–212, 221, 226, 228–230, 238–239, 264, 294–295; *criollo,* 151, 174–179, 182
ethnography, 18, 24, 29–32, 34, 36, 49, 71–76, 108, 143, 213, 309n.21, 310nn.23, 24; feminist, 33, 49, 73–75
ethnographer, roles of, 29, 33, 46–47, 49–52, 71–77, 140–144, 146, 153–154, 181–184, 187, 198, 211–213, 241–245, 267–268, 286, 295–297
Europe, 79, 83, 84, 92, 110, 167, 176, 209–210, 271, 272, 274, 321nn.2, 5
exchange, 13, 34, 109, 154, 161, 163–174, 180, 244–250, 254, 262–266, 267–297, 320nn.1, 2, 5, 9, 321nn.13, 18

fashion, 15, 25, 33, 57, 105, 106, 108, 115, 126–130, 137, 143, 157, 158, 161–162, 176–177, 179, 250, 262–264, 270–280, 289–293, 307n.19, 312n.8
father, 31, 155, 157, 162, 165–166, 175–179, 215–219, 246, 252, 256, 258–259
Femenías, Blenda, 80, 83, 110, **142,** 167, 307n.14, 310n.22, 311n.2, 313nn.1, 15, 314nn.11, 18, 318n.12, 319n.21
Femenias, Ramona, 54
feminism, 49, 73–74, 211, 220, 317nn.2, 3
Feria, Eufemia, 121
festival, 17, 19, 33–34, 42, 51, 94, 98, 103–104, 108, 109, 112, 119–120, 124, 144, 146, 172, 174, 185–214, 252, 266, 268, 281, 286, 288, 290, 315nn.1, 3; sponsor, 54, 123, 191–193, 195, 196, 199, 211, 213–214, 308n.12, 315n.4
fieldwork, 2–3, 30, 36–44, 46, 49–60, 71–77, 108, 116–118, 147–154, 196, 212, 241–245, 261, 308n.7, 315n.5; dressing for, 35–36, 41–42, 104–108, 140–144, **142,** 187, 190, 196, 198, 200, 210–212, 311n.15
flowers, 21, 131, 132, **133,** 138, 200, 273–275
folklore, 23, 116–118, 120, 130, 185–186, 189, 199, 203, 207, 208, 212–214, 270, 288–289, 294–296, 312n.5
food, 1–3, 11, 40, 43, 51, 56, 58–60, 62, 124, 164, 170, 173, 193, 194, 196, 198, 199, 211, 222–223, 226, 250–251, 253, 277, 282, 284
friendship, 32, 46–47, 51, 72, 77, 274–278
Fujimori, Alberto, 9, 12–13, 100, 232, 306n.7, 311n.11, 319n.22

Garber, Marjorie, 25–26, 315n.2
García Pérez, Alan, 12, 84, 318n.9
garments: female, 35–36, 41–42, 61, 94–98, 104–118, 123, 126, 140, 145, 150, 156, 160, 245–250, 253–258, 263, 267–268, 271–273, 276–277, 281–286, 290–294, 320n.5; male, 98–100, 121, 147–151, 158–161, **159,** 163, 164, 176, 198–201, 274, 312n.10; Spanish, 109–110
Gatens, Moira, 220–221
gay activism, 188, 207, 317n.18
Gelles, Paul, 70, 90, 92–93, 305n.2, 308nn.3, 6, 10, 309nn.15, 17, 18, 20, 317n.16
gender, 16–18, 21, 73–74, 79, 137, 142–145, 186–204, 207–214, 244–248, 253–255, 258, 261–266, 300–301, 307n.20, 315n.2, 317n.17; and culture, 24; ethnic qualities, 80, 94–100, 145–146, 152–153, 161–162, 186–188, 198–199, 202–204, 208–209, 212–214, 219–222, 233–239, 292–295, 299; exchange and, 269–270, 276, 279–285, 292–295, 320n.1; historical importance

in Caylloma, 152–153, 155–156, 167–168, 170–183, 189, 202–209, 212–214; theory, 26–27
generation, 121, 137, 150, 152–153, 157, 162–166, 170, 176, 178, 181, 194–195, 203–204, 213–214, 255–258, 265
globalization, 20, 33, 48, 83–84, 93, 127, 138–140, 146, 154, 161, 167, 180, 183, 227, 231–232, 236, 239, 287, 321n.4
Good Friday, 268, 270, 271, 274, 278–280
Guillet, David, 79, 308nn.3, 10, 309nn.13, 20, 310n.4, 311n.11

Harrison, Faye, 85, 93, 311n.6
hat: cap (*ch'ullu*), 98–100; embroidered, **3**, 112, **114**, 119, 131, 135–136, **231**, 267, 281, 283, 284, 292; *montera, sombrero,* 2, 3, 19, **42**, **53**, 54, **96**, 98–100, 109–110, 112, 119, **120**, 126, 130, 134, 141, **142**, 144, 148, **149**, 151, 157, **159**, **160**, 162–166, 174, 176, 180, **186**, 200, 201, **216**, 223–224, **225**, 233, **234**, **242**, 272, **273**, 289, 292, **293**
hatband (*anqoña, cinta*), 112, 186 fig. 26, 199–200, 272, 280
health, 41, 46, 92, 222, 287, 308n.5
heirloom, 13, 152, 156, 181, 271, 276–280; inheritance, 57–58, 174–179, 182–183
Hendrickson, Carol, 139, 307n.19
heritage, 22, 31, 88, 92, 154, 156, 186, 188, 195
Herrera, Leonor, 162, 171, 173
Hobsbawm, Eric, 181, 307n.18
Hollander, Anne, 126, 272, 290, 307n.19
home, 33, 45, 47–60, 74–77, 108, 117, 125, 142, 144, 146, 156, 167, 182, 192–195, 198, 203–204, 210–213, 244–250, 252–253, 256, 261, 264–265, 316nn.13, 14
house and house compound, 55–60, **56**
household; 221, 223, 226, 245–248, 252, 309n.13, 319n.3
Huanqui, Dionisia, 164, 173
Huaracha, Florencia, 78–79, 98, 101, 124, 145, 165
Huaraya, Cecilio, 164–165
Huaraya, Ramón, 165
Huaraya, Seferino, 206
Huayapa, Jerónimo, 160, 167, 169, 170, 176
Huaypuna, Fermín, 139, 312n.10
human rights, 16, 219, 233, 306n.9, 317n.2
Hurley, William, 91–92, 94, 308n.3, 309n.20, 315n.1
Hurston, Zora Neale, 24–25, 302

Ichupampa, 44, 61
identity, 17–22, 33–34, 45–46, 50, 101, 106, 116–118, 140–144, 244, 246, 264, 267–270, 286–297; Andean, 80, 85–89, 92; Arequipeño, 85, 99, 174–179; black, 86, 90, 307n.16, 312n.5; *chileno,* 31–32, 45; *cholo,* 95; *costeño,* 82; *gringo,* 31–32, 46, 48, 54, 64, 128, 140–144, 150, 286, 289; Hispanic and Latino/a, 32, 46, 75; homosexual, 188, 207–208, 307n.20, 315n.2, 317nn.17, 18; national and Peruvian, 22, 80, 85–89, 102, 118, 176, 189, 212–213, 235–236, 299, 307n.16; native, 22, 86, 90, 168, 174–179, 181–182, 188–190, 202–204, 212–213, 222, 235–237, 239, 271, 286, 291–297; Native American, 86, 292, 317n.17; *originario,* 86, 203; peasant, 86, 89, 92, 102, 124, 227–230; *serrano,* 82, 84, 88, 101; Spanish, 31, 83, 85, 90–91, 168, 174–175, 177, 203–204, 208–209, 212; white (*blanco*), 22, 34, 74, 82–83, 85, 87–88, 97, 150–151, 158, 168–170, 174–180, 182, 203–204, 208, 212, 236–237, 239, 287, 290, 293–294, 317n.2
Indian (*indígena, indio/a, runa*), 1, 12, 19, 22, 31, 33, 34, 47, 79, 82–95, 97–98,

101–102, 110, 120, 125, 147, 150–151, 154, 155, 158, 162, 163, 168–170, 174–180, 183, 184, 190, 203–204, 208–209, 212–213, 221, 229, 233, 235–237, 239, 270, 286–287, 291–297, 307n.16, 311nn.7, 9, 10, 314n.11
individuality, 130–131, 135–138, 144, 154–155, 182–183, 190–193, 198–199, 205–209
Inkas, 79, 83, 85, 92, 101, 157, 200, 202–203, 212, 307n.15, 316nn.9, 11, 322nn.14, 16
invention, 23, 137, 152, 154–158, 162–167, 180–184, 307n.18

jacket: female (*jubón, saco*), 2, 3, 106, 109–115, **111,** 131, 159, 164, 224, 233, 272; male, 148, 158–159
Jiménez, Melania, 230, 319n.19
Johnson, George R., 148, **149, 160**
Jurewicz, Patricia, 54, 267–270, 278, 290–291, 322n.17
justice, 209, 212, 215–218, 235

Kingsolver, Barbara, 274, 277–278
kinship, 15, 22, 34, 45, 52–60, 87, 95, 152–155, 174–183, 193–195, 221–224, 230, 238–239, 243–250, 254–266, 269–270, 281–285, 294, 308n.9, 319n.2, 320nn.5, 10; *compadrazgo,* 30, 32, 46, 52–55, 90, 119–121, 129, 141–142, 169, 175, 177, 192, 194, 196, 213–214, 267–268, 274–278, 308n.10, 309n.11
knitting, 13, 99, 226
knowledge: cultural, 70, 85–86, 106, 112, 132, 140, 141, 143, 166, 230, 238, 245–248, 254–255, 258–260, 264–266, 270, 280–282, 291; epistemology, 29–32, 73
Krutch, Joseph Wood, 51

landscape, 40, 66–71, 79, 129; embroidered, 108, 130–140, 145–146
land use and land tenure, 38, 154–157, 169–170, 175–181, 191, 195, 206, 213–214, 230, 318n.5; *hacienda* and *estancia,* 83–84, 93, 164, 204, 310n.4
language, 29, 79, 93; Aymara, 79, 314n.1, 316n.13, 322n.13; bilingualism, 31, 57; Quechua, 29, 31–32, 39, 57, 79, 109–110, 128–129, 206, 223, 230, 275, 308nn.9, 23, 309n.14, 311n.12, 312n.9, 314n.1, 321n.10, 322n.13
Lari, 68, 112, 158–159, **159,** 176, 309n.13, 311n.11
Larico, Margarita, 29, 150
law, 119–120, 218–220, 227–229, 233, 318n.5
learning, 30, 106, 130, 165, 166–167, 241–245, 248, 254–261, 266
Lederman, Rena, 74
life course, 18, 21, 33, 105–109, 116–125, 144, 187, 191, 195, 199, 208, 291
Lima, 8, 9, 57, 80–82, 101, 186, 207, 226, 284, 288, 305n.1, 314nn.13, 14, 317n.2; identity, 82, 176; migration, 57–59, 95, 120, 165, 190, 192, 195, 213
llama train (*trajín*), 81, 147, **149,** 151, 163, 183, 310n.2
Lobo, María Luisa, 279

Maca, 2–3, 17, 91, 110, 121, 124, 210
MacLeod, Arlene, 28
Madrigal, 63, 81, 117, 130, 163, 172, 189
Majes River and Project, 69–70, 81, 84, 91, 93, 101, 123, 166, 172–173, 180, 287, 309n.20
Malcohuaccha, Fernando, 39, 46–47, 52–53, 308n.2
Mamani, Eleuterio, 283
Manrique, Nelson, 81, 83, 93, 170, 172, 305n.2, 307n.16, 308n.6, 310n.3, 316n.11
Maqui, Clorinda, 92, 255
Markowitz, Lisa, 84, 93, 101, 159, 161,

305n.2, 307n.15, 308n.1, 309n.13, 310n.4, 313n.9, 317n.3, 318n.13
marriage, 121, 154, 157, 165, 174–179, 190–192, 213, 215–218, 223, 227, 229, 308n.2, 316nn.11, 13, 319n.17; courtship, 120, 194–195, 202–205, 208, 211; role of wife in, 76, 190–192, 215–218, 246, 254–265, 315n.4, 319n.20
masculinity, 98, 100, 174, 177–178, 187–189, 198–205, 207–210, 212–214, 218, 220–221, 234–235, 316n.9, 317n.18
materials, 57, 62, 97, 105–107, 112–115, 128–130, 138–140, 154–155, 158–162, 164–165, 171, 173, 179–181, 244, 249, 250, 259–261, 283–285, 314n.15; foreign, 20, 127, 138–140, 146, 155, 158–162, 169–172, 281, 283–284, 290, 314n.13; thread, 112, 115, 130, 135–136, 145, 313n.12; yarn, 112, 128–129, 136, 138–139, 257 fig. 35, 272–274, 283, 290, 292, 313n.14
meaning, 14, 21, 109, 127, 157–162, 180, 246–248, 254, 291, 297, 306n.8, 321n.2
Meisch, Lynn, 294, 307n.14, 321n.7
Mejía, Leonardo, 17, 28, 62, **99,** 103–108, **104,** 125–126, 134–135, 137, 244, 245, 256, 248–253, 256, 266, 281–282, 286
Mejía, Vilma, 36, 110
Mejía Taco, Carmela, 178–179
memory, 32, 35–36, 147–184, 202–207, 209, 214, 274–280, 296; visual, 38, 131
men, 18, 21–22, 134, 158–159, 159 fig. 24, 162, 168, 171, 173–178, 185–187, 190–191, 195–198, 200, 205–213, 245–246, 254–258, 261–265, 315n.4, 316n.10
merchant, 93, 101, 148, 283–285, 294–295
mestizo, mestizaje, misti, 22, 33, 34, 64, 84–94, 98, 154, 162, 163, 167–179, 182, 188–189, 203, 212–213, 229–230, 233, 235–239, 294, 310n.10, 311nn.9, 12
metaphor, 24, 25, 108, 130, 143, 144, 187, 204–205. *See also* synecdoche
methodology, 29–32, 49, 108, 138, 140–144, 146, 150–156, 162–163, 168, 173, 181–184, 187–188, 196, 206, 210–213, 233, 241–245, 307n.22; survey, 29, 125, 137, 241, 245–246, 249, 254–257, 262, 307n.22, 320nn.4, 5
migration, 1–13, 84, 95, 120–121, 125, 144, 153, 189, 190–195, 211–214, 258, 261, 305nn.1, 2; Provincial Association of Caylloma, 13, 116–118, 312n.3
military occupation, 9–10, **9,** 12–14, 16, 48, 64, 232, 306n.9
mines and mining, 79, 81, 90–91, 170, 172, 263
modern and modernity, 23, 28, 94, 95, 100, 101, 126, 137–139, 171, 233, 235, 287
modernization, 1–2, 8, 83–85, 89, 138, 148, 172–173, 289
money, 57, 62, 84, 87, 93, 109, 122–125, 166, 172, 192, 194, 199, 211, 254, 256, 266, 268, 284, 286, 296, 313n.9
Monroy, Miguel, 52, 116–118
Morris, Rosalind, 27, 32, 303, 307nn.20, 21
mother, 19, 31, 33, 52–55, 57, 123, 156–157, 162, 174–179, 182–183, 215–219, 221–224, 227–230, 238–239, 257, 263, 272, 274–278, 282, 291–292, 294, 304; Madres de Plaza de Mayo, 318n.6
Mothers' Club, 13, 43, 215–219, 222, 226–229, 233, 318nn.9, 10, 319nn.7, 19
mountains, 11, 37, **37,** 38, **41,** 47–48, 60–71, 81–82, 87, 101, 161, 271, 287–288, 309n.18, 312n.10, 322n.14
mourning, 34, 122, 268, 270–280, 289–291, 296–297, 321nn.3, 5, 7, 8
Moyano, María Elena (Malena), 317n.2
music, 54, 190, 193, 196, 198, 206, 211, 283

nation, 9–10, 19, 22–23, 62, 79, 80, 88, 91, 100–101, 127, 138–140, 153–154, 189, 199, 211–212, 218–221, 227–229, 235–236, 239, 316n.16. *See also* Peru
national symbols, 131, 212
Nelson, Richard, 77
Ness, Sally, 14
NGOs, 43, 63, 215, 219, 224–230, 233, 263, 281, 284–285, 309n.16, 318nn.7, 11

objects, 21, 24, 106, 109, 152, 154, 270–272, 279–280, 286–287, 291–297, 306n.8, 321n.2
Ocsa, Tiburcio, 36, 110
Orlove, Benjamin, 80, 81, 160, 161, 294, 313n.14, 314n.12, 316n.15

pants, 21, 35, 55, 94–95, 116, 142, 156–163, 176, 183, 222, 224, 230, 276, 292
pastoralism, 65, 79–82, 112, 160–161, 164, 168, 172, 305n.2, 308n.1, 320n.8
patriarchy, 153, 154, 174–179, 202–204, 208–210, 214, 226, 232, 246
Paz, Octavio, 213
Pelto, Gretel H. and Perti Pelto, 140–141
performance, 30, 33, 116–118, 144, 153, 185–214, 215–219, 224–238, 288–289; theory, 22, 24–29, 32
person, 19, 24–28, 146, 220–221, 254, 306n.13
Peru, 15, 22, 23, 33, 70, 72, 99–100, 138–139, 188, 189, 207, 211–213, 228, 232–233, 272, 274, 294, 301–304, 305nn.1, 2, 315n.9, 316n.16, 317n.18, 320nn.1, 4, 322n.15; Apurímac, 170, 284; Ayacucho, 9; crisis, political-economic, 12–17, 62, 224, 250; education, 119–121, 309n.14; history, 80–85, 203, 306nn.5, 6; Mollendo, 81, 124; 1992 coup, 12–13, 232, 311n.5; politics, 9–10, 12–13, 16–17, 30, 239, 306n.5, 306n.7, 317nn.1, 2, 318nn.7, 9; southern, 2, 10, 31, 80–85, 100–101, 160–164, 167–173, 227, 318nn.10, 12, 321n.6; Tacna, 124; tourism, 179, 287–290, 293, 322nn.14, 16
petty commodity production, 20, 34, 245–248, 266, 319n.2
photographs and photography, 29, 38, 39, 59, 60, 140, 142, 148, 149 fig. 22, 149 fig. 23, 150–153, 155–156, 158–161, 162, 163, 164, 168, 172, 176–177, 181–182, 184, 275–276, 279, 292, 313n.1
Picha, Melitón, 155, 166, 313n.12
place, 18, 50–51, 66–71, 74–77, 88, 125, 130, 156–157, 167, 174–175, 180
plant: motifs, 131; native, 309n.16
play, 185–186, 192–195, 202, 207–210
political economy, 33, 48, 71, 80–85, 93–94, 154, 167–181, 244, 246–247, 265–266, 271–272, 280–295, 306n.8, 319n.2, 320n.4, 321n.2
political organization, 34, 50, 67, 80–85, 191, 193, 207–209, 215–219, 222–224, 226–230, 233–235, 252, 263, 305n.3, 308n.8, 310nn.1, 5, 313n.3, 314n.17, 315n.4, 319n.22
politics, 22–23, 90, 98, 100, 152–154, 168–170, 177–179, 182, 183, 207, 215–240, 286; democracy, 12–13, 89, 213, 220–221, 224–228; elections, 98, 218, 223–224, 228–230, 233–235, **234**, 317n.2, 319nn.14, 22; gendered dimensions, 34, 43, 215–240, 307n.17, 314n.17, 317n.1–319n.22
polleras, 2, 27, 31, 54, 55, 62, 78, 80, 94–98, 100, 102–103, 125–130, 136, 140–146, 152, 155–161, 184–187, 196–201, 207, 210–211, 214, 243–245, 258, 259, 264; agricultural use, 41–43, **42**, 108; black, 272–276, **276**, 290–291; Cabanaconde-style, 112, **113**, 131, 136–137, 276; Chivay-style, 112, **113**, 128,

136–137; doll and miniature, 292–293, **293**; history, 164–166, 172, 174, 176–180; kinship gifts and loans, 294; male use, 21–22, 185–214, 293, 299–300; negative connotations, 78–79, 97–98, 102, 119–120, 125, 144, 174, 299; political use, 23, 34, 215–240. See also *bordados;* mourning
poncho, 41–42, 98–100, **99**, 272, 274, 279, 290–291, 295, 311n.13
Poole, Deborah, 87, 190, 306nn.5, 11
power, 16, 19, 21, 22, 25, 28, 47, 49, 75, 80, 85–89, 101, 134, 141, 146, 153, 156, 167–179, 180, 182–192, 197–198, 202–204, 208–214, 220, 225–226, 229, 232, 235–240, 306n.12, 316n.9
practice(s), 34, 85–86, 92–93, 101–102, 124–125, 144; ethnic, 22; political, 219–220, 228, 237–238; theory, 25–27
pre-Columbian societies, 10, 22, 36, 44, 79, 81, 88, 90, 189, 201, 202–203, 222, 271, 287, 309n.18, 322nn.14, 16
pride, 17, 18, 33, 78, 86, 92, 94, 98, 102, 122–123, 125, 145, 150, 157, 162, 166–167, 168, 170, 180–181, 183, 189, 190, 195, 212, 224, 236, 243, 258, 259; shame, 78–79, 94, 98, 124
production, 13, 19, 23, 28, 33, 34, 57, 84, 104–105, 137, 162–166, 170–174, 180, 241–266, 306n.12; cultural, 190, 207, 306n.11, 312nn.4, 5
Puno, 9, 81, 97–98, 101, 161, 163, 167, 170, 233, 284, 316n.9, 318nn.10, 12

Quinto, Froylán, 283, 285
Quispe Ticona, Sebastián, 122–123

race: biological, 87; categories, 79, 85–95, 150–151, 237, 311n.7
race and racism, 10, 12, 17–19, 22–23, 33, 34, 85–90, 97–98, 101–102, 146, 179, 186, 188–191, 208–209, 212–213, 219, 307n.16, 311n.6, 312n.5; history in Caylloma, 168–170, 174–179, 180, 202–209, 212–214; relationship to gender, 202–204, 208–209, 212–214, 219, 221, 229, 235–239
Ramos, Leandrina, 255
Ramos, Ricardo, 286
Ranger, Terence, 181
Rasnake, Roger, 190, 191, 193, 315nn.4, 7
regional fair, 63, 129, 165, 171, 270, 280–285, 287
regionalism, 33, 34, 78–85, 100–102, 126, 139, 152, 154, 167–174, 180, 186, 189, 199, 212, 220–221, 227–230, 310n.5
representation, 18, 19, 21, 29–33, 46, 49, 72–74, 80, 99, 107–108, 122, 130, 144–145, 147–184, 190, 295; public, 187, 190, 193, 195–199, 207, 209, 215–240
reproduction, 194, 208, 219, 221–222, 245–249, 258–261, 264–266
resistance, 18, 70, 83, 89, 110, 146, 154, 169–170, 173, 180–183, 184, 193, 202, 208–214, 225, 310n.3, 314n.11
ritual, 18, 26, 27, 28, 93, 122, 185–214, 268–280, 289–297, 309n.15, 315nn.3, 6, 15, 320n.7, 321n.3; calendar, 192, 194, 315n.3
Rodríguez, David, 131
Rojas, Fermina, 116–119, 125
Rosas, Dionisio, 85, 203, 276, 316n.12
Rowe, Ann P., 95, 307n.14, 312n.2

Salinas: Luis, 147, 168–171; Manuel, 168–177; family, 148. *See also* wool trade
Sarayasi, Damiana, 243, 255
Schneider, Jane, 290, 321nn.2, 5
sewing, 11, 19, 30, 35, 104–105, 128, 134, 194, 222, 250, 253–268; machine, 2, 14, 45, 57, 104, 115, 131, 132, 136, 155, 162, 164, 166, 169, 171, 181, 194, 196, 226, 241–243, **242**, 249–254, **257**, 259–260, 314n.12, 320n.5

sex and sexuality, 26, 28, 30, 97, 153, 185–189, 194–195, 198–210, 212–213, 307n.20, 315n.2, 316nn.9, 14, 317n.18
Seyco, Mario, 131
shawl (*manta, phullu*), 41, 100, 132, **133**; black, 270–273, **273,** 276–277, **276,** 280, 290
Shining Path, 10, 13, 306n.6, 317n.2
Shippee-Johnson Peruvian Expedition, 30, 147–149, **149,** 150, 158–160, **159, 160,** 163–164, 168, 176, 313n.1
shoes, 109–110, 118, 148, 151, 163, 176
Sibayo, 161, 259
skill, 34, 115, 132, 145, 157, 166, 171, 183, 243–245, 249, 254, 257–266, 281, 320n.9
skirt, 2, 3, 18, 21, 41–42, 94, 95, 105, 107, 109, 112, 117–119, 123, 140–144, 150, 155, 156, 159, 176–177, 184, 185, 187, 198–201, 208, 214, 235
sling, braided (*honda, waraka*) and slinging, 200–201, 205–206, 315n.9
social movements, 10, 89, 306nn.6, 7, 311n.10, 314n.11, 317n.3
social organization, 15, 187, 189–193, 202, 204, 247, 254–265; hierarchy, 185, 192–193, 213; civil-religious (*cargo*), 190–191, 194–195, 199, 207–209, 309n.2, 315n.4; *saya,* 11, 193, 205, 209
souvenir, 62, 271, 285–297, **293,** 303
space, 1–2, 10–11, 45–47, 71, 76, 87, 147–148, 170–172, 183, 246, 248–253, 296–297; domestic, 55–58, 249; public, 33–34, 189–190, 198, 202, 215–221, 224–225, 227, 231–232, 237–240, 250–253
Spanish: colonialism, 10, 71, 80, 83, 88, 90–91, 100, 132, 148, 150, 159–161, 189, 202–204, 208–209, 213, 271, 272, 287–288, 308n.6, 313n.14, 321n.11; invasion and conquest, 44, 79, 82–83, 202–203, 204, 209, 212–214, 316n.10; language, 29, 31–32, 39, 57, 94, 109, 128–129, 223, 225, 229–230, 237, 275, 293, 308n.9, 309n.14, 312n.9, 314n.1, 321n.10, 322n.13
spinning, 159–161
star, **114,** 131, 135–136
state, 9, 12–13, 83, 101, 118–120, 122, 146, 206, 209, 220–221, 224–229, 235, 239–240, 311n.10, 316n.16, 320n.4
status and prestige, 23, 87, 90, 91, 123, 139, 151, 154, 176–179, 183, 190, 195, 199, 211, 245, 261–266
Stegner, Wallace, 66–67, 70
Steiner, Christopher, 21, 287, 306n.11, 313n.5, 321n.2
Stephenson, Marcia, 97, 218, 318n.4
Stewart, Susan, 286
Stoner, Bradley, 92–94, 308n.5
stories, 29–32, 45, 77, 152–154, 177–178, 182, 189, 195, 202–210, 316n.10
Strathern, Marilyn, 75, 265, 310n.23
street market, **11,** 48, 148, **149,** 150, 171, 270
style, 22–23, 33, 94–100, 105–115, 122–124, 127–140, 144, 157, 198–199, 201, 221, 224, 230, 232, 236, 310n.1
subjectivity, 29, 34, 49, 73–76, 141, 144
suit, 121, 158–161, 176, 235
Sullca, Livia, 123, 138, 292–293
Sullca, Margarita, **96,** 122–123, 157, 162, 163–165
Sullca, Tiburcio, 157, 163–167, 170–171
Supo, Bernardo, 165–166, 173, 260
Surco, Felipe, 157, 158, 169, 180
Suyo, Natalia, 121
symbolic economy, 10, 14–16, 71, 155, 174, 180, 306n.11
symbols, 10, 21, 28, 34, 89, 93, 98–101, 151–152, 171, 172, 174–179, 184, 186, 202, 214, 218, 220, 230, 235–239, 293, 296; key, 18, 187
synecdoche, 25, 95, 220–221, 232

Taco Apaza, Alejandro, 205–206, 209
Taco Inca, Zenobia, 222–224, **225,** 229–230, 238, 318n.13
Tahuantinsuyo movement, 168, 314n.11
tailor, 34, 159, 161–162, 163, 164, 171, 313n.10
teaching, 30, 125, 134–135, 162, 164, 166, 173, 243–245, 249, 252, 254, 256–261, 263, 266, 320n.9
technique, 112, 115, 132–136, 154–155, 241–244, 254, 256–266, 257 fig. 35
Tejada family: Antonio, 162; Emilio, 155, 162, 171; Juan, 121, 125, 155, 162, 166, 284, 313n.12
Terán family: Edilberto, 178–179; Hernán, 178; Juan Zoilo, 178; Marcelina, 274, 277; Maximiliana, 38–46, 42 fig. 6, 52–53, 227, 308n.2
textiles, 13, 57, 79, 81, 83, 84; Andean, 20, 95–97, 132, **133,** 271, 272, 307nn.14, 15, 311n.2, 321nn.4, 8, 11; industrial production, 139, 162, 172–173, 290, 314nn.13, 15, 322n.17; ritual, 55. *See also* cloth; weaving and woven textiles
theory: feminist, 24–29, 32–33, 49, 72–77, 87–188, 211, 220–222, 245, 247–248, 265, 309n.21, 310nn.22, 23, 317n.3, 318nn.4, 6, 319n.3; political, 220–222, 318n.4; queer, 187–188, 315n.2, 317nn.17, 18
t'inkachiy and *tinku,* 194, 316n.15
Toledo, Alejandro, 100, 306n.7, 314n.19
tourism, 62, 138, 245, 267–272, 278–281, 286–297, 312n.10, 322nn.13, 14, 16
trade and trading, 20, 34, 40, 81, 83, 129, 147–151, 159, 163–175, 267–297
tradition, 18, 23, 28, 33, 94, 127, 137, 139–140, 152–160, 180–185, 188–189, 195, 203–204, 206, 209, 212–214, 218, 220, 228, 238–239, 268, 272, 278, 280, 290, 292–294, 296, 307n.18, 315n.3
transportation, 10, 36, 48, 60–66, 81–83, 101, 163, 172, 193–194, 241–242, 252, 267, 283, 286, 288, 310nn.2, 3
transvestism, 25–26, 28, 33, 143, 185–214, 215–219, 233–237, 293, 315n.2, 317n.17; Witite, 33, 116–117, **186, 197,** 293, 314n.1
travel, 32–34, 35–77, 78, 95, 123–124, 241, 253, 262–263, 270, 280–288, 322n.16
Treacy, John, 46–47, 53, 68, 69, 275–278, 305n.2, 308n.3, 309nn.16, 17, 20, 312n.9, 315n.3, 316n.11
Tupac Amaru Revolutionary Movement, 10, 306n.6. *See also* Shining Path; war
Turino, Thomas, 17, 190, 315n.7
Turner, Victor, 26

uniform, 119–120, 122, 146, 200, 224, 235, 238, 239
urban centers, 1–16, 49–50, 61, 147–150, 249, 260; *pueblos jóvenes,* 10–13

Valera, Rosalía, 54, 123–124, 128–129, 146, 255, 285, 294, 304
Valero, Francisca, 156
Van Keuren, Victor, 148, **149, 159**
Vargas, Cecilio, 132–133
Vargas, Edgar, 132–133, 138
Vargas Llosa, Mario, 12, 79
Vega, Grimalda, 133 fig. 20
vendors, **3,** 16, 17, 78, 96–97, 147–148, **149,** 156, 160, 162–165, 167–174, 241–244, 250–253, 255, 267–271, 280–296, 307n.22, 322n.13; *ambulantes,* 1–3, 8, 270, 305n.1
vest: female (*corpiño*), 2, 105, 109, **111** 124, 132, **133,** 141, 224, 261, 263–264, 267–270, 269 fig. 36, 272, 281, 290–291; male (*chaleco*) 158, **159,** 164, 312n.10
Vilcape, Hugo, 113, 131, 135–137, 166, 290

Vilcasán, Gerardo, 51, 119, 128, 143, **242,** 261
Villavicencio Condori, Marcial, 130, 132, 135, 136, 138, 172
violence, 8–10, 12–14, 16–17, 71, 153, 154, 168–170, 180–183, 186, 188–189, 200–207, 209, 211–213, 215–217, 227, 231–233, 306n.10, 317n.2; nonviolence, 34, 207, 216–217, 231–234, 231 fig. 30, 234 fig. 31
vision and visual qualities, 29–31, 33, 66–68, 80, 87, 106–107, 126–127, 135–137, 151–154, 181–182, 222–224, 238, 263–264, 302, 304

war, 16, 201, 212, 279, 306n.10; civil war, 9–10, 12, 14, 48, 187, 287; War of the Pacific, 175, 177, 316n.10
wealth, 81, 83–84, 91–92, 123, 157, 172–173, 175–177, 183, 195, 214
weaving and woven textiles, 13, 20, 44, 55, 57, 93, 99, 132, **133,** 141, 159–164, 171, 183, 200, 259–261, 271–278, 290–291, 307n.15, 311n.2, 312n.9, 320n.5, 321nn.4, 8, 11; loom, 20, 161
Weiner, Annette, 295
Weston, Kath, 25, 27, 307n.20
widow, 46, 75, 122, 291, 308n.7
Witite. *See* transvestism
Wolf, Diane, 75, 310nn.23, 24
women, 2, 12, 13, 18–19, 21, 28–29, 33–34, 41, 58, 62, 73–74, 105–107, 152–156, 167, 168, 170–171, 173–179, 180, 182–183, 247–248, 254–255, 261–264, 271–273, 291, 294–295, 301–304, 308n.2, 309n.21; organizations, 219, 220, 224–233, 238–240, 263; unruly, 185–186, 196–199, 202, 207–212; Women's Federation, 43, 217, 219, 222–233, **225, 231,** 237–240, 318nn.12, 13, 319nn.14, 18, 19
wool, 20, 81, 99, 101, 112, 115, 158–161, 167, 176, 277, 283, 284, 290–291, 313nn.7, 13, 314n.15, 321n.11
wool trade, 20, 81–84, 93, 147–151, **149,** 163–164, 167–174, 180
work, 15–16, 34, 76, 85–86, 155, 163–166, 192–195, 222–223, 226–227, 245–248, 251, 254–255, 261–266, 268–270, 280–286, 320nn.9, 10; labor, 34, 80, 85, 93, 129, 223, 243–244, 246–249, 254–265, 310n.3; labor, division of, 21, 57, 134–135, 220, 245–246, 254–265; labor draft (*mita*), 90–91, 101
workshop, 13–15, 19, 20, 22, 57, 58, 103–104, **104,** 118, 125, 134–135, 154, 160, 241–266, **242, 257,** 267, 282–283, 288–291, 296, 307n.14, 312n.4, 320n.8; history of, 162–167, 171–173
writing, 23–24, 72–73, 77, 196

Yajo, Elías, 121
Yanque, 39, 49, 61, 91, 92, 120, 278–279, 310n.4, 316n.10

Zapater Neyra, Manuel, 176
Zavala, Adrián, 110, 176
Zorn, Elayne, 95, 308n.10, 312n.2, 313n.14, 316n.9, 321n.6